The Menopause Manifesto

BY DR. JEN GUNTER

The Preemie Primer
The Vagina Bible
The Menopause Manifesto

THE MENOPAUSE MANIFESTO

Own Your Health with Facts and Feminism

DR. JEN GUNTER

PIATKUS

PIATKUS

First published in the United States in 2021 by Citadel Press Books,
an imprint of Kensington Publishing
First published in Great Britain in 2021 by Piatkus

A CIP catalogue record for this book is available from the British Library.

ISBN: 978-0-349-42760-7

PUBLISHER'S NOTE
The reader is advised that this book is not intended to be a substitute for an
assessment by, and advice from, an appropriate medical professional(s).

Printed and bound in Great Britain by Clays Ltd, Elcograf S.p.A.

Papers used by Piatkus are from well-managed forests
and other responsible sources.

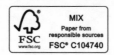

MIX
Paper from
responsible sources
FSC® C104740
FSC
www.fsc.org

Piatkus
An imprint of
Little, Brown Book Group
Carmelite House
50 Victoria Embankment
London EC4Y 0DZ

An Hachette UK Company
www.hachette.co.uk

www.littlebrown.co.uk

For every woman.
Your awesomeness is unrelated to your estrogen.

Contents

The Manifesto

IF MENOPAUSE WERE ON YELP it would have one star.

> *This establishment has temperature control issues. Drenching heat followed by terrible chills. Defies the laws of thermodynamics. Would not recommend.*
>
> *Awful, awful, awful! Bleeding was scheduled, but was rebooked without notification so arrived 3 weeks later than expected while I was in an Uber and I flooded the car. The driver gave me a terrible review!*
>
> *The sex was dry.*

And it's no surprise. Most women have no idea what to expect when they are no longer expecting a period, and it's uniquely awful and disempowering to not understand what is happening to your body and why. Menopause is like being sent on a canoe trip with no guide book and only a vague idea where you are headed—although the expectation is it's awful. There will be no advice on how to get there or how to manage any of the obstacles, such as rapids. That is if any exist. Who knows? Have fun figuring it out! Good times. Oh, and don't write. No one wants to hear about your journey or what it is like when you arrive.

Fear? Check. Uncertainty? Check. Medical ramifications? Check. Unpleasant symptoms? Check. Societal irrelevance? Check.

No wonder menopause receives such awful reviews.

The culture of silence about menopause in our patriarchal society is something to behold. Menopause doesn't even rate the shame that society gives to the vulva and vagina. Apparently there is nothing of lower value than an aging woman's body, and many in our society treat menopause not as a phase of life, but rather as a phase of death. Sort of a predeath.

What little that is spoken about menopause is often viewed through the lens of ovarian failure—the assertion that menopause is a disease that exists because women and their ovaries are weak. The only grounds for this claim are that men don't experience menopause. But comparing women and men in this way is the same as comparing the liver with the heart. The liver isn't weak or diseased because it doesn't beat like the heart, and women aren't diseased because the ovaries stop making estrogen.

The absence of menopause from our discourse leaves women uninformed, which can be disempowering, frightening, and makes it difficult to self-advocate. Consequently, many suffer with symptoms or don't receive important health screenings or therapies because they have been dismissed with platitudes like "This is just part of being a woman" or "It's not that bad." But the issues with menopause even go beyond these knowledge gaps and the medical neglect. Women tell me that menopause is lonely; that there are no stories or culture. And so there is no whisper network to take up the slack from medicine. Nothing to offer comfort.

But many women are desperate to know more about menopause so they can understand how and why their body is changing, and they want information so they can make decisions that work for them. They also want to talk about what is happening to their body.

I contrast these experiences with my own. Having started medical school when I was twenty years old and my OB/GYN training when I was twenty-four, I can't remember back to a time when I didn't have a detailed understanding of the hormonal changes of both the menstrual cycle and menopause. And not just the biology, but how to apply it practically to my own body. I never once thought, "Wow, that is unexpected," or "Why am I sweating so much at the age of forty-five?" or "WHAT IS GOING ON— WHY AM I BLEEDING EVERYWHERE!?"

My medical knowledge didn't prevent me from having menopause acne, hot flushes, or those "special" heavy periods that are all typical of the menopause transition. But because I knew exactly what was happening and when to seek care, it made the whole process feel routine. Because I knew the tests that were indicated and those that were not, and because I understood the medicine, it was much easier for me to navigate the treatment options and choose the safest most effective therapy and avoid the snake oil. By the time I entered my own menopause transition, I had spent over twenty years speaking with women about their menopause and helping them manage their symptoms and any health concerns, so I had heard many stories and had knowledge of the range of experiences as well as the treatment options. It was fortunate that my view of the subject wasn't confined to what I saw at home. My mother's menopause was volcanic, and if that was all I had to go on, I would have been quite frightened.

Online, on book tour for *The Vagina Bible,* and during many interviews with reporters I often heard (and still hear today) "What do I do?" and "Where do I turn?" from women about menopause. I remember one interview in particular that had nothing to do with menopause or even menstruation and when for some reason I tangentially mentioned I was using an estrogen patch the conversation derailed and all the reporter wanted to discuss was menopause. Hearing over and over again from women from many countries about this need for knowledge made me obsessed with the idea that every woman should know about menopause like a well-informed gynecologist and so that is what I have set out to do in these pages.

For women to navigate menopause, they need facts because empowerment requires accurate information—but they also need feminism because our bodies, our medical care, and even our thoughts have been colonized by the patriarchy. The cultural absence of menopause from our discussions isn't because that's what women want. The often pejorative language about menopause and the medical neglect also aren't up there on the meno wish list.

Women often only hear the awful stories about menopause, but the truth is the menopause experience is a vast diaspora. Many women have mild symptoms, some moderate, and others severe. Often these symptoms are temporary, but occasionally they're long lasting. Menopause does start a series of biological events that increase a woman's risk of several medical conditions, such as cardiovascular disease and osteoporosis. But menopause isn't the only paint on a woman's canvas. Age, other medical conditions, diet, exercise, and even adverse childhood events are also adding color to her portrait. So when a woman wants to consider what she should do, it's important to step back and look at the whole picture. Managing menopause is the ultimate exercise in whole body or holistic medicine.

Menopause is not a disease. It is an evolutionary adaptation that is part of the survival of the species, like menstrual periods or the ability to suppress the immune system during pregnancy so the body doesn't attack the fetus. Like these other biological phenomena, menopause is associated with downsides—in this case its bothersome symptoms for some women and an increased risk of several medical conditions. But menopause also occurs while a woman is aging, so it's equally important not to brush off every symptom as hormone related. It's vital that women know about menopause, but also everything that is menopause adjacent, so they can understand what is happening to their own bodies, put that in perspective, and advocate for care when indicated.

A manifesto is a public declaration or proclamation and we are well past due for a manifesto on menopause as 2021 is the 200th anniversary of the introduction of the word. My manifesto is for every woman to have the knowledge that I had to help them with their own menopause. I demand that the era of silence and shame about menopause yield to facts and feminism. I proclaim that we must stop viewing menopause as a disease, because that means being a woman is a disease and I reject that shoddily constructed hypothesis. I also declare that what the patriarchy thinks of menopause is irrelevant. Men do not get to define the value of women at any age.

If you are years from menopause, this book will hopefully help you understand the road ahead. My hope is that it allows you to view menopause as a phase of life, as well as inform you of the preventative care that can be taken to lessen any impact of menopause on your health. In addition, may this book provide the knowledge to best manage your menopause with a view to your unique concerns.

If you are already on Team Menopause, I hope this book helps you understand how you got here—biologically speaking—and informs you of important health considerations that may still lie ahead. It's never too late for preventative health care and many symptoms and medical conditions may still need managing.

And if you are in your menopause transition and experiencing that hormonal chaos, know for many women this is the rockiest phase. Often just that acknowledgment can help. I hope the information here helps you reframe what is happening to your body, and if you are suffering I hope you take comfort knowing there are many explanations for how and what you are feeling, as well as therapies—and these rapids won't last forever. My hope is that this book helps to hold your canoe steady so you can catch your breath.

Facts can bring order to the chaos and uncertainty of menopause, because knowledge can dispel fears and open up treatment options. Even if the option is to take no action, it is still a position of power because it is an act of self-determination. Feminism can help women see the biases that may have informed previous beliefs and reframe their menopause not as a terminal event, but as another phase of life.

Women want more information about menopause and that knowledge can reduce suffering. Knowing what's happening to your body and that you're not alone in your experiences is powerful medicine. Facts empower women to make the health decisions that work for them—you can't be an informed patient with inaccurate information.

It shouldn't require an act of feminism to know how your body works, but it does. And it seems there is no greater act of feminism than speaking up about a menopausal body in a patriarchal society.

So let's make some noise.

Part 1

Reclaiming the Change:

Understanding Your Body as an
Act of Feminism

A Second Coming of Age:

Why Menopause Matters

MENOPAUSE IS PUBERTY IN REVERSE—a transition from one biological phase of ovarian function to another, but the way we view these two events couldn't be more different.

Puberty is frequently a subject, or at least a costar, in teen and young adult novels. (Thank God for Judy Blume!) It's often covered—the basics at least—in school biology curriculums and in sex education (although it's an unfortunate truth that sex education isn't universal or always accurate). Medical providers also check puberty milestones, such as breast development and the appearance of pubic hair, to make sure it's progressing correctly, and even the simple act of measuring height with a pencil on a door frame during a growth spurt is a basic affirmation of the existence of puberty. A coming of age—transitioning from childhood to teen or adult—is commonly celebrated or at least acknowledged in multiple cultures and/or religions (although as an aside it's important to note that having menstrual periods does not magically transform a girl into a woman). Puberty is also a trigger for medical conditions. For example, acne, painful periods, and depression and puberty even starts the chain of events that could one day lead to breast cancer.

While the degree and accuracy of puberty 101 may vary culture to culture, school to school, and family to family, almost everyone is able to acknowledge its existence and generally manages to discuss puberty without making it a disease or framing being a child—the time of life when these conditions didn't occur—as the gold standard for health.

Even though menopause is a universal experience for every woman with ovaries who lives long enough, unlike puberty menopause is shrouded in secrecy. There is no menopause curriculum in schools, and providers rarely discuss it in advance. Typically it's only after a woman has mentioned concerns that the *It might be menopause* conversation is raised. When menopause is discussed in Western society, it's often viewed negatively, as a cruel joke or even as a disease. This stems from the harmful belief that women lose value once they are no long able to reproduce and the false hypothesis that menopause is a biological flaw as there is no equivalent for men who can make sperm into their old age. But if we looked at that argument from another angle we might as well say that men are biologically flawed because they can't get pregnant or because they develop heart disease earlier than women. Also, let's be real. While theoretically men have the biologically machinery to reproduce until they die, aging significantly impacts male fertility and a man's physical ability to be sexually active.

When a cisgender male body is used as a so-called standard, it's easy to view the female body as flawed. This is a core tenet of the patriarchy.

So let's set the record straight. Menopause deserves at least the same attention as puberty (I'd even argue more), and menopause is no more a disease than being a man is a disease.

What Is Menopause?

The word has nothing to do with men. It was conceived in 1812 by Dr. Charles De Gardanne, a French physician, who started with the word *ménèpausie*, a combination of *menes*, from the Greek for month, and *pausie*, from the Greek for cessation (a common term for this phase of life). In 1821 De Gardanne updated the term to *ménopause*, and then somewhere along the way the accent was dropped in the medical literature.

Menopause occurs when there are no more follicles in the ovaries capable of ovulating, meaning there are no more eggs. The average age

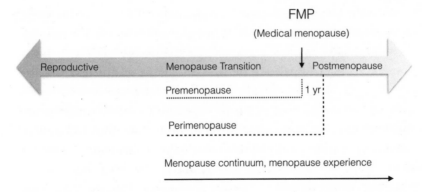

Figure 1: Phases of Ovarian Function

when this happens is fifty to fifty-two years. One of the defining features is the dramatic drop in estrogen levels as the follicles are the main source of estrogen. It's the drop in estrogen that causes many of the symptoms and medical concerns unique to menopause; however, there's new research that suggests other hormone changes (that we'll discuss later) are also important.

Medically speaking, the menopause transition is the time leading up to the final menstrual period (or FMP), the FMP marks menopause, and everything after is postmenopause (see figure 1). As it isn't possible to know which period is the final one until, well, it's final, menopause is formally confirmed twelve months *after* the FMP.

The menopause transition is the period of time leading up to the FMP that's characterized by hormonal fluctuations that result in irregular periods and symptoms, such as hot flushes. There are two other common terms for the menopause transition: *pre*menopause, which is interchangeable with menopause transition; and *peri*menopause (not to be confused with premenopause, which is indeed a separate term), which is the menopause transition as well as the first year after the FMP.

The length of the menopause transition (or premenopause) can vary significantly woman to woman, and a hard start date isn't always possible to determine. During the menopause transition there may be a lot of false finishes or gotchas where a woman thinks she's had her last period and, nope, not yet, and for others the menopause experience can feel more like a gradual meandering process. Or both. The only predictable thing about the menopause transition is its unpredictability.

Adding to the confusing terminology is the colloquial way in which we discuss menopause. Many women and their providers often use the word "menopause" more liberally, for example, "I'm going through menopause" for the menopause transition or "I'm in menopause" for the postmenopausal phase. I'm a fan of using the term "menopause" to encompass the whole continuum or experience from the menopause transition onward, as symptoms and medical conditions linked with menopause don't magically start or stop with the final period. The timing of the FMP matters for research, fertility, and in evaluating abnormal uterine bleeding, but otherwise it's more of a footnote than the lede. Using the term "menopause" generally, and being more specific about the relation to the final menstrual period when it matters medically, feels like the best way to facilitate communication.

The Knowledge Gap

Despite the universal nature of menopause, many women aren't well informed about the symptoms, the physical changes, the medical concerns, or their treatment options. This information vacuum has been created by a toxic combination of medical providers being unable to meet the educational needs of their patients (medicine has some serious communication issues) and medical misogyny, meaning medicine's long history of neglecting women. Consequently, women have their symptoms and health concerns related to menopause dismissed as being fabricated, unimportant, or just "part of being a woman"—meaning something to endure.

But the societal shame extends beyond any provider's office. There is the general disdain for women as they age. Maybe disdain isn't the right word since the concerns of women as they age are often so unimportant that they aren't even worth that minimal effort... they're simply ignored.

As a teen I read books where the character had her period or wrestled with bras, and there were a few cool moms in my group of friends who were willing to talk with us about menstrual products. My friends and I talked about periods among one another. It was exciting. I wasn't exactly sure why, but I was aware it was a marker of my relevance in society. I was reminded about these conversations on a recent trip home to Winnipeg when I had lunch with Tiffany, a friend from junior high school. What was our strongest shared memory? We were the last two girls in our group to get our periods. Me in the early spring of 1980 and Tiffany a month later.

In contrast there are no coming of age stories for women in menopause, and the rare times when menopause is alluded to it seems ubiquitously negative. Women often don't discuss menopause even among themselves. Possibly they are unsure of the facts so are less likely to share, or they falsely assume most of the therapies are ineffective or unsafe or even that there are no treatments available, so why bother? In addition, unlike your first period, the final menstrual period feels like a dotage date—and who wants to be forty-eight and making plans for either graduating to a plucky lady detective who is forced to pass off her competence as a series of fortunate breaks, a vindictive matriarch exacting retribution for her societal impotence on all who cross her path, or an asexual homebody with an ever-increasing assortment of cats with questionable litter box skills?

In the more than twenty-five years that I've been a gynecologist, the science on menopausal hormone therapy (MHT) has changed significantly, and effectively communicating how the science evolves is challenging. We're all comforted by certainty, but the truth is medicine largely operates in shades of gray, and what we in medicine believe to be true today could change when more research becomes available or new technology is developed to answer questions we never dreamed of asking. And then there are the headlines. Fear sells and it seems as if much of what is covered in the lay press overamplifies the risks seen with some therapies. In addition to the traditional news and magazines, women must also navigate the information of varying quality on social media.

There is another matter of misinformation and even disinformation as the unfortunate silence about menopause and the gaps in knowledge are exploited by both the pharmaceutical industry and those who sell supplements and other so-called natural products.

Menopause: The Basics

Most women will spend one-third or even one-half of their lives post-menopausal. If you include the menopause transition, then it's definitely one-half. Currently there are seventy million women in the United States who are forty-five years or older, and worldwide that number is over one billion. As the population is aging because of lower birth rates, percentage-wise the number of women in the menopause transition or who are postmenopausal is only going to increase.

The hormone fluctuations that start in the menopause transition can trigger a variety of symptoms. For some women these may be bothersome enough to treat; for others having the knowledge that what's happening is typical may be enough. Thinking a weird body thing is uniquely yours is very disempowering, and many women are relieved simply to know their experiences are common and expected. It's also important women know what symptoms might be a sign of a more serious concern and what's annoying, but not dangerous.

For example, I was headed to Europe eight months from my last period, and as I'd had some significant hot flushes I was sure I was done. I was stoked not packing pads and tampons. Then five minutes into the ten-hour flight—the seat belt light was still on—bam! I felt a gush and my underwear was soaked with blood. I felt like Michael Corleone (*Godfather III)* sitting on the airplane toilet muttering to my ovaries, "Just when I thought I was out, they pull me back in!"

Changing underwear in an airplane bathroom (just another space not designed for menstruation) and using cheap airplane menstrual pads for ten hours that resulted in an irritating vulvar rash at the start of my vacation was very bothersome—the amount of blood was not. Had I been embarking on a lot of international travel, I might have considered medication to help regulate my periods because menstrual hijinks at cruising altitude are not my jam. That's why it's important for women to know all their options, so they can choose if they want treatment or not. Quality of life concerns aren't trite; it's medicine.

Common symptoms that may be experienced over the menopause continuum are listed in table 1 and will be discussed in detail throughout the book. Quality of life aside, menopause is also important because it's associated with a variety of health concerns (also in table 1), and these aren't a fringe part of women's health care, they're a central concern. Cardiovascular disease, which is linked with menopause, kills almost four hundred thousand women in the United States per year or one out of every three women. For comparison, breast cancer kills approximately forty thousand, and yet many women at average risk for both cardiovascular disease and

Table 1: Common Symptoms and Medical Conditions
         Associated with Menopause

SYMPTOMS	MEDICAL CONDITIONS
Abnormal menstrual bleeding (heavy and/or irregular periods, bleeding in between periods)	Heart disease
Hot flushes and night sweats	Osteoporosis
Sleep disturbance	Dementia and Alzheimer's disease
Temporary cognitive changes (brain fog)	Depression
Vaginal dryness	Metabolic syndrome
Pain with sex	Type 2 diabetes
Decreased libido	Genitourinary syndrome of menopause
Joint pain	Urinary tract infections

breast cancer are far more frightened by breast cancer even though cardio-vascular disease is more likely to kill them. This isn't about disease favorites, for lack of a better expression. Rather, for perspective, it's about stepping back and looking at the entirety of the diseases that affect women.

Sometimes I hear people talk about medical schools needing a menopause curriculum, but you can't separate women from menopause. The answer isn't to put menopause into a silo, because that forces women into silos. Instead, studies of medical conditions and medications need to include women of all ages so we understand how to manage women's health across the menopause continuum.

Menopause Doesn't Happen in a Vacuum

One of the complexities of menopause is that it happens as we age, so sorting out hormone-related from age-related can be hard. In addition, we accumulate medical conditions over the years, and many of them have symptoms that can overlap with the symptoms of menopause.

Let's consider a common menopause experience—difficulty sleeping. Sleep issues can also be age-related or due to a medical condition, such as sleep apnea or depression. To add to the complexity, the menopause transition can trigger depression, and lack of sleep can worsen depression. And sleep apnea is also linked with depression. It's a medical Gordion knot. So a medical provider and patient must ensure they've considered all the contributing factors and how they may be interrelated before assuming a symptom that develops during the menopause transition or during postmenopause is truly hormonally related. It's important that women are not brushed off with a "that's just menopause," or told hormones will "fix everything," when in reality there are other medical conditions—some potentially serious—that are the root cause.

There is another layer of complexity. Our health and how we age—not just the ovaries, but everything—are related to our macroenvironment. For example, diet, exercise, stress, personal relationships, or whether we've had children and if so, did we breastfeed? Some people refer to these as lifestyle factors, although I personally dislike that term as this isn't about choosing between gym memberships.

Other important considerations are social determinants of health, which are social and economic conditions in which people are born, grow, live, work, and age that affect health and quality of life. I often think of these factors as the microenvironment. They produce unfair and preventable differences in health status via many mechanisms, such as lack of access to adequate medical care and education, unsafe work conditions, crowded living conditions, racism, and poor nutrition. How these socioeconomic factors affect health is complex because these are often intertwined and may be additive. Social determinants of health are linked to the age of menopause as well as many of the symptoms and health conditions associated with menopause.

A very important social determinant of health is exposure to childhood adversity, known as ACEs (adverse childhood experiences). ACEs include traumas such as emotional or physical abuse from a parent, insufficient food or clothing, loss of a parent, living with anyone who had a problem with drinking or drugs, witnessing violence in the home, and sexual abuse.

ACEs influence some behaviors that may impact menopause, for

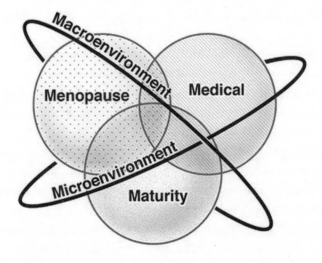

Figure 2: M Diagram: Menopause in Perspective

example, whether a woman starts smoking or the age of her first pregnancy. But it's so much more. There's a growing body of literature that shows adverse childhood experiences lead to many negative health outcomes by triggering a dysregulated stress response that affects the developing brain as well as the endocrine and immune systems. This is known as the toxic stress response, and it can have profoundly negative complications. Exposure to four or more adverse childhood experiences increases the risk of many conditions intertwined with menopause such as heart attack, stroke, sleep disorders, Alzheimer's disease, diabetes, depression, and breast cancer. Trauma literally rewires the brain and the body.

I find it helpful when evaluating any health concern to consider what I call my M diagram—a Venn diagram (or Jenn diagram™) of menopause. The nucleus is menopause, medical conditions, and maturity (age-related), and circling around this nucleus are the macroenvironment and the microenvironment (see figure 2).

Women are so much more than just their ovaries, so it's important to sit back and look at the whole picture for perspective.

BOTTOM LINE

- Menopause is a transition from one phase of ovarian function to another—it's essentially puberty in reverse.
- The hormonal changes of menopause can have cascading biological consequences that may lead to distressing symptoms and health concerns for many women.
- Many women will live one-third to one-half of their lives in the menopause continuum.
- There is a huge disconnect between what we know medically and the information that's accessible for women.
- Age, medical conditions, environmental factors, and social determinants of health all influence the menopause experience.

The History and Language of Menopause:

From a Critical Age to the Change

DID THIS WORD "MENOPAUSE" START the medicalization of a normal, physiologic process or is naming the experience the ultimate act of matriarchy—validating symptoms and drawing attention to a much neglected aspect of women's health?

It turns out it may be both. With menopause, the answers are never that simple.

Menopause in the Eyes of Medicine, from Ancient Times to the Early 1800s

The loss of menstruation with age is noted in both ancient Chinese and Greek medical writings, and there was an understanding that this signified an end of fertility. In traditional Chinese medicine, the time after the last period wasn't viewed as different from old age, and just as women stopped menstruating men developed scanty semen. The ancient Greeks were extremely interested in menstruation as a vital sign. According to the thinking of the time, men were in balance with the world and women were overly moist as their flesh was loose-textured and spongy, so they absorbed excess fluid from their diet. To compensate, women released fluid once a month from their uterus. Whenever anyone holds out Hippocrates or uses "ancient" as being aspirational in health, I think of ancient Greek physicians believing women were walking defective plumbing.

Missed menstrual periods in ancient Greek medicine—the foundation that led to ancient Roman, Persian, Arabic, and then to modern Western medicine—were considered concerning as they were a sign of a potential fertility problem as well as a dangerous buildup of fluid. This helps to explain much of the ancient medical obsession with menstrual periods—many of the 1,500 pharmaceutical recipes in the Hippocratic corpus, 80 percent of them are related to menstruation. It also sheds light on why there is such a thorough detailing of the expected age of the final menstrual period in most ancient Western medical writing. Ancient Greek and Roman physicians were very accurate with their recordings of the average age of menopause—the loss of fertility was a sentinel event.

Ancient physicians were well aware of the concept of a final menstrual period; it's just the symptoms—if they existed—and what happened afterward seem to not have been of interest. It's important to remember that medicine, like everything else, primarily existed to satisfy the needs (and hence secure the patronage) of the male elite who were likely not interested in the aging female body. Interestingly, in some ancient Greek societies postmenopausal women were appointed as priestesses (menopause was viewed as a renewed virginity affording at the level of purity a woman needed for priesthood).

The first mention in Western medical literature of symptoms that we can identify today as related to menopause is in 1582. Dr. Jean Liébault, a French physician, described *petites rougers* or small reds—what today we would call hot flushes—that typically occurred in the face and often ended in *moiteurs* or profuse sweating. These words are no different from what I might hear in the office today.

Dr. Liébault was a specialist in women's diseases and the physician of Catherine de Bourbon (sister of Henri IV, king of France), supporting the concept that patronage plays a role in medical discoveries. However, Liébault was also ahead of his time in many ways. He wrote that "a woman is not an imperfect male," was against forced marriages for women, believed that menstrual discharge was blood not toxic fluid, described bloating before menstruation, and believed that pleasure during sex was important for women as well as men! He was married to Nicole Estienne, who wrote the manifesto *The Woes of the Married Woman,* an indictment of the institution of marriage and of men. Whether their union was happy or not is beyond the scope of this book.

While Liébault was clearly a medical Renaissance man with his observations about women's health, most physicians of the day were hampered by their belief that women were an inferior version of men as well as by their lack of knowledge of female anatomy and a complete lack of understanding of menstruation. Although the loss of menstruation with age was expected, it was blamed for most ailments that affected women after their final menstrual period. Menstrual blood was considered toxic, the cause of a vast array of illnesses from miscarriages to cancer to consumption to rabies. Menstrual blood could also kill plants and ruin mirrors. Women's health worsened as they aged because they became too feeble to expel this toxic substance, so it accumulated in the body.

The first formal dissertation on what we now call menopause was written in 1710—the Latin title translates to *Final Menstruation, Beginnings of Disease,* which is an accurate summary of the thinking of the time—the title may as well have been *Being a Woman, from Bad to Worse.* Medical illness increased with age, this was known, but when men had an ailment there was a reason, not one we might think of today, but an explanation that fit the understanding of the human body of the day. For women it was the uterus. If you see women as inferior or weak or dirty or damaged, it's easy to make the medical knowledge, such as it was, fit your world order. It is a very important lesson that we in medicine should never forget.

Shortly after the first dissertation on menopause, writings on the subject—for both physicians and the general public, began to appear in Europe and England. *The Ladies Physical Directory,* first published in 1716 by the anonymous A Physician, had multiple printings—by 1727 it was in the sixth edition, and included information on how to treat many conditions that would have been common for women in their late forties and beyond—heavy periods, missed periods, and uterine prolapse. So clearly there was interest. Most of the therapies of the day involved bloodletting, leeches, and purgatives (laxatives)—methods for removing "toxins" and/or fluid that had accumulated due to a lack of menstruation. Looking at the recipes, they could not possibly have been effective medically, although many likely triggered diarrhea and possibly uterine contractions, possibly leading to some bleeding for women in the menopause transition (not normal menstruation, rather a sign that a bad thing has happened to the body!). These effects were courtesy of the dangerous ingredients, such as oil of savin, arum root, and iron filings. Other recipes were likely benign and ineffective, possibly producing results via a placebo effect or more likely the wine chaser and long walk that was often recommended as part of the therapy. There was also a range of vaginal potpourri that would make Gwyneth Paltrow jade with jealousy.

A variety of terms to describe symptoms of menopause can be found in these texts; many are similar to what we use today and some are even better. What we now call the menopause transition was known in England during the eighteenth and nineteenth centuries (and possibly earlier) as *the dodge* or *dodging, a*s women were dodging between irregular periods. During the dodge women might experience headaches, back pain, vasomotor symptoms (what we now call hot flushes and night sweats), wandering pains, and general unease. The terms for hot flushes were feverish heats, flushing heats, and hot blooms.

The dodge is so perfectly descriptive it's delightful. I now use it in the office when I explain the menopause transition, and almost universally I get a smile. The term "hot flushes" seemed acceptable until I started experiencing them. To me a flush is in your cheeks, and while my face definitely feels hot, it's not just my cheeks. Flushing also sounds demure, as if I were one of Jane Austen's protagonists turning red and feeling faint under the gaze of some man with £4,000 a year. A "hot bloom" is wonderfully apt because the heat feels as if it starts internally and blooms upward and outward to my head, face, neck, and arms. (As an aside, I dislike the term "hot flashes," which is used interchangeably with hot flushes, because a flash evokes a sensation that lasts for a second or two, and that isn't accurate—and for me that can downgrade the severity of the experience.)

As most of what women experienced was passed down by oral tradition, it's hard to know how many words in how many cultures have been lost due to disinterest or medical mansplaining—meaning let me listen to you, interpret your experience with my narrow view and the biases of society and religious beliefs, and explain it back to you in my medical textbook.

Western medicine was aware of the medical concerns experienced in the menopause transition, but these symptoms were viewed primarily as a consequence of the main pathology—retained toxins. As such, menopause was viewed as just another female fault and something to fear. In 1776 John Fothergill, an influential and astute English physician, challenged this notion in his paper *On the Management Proper of the Cessation of Menses*. Dr. Fothergill asserted that women were taught to look at menopause with "some degree of anxiety" and "The various and absurd opinions relative to the ceasing of the menstrual discharge, and its consequences, have propagated the hours of many a sensible woman."

Dr. Fothergill did not believe that menstrual blood was toxic, and while it may contain some "morbid humours," men, too, according to Fothergill had those same humours and released those via their hemorrhoids. He also noted that women who are taught to fear menopause are more likely to suffer with symptoms. To Dr. Fothergill menopause was a normal progression, and for many women he observed that it occurred without major consequences. Furthermore, he also correctly noted that those women who suffered from heavy or painful periods found relief in menopause. In addition he acknowledged that some women do have bothersome symptoms, such as hot flushing followed by "instantaneous sweats," difficulties sleeping, mood disturbances, and joint pains—although often they were temporary. Many of his therapies were typical of the time: bleeding and laxatives (his were far more gentle, and many that we still use today, such as senna and magnesium), but what is different is none of his prescriptions appear to contain any poisonous plants, possibly because he was also an accomplished botanist. He also recommended modifications in diet and the standard wine o'clock.

Until Dr. Fothergill's paper much of the language of menopause was about doom, as if there were no greater horror than a woman in menopause, and unfortunately his work didn't put an end to those negative attitudes. In 1787 Claude Jeannet des Longrois, a French physician, referred to women in menopause as dethroned queens. Many of the texts of the day that are applicable to women in menopause have fairly large sections on cancers of the cervix, uterus, and breast, and even though those were almost universally fatal conditions with awful deaths, the language is less depressing than that used for menopause. Nevertheless, over time Dr. Fothergill's paper was translated into several languages and began to attract attention. This also coincided with a shift in general changes in attitudes toward aging.

The Birth of the Menopause

As discussed earlier, the words *"la ménèspausie"* first appear in 1812 in a dissertation written by Dr. De Gardanne. He subsequently published a book on la ménèspausie in 1816 titled *Advice to Women Entering the Critical Age* or *Avis aux femmes qui entrent dans l'âge critique*. The second edition, published in 1821, has an updated title—*Menopause: The Critical Age of Women* or *De la Ménopause, ou de l'âge critique des femmes*.

De Gardanne explains in his 1812 paper that a new term was needed as there were so many words in use. Some of the classics of the day include the not so bad: climacteric, critical time, critical stage, and change of life; the not great: middle-age decline; and the simply awful: women's inferno, women's winter, and the death of sex. Can you imagine saying, "Just have to pop down the street to see my Woman's Winter specialist for some advice…shall I pick up a baguette on the way home?" Right. My best guess is being the first with a new name that didn't sound pejorative and was specific to women—terms like "climacteric" and "change of life" were also applied to men—was good for business and likely made it sound as if he had something new to offer.

In his dissertation in 1812 De Gardanne explains his origin of *la ménèspausie* as a portmanteau of two Greek words, μήνας or *mois* in French (month in English), and παῦσις or *cessation* in French (cessation in English), which he states is taken from παύω that he translates as *je finis* or *je cesse*—I stop or I cease in English. To De Gardanne these two Greek words may have come together phonetically in French as *ménèspausie*. Perhaps his final word choice was also influenced by the French word *menstrues* (menses in English, from the Latin *mēnsēs*, which according to the Oxford English Dictionary is "a specific application of the plural" for month).

While today we think of the word pause as a temporary break, it is clear from De Gardanne's writing that he didn't expect menstruation to start up again and the "pausie" of his *ménèspausie* was meant as final.

What De Gardanne doesn't explain is why he shortened *la ménèspausie* to *ménopause* in the second edition of his book in 1821? And why did he use it for the title of this second edition? Had his word become that popular or was it so associated with him that it was branding and would help his work stand out from other works on the subject?

I read De Gardanne's book in French, but my junior high Canadian French Immersion felt like an entirely different language than nineteenth-century French. To be certain to understand the book, I received a generous assist from Dr. Martin Winkler, a French OB/GYN who wrote the introduction for the French edition of *The Vagina Bible*.

De Gardanne's book is best summed up as a lamenting of the fate of women as they age, so not a revolutionary work. He doesn't discuss symptoms of menopause in any detail, and like many physicians of the day and those before him, he blames many illnesses that affect women as they age on menopause. How the uterus causes gout or problems with digestion for women and yet men get these same conditions is never explained. It's a tired trope—men age and women are betrayed by their womb. (I despise that word, but I'll allow it here.)

De Gardanne's book is filled with dietary advice, such as eat starchy foods and avoid all alcohol except watered-down wine, what bed to choose, and hygiene recommendations—there are pages and pages on the perils of hair dye and makeup (blush being specifically problematic). Clothing is also discussed, although not what fabric might help to keep one cool, rather how it was so tragic to see women older than fifty dressing as if they were younger, especially if they were showing their bare arms. And this nugget: "At the menopausal era, one would think that age made the woman wise; on the contrary, habit, added to need, means that she consults her fashion merchant more often than her doctor."

Given the patriarchal advice and the quality of the medical therapies (vulvar leeches anyone?), no wonder retail therapy was popular. And I hope there were plenty of short sleeves and prominently displayed breasts. De Gardanne's book was not well received by his peers, who correctly pointed out that he offered very little information and simply blamed most illnesses of age on menopause.

Many medical textbooks from the time of De Gardanne were like his—short on medicine, but dripping with patriarchy. One notable exception is Dr. Edward Tilt's 1857 text, *The Change of Life in Health and Disease*. It was popular, scientific, and forward-thinking for the time. Tilt used the word "menopause" once and then only to indicate that others have used the word and he found it unnecessary—it seems to have been a very specific callout of De Gardanne (I do love some good medical shade). He preferred the term cessation or c. for short. Dr. Tilt's book is fascinating.

Like Fothergill, he doesn't view menopause as a disease and includes data on women he surveyed about their symptoms. Dr. Tilt uses the term "flushes" as it is "short and expressive," but mentions "hot blooms" and states that term, more "faithfully indicates what really occurs." He made many medical observations that hold up today. While a lot of the therapies are awful, they were based on the science, such as it were, and in general medical therapies of the day were universally dreadful.

Before De Gardanne introduced the term "menopause," the most common terms found in textbooks were "climacteric," "critical age," and the abbreviation "c." for cessation of menses, but menopause soon made its way into the medical lexicon. It appears in the *New England Journal of Medicine* in 1871 and over the years was used interchangeably with climacteric to describe the time around the final menstrual period and the years afterward.

After reading Dr. Tilt's book and many articles on menopause in medical journals from the 1920s to the late 1940s, I'm struck by the moments of distress and suffering that have been captured given the expository style of the day—snippets of lives instead of the de-identified tables and charts of today. Such as: "H.L., aged 31, married, artificial menopause November, 1925 (intrauterine and vaginal radium for endometriosis) who has hot flushes every 5 minutes" as well as "headaches, and backaches who was admitted to hospital in 1929 and discharged with no diagnosis who finally found her way to a menopause clinic for treatment in 1932."

Article after article from before Big Pharma detailed symptoms identical to what I hear today—hot flushes, sweats, insomnia, joint pains, and mood disturbances. Although, tragically many women in these papers suffered from premature ovarian insufficiency due to radiation therapy, surgical menopause, or reasons that are unknown. Many had also been erroneously labeled as hysterical or "nervous."

There were even clinics dedicated to menopause as it was considered so medically challenging—this was a time before reliable menopausal hormone therapy (MHT) existed. Drs. Samuel Geist and Frank Spellman from Mount Sinai in New York wrote the following in the *American Journal of Obstetrics and Gynecology* in 1932:

No symptom complex has been more resistant to treatment and none so wrapped in obscurity from an etiological standpoint as a group of manifestations characterized as the menopause.

Drs. Geist and Spellman note in their clinic that simply being listened to and having contact with a doctor may have been equally if not more therapeutic than what they had to offer.

Having your experiences validated is powerful medicine.

The term "menopause" supplanted "climacteric" as the go-to term in the United States by the 1960s. What changed? While hormones had been prescribed for more than thirty years, they were messy, expensive affairs that typically required injections, which would have produced wild swings in hormone levels. What happened in the 1950s was a new method of production, so hormones could be taken as a pill. Now there was a far better product to sell. The PR firms knocked themselves out—Are you in the menopause? You can transition without tears! Why the pharmaceutical industry settled on menopause and not climacteric or the change probably reflects a greater public familiarity with the term, but there may have been other reasons. My personal belief is that "pause" tied into the marketing—that with these new hormones menopause could truly be temporary.

Fortunately, the pendulum has swung away from the disease model and in the 2020s we're back to the concept of menopause as a phase or change of life that can be helped with preventative care and may or may not require medical intervention, but for the present time the word "menopause" in North America seems here to stay.

Does the Word We Use Matter?

Dr. Lera Boroditsky's TED Talk "How language shapes the way we think" has over ten million views and with good reason. It's a fascinating look at how language isn't a passive descriptor; rather, it's an active participant. Words influence our thoughts.

Many languages have gendered nouns—masculine and feminine—so a word may be feminine in one language and masculine in another. When researchers studied native speakers of languages with different genders, they found people thought of a noun differently based on its gender. One example given by Dr. Boroditsky in her talk is "bridge," grammatically feminine in German and masculine in Spanish. Native German speakers are more likely to describe a bridge with stereotypical feminine words, for example "beautiful," and native Spanish speakers in masculine terms, such as "strong."

What if we apply that same concept in medical terminology? For example, the word "pudendum"—a general term for external genitals of women comes from the Latin *pudor,* which means shame or the clitoris, which is from the Latin *kleio,* meaning to hide. Might these Latin origins have affected how physicians viewed these body parts, reinforcing general societal misogyny?

And how might the word menopause affect what we think of the experience?

The first issue is the *pause,* which in today's world feels negative given the general societal view that women should hold back, reflect on how they present themselves, or that they should diminish as they age. Pause is also not permanent, but the final menstrual period is really the final menstrual period. Another issue is that the end of menstruation is a symptom, not the cause, and focusing on the final menstrual period ignores the fact that many women have symptoms and health conditions associated with menopause starting years before menstruation ends. It's also misogynistic to tie a description for one-third or possibly even one-half of a woman's life to the function of her uterus and ovaries. We don't define men as they age by an obvious physical change in their reproductive function. Yes, the menopause continuum is a marker for an increased risk of heart disease for women, but so is erectile dysfunction for men— in fact many medical experts consider erectile dysfunction the "canary in the coal mine" for men's heart health.

Now imagine a world where we said men were in *erectopause?*
Right.

Many cultures manage just fine without the word menopause. In Dutch the word is *overgang,* meaning the passing way or road from "A to B." In Finnish the term is *vaidhevoudet, c*hange of year, in Swedish it's *klimacterium,* change or stages of life, and in Japanese the word is 閉経期 or *kōnenki,* which translates to change of life. There is some research that suggests women in cultures that don't use the word menopause may suffer less during their menopause transition. This doesn't mean that changing a word will change whether a woman has hot flushes or vaginal dryness, but perhaps when a society publicly embraces menopause as a change as opposed to a dreadful disease there are downstream effects. This isn't any different from what Dr. Fothergill proposed in late 1776. After all, it's harder to feel positive about yourself when everyone is telling you how much you suck.

It's clear that many women want to talk about the changes happening to their bodies, so a word is needed. But menopause? If we can manage to look after women in their twenties and thirties without tying them to their first menstrual period, surely we can do the same for women after their final menstrual period? When I'm sixty it will feel ridiculous to describe my health based on my last menstrual period. It feels ridiculous now at fifty-four, especially given the final last menstrual period is only of significance regarding the ability to get pregnant and in evaluating abnormal menstrual bleeding.

Medical thought leaders have considered other language of menopause to be problematic and consequently made changes. Genitourinary syndrome of menopause or GUSM, the changes that happen to the vagina during menopause transition, used to be known as vaginal atrophy or atrophic vaginitis. But vaginal atrophy led people to forget other genital tissues can also be affected. In addition, the word "atrophy" is pejorative—women are already diminished enough as they age, so they don't need words that evoke shrinkage. Primary ovarian insufficiency—ovulation that stops before age forty—used to be called premature ovarian failure, an awful term. Medical terminology is constantly changing as new information is gathered, so the idea that it's too difficult to change the word menopause just doesn't fly.

While menopause transition is acceptable for the time leading up to the final menstrual period that is characterized by erratic hormones, transition works just as well and takes the focus away from menstruation, although I could totally be convinced to go with the dodge. Climacteric feels most appropriate for when a more steady state is achieved—after the final menstrual period—and this was the term used for centuries for both women and men to describe the phase of middle age and beyond. The earliest writings from both Western and Eastern medicine described life in phases, so climacteric also honors that commonality.

The term menopause came to be before science knew hormones existed. It was never meant to signify a pause. It was invented by a man who felt women should cover their arms and not wear blush—whose book on the subject contributed nothing valuable to the body of knowledge except it left a term that ties women forever to menstruation. The word menopause was then weaponized by the pharmaceutical industry and transformed from troublesome phase of life into a lifelong disease that affected every woman. And not just any disease, the worst kind of disease—one that made women undesirable to men. It's not a great origin story. The word menopause is due for an update.

With menopause it is as much about perspective and branding as it is about hormones and science.

BOTTOM LINE

- Menopause was not recently uncovered due to increases in life span
- Symptoms of menopause have been recorded in Western medicine since the 1500s
- The word menopause was coined by French physician Dr. De Gardanne
- Words influence our perceptions
- Women who live in cultures that use terminology that references a change of life instead of menopause tend to be less bothered by common symptoms of menopause.

Chapter 3

The Biology of Menopause:
The Brain-Ovary Connection

To UNDERSTAND MENOPAUSE LIKE A gynecologist we need to begin at the beginning—as in fetal development, all the way to the first trimester (around nine weeks into the pregnancy). At this point the fetal ovaries and testicles (also called testes) are identical structures. If there's a Y chromosome the tissue receives signaling to develop into a testicle, and without the Y chromosome the tissue becomes an ovary. *Yes, the ovary is the default.* There is a lot of irony here as many "origin of man" stories, whether it is Eve or Pandora (the first woman in Greek mythology), have women coming after men and/or being made from man.

Primordial follicles are immature eggs and their surrounding tissue. They develop and multiply in the early stages of fetal development, and by twenty weeks of fetal life there are six to seven million primordial follicles. At this point no more can be made. This is an important fact, because menopause occurs when there are no more follicles capable of ovulating, meaning producing a mature egg. The basic plan for menopause is laid before birth.

A very cool and sort of mind-blowing fact is when your grandmother was pregnant with your mother she also contained the primordial follicle inside one of your mother's ovaries that was destined to become you.

The number of primordial follicles at twenty weeks before birth is often described in medical texts as zenith or peak, and while technically those words are synonyms for greatest number, zenith also means most powerful or most successful and peak implies success. I wasn't at my peak or my zenith when I was a twenty-week fetus. We must not assign value judgments to a normal physiological process, especially when discussing women's bodies that have long been prized for youth and childbearing.

After twenty weeks, millions of the primordial follicles start to disappear, a process known as atresia. This process continues after birth until puberty when approximately three hundred thousand primordial follicles remain. Think of sowing seeds in a plant pot. If the conditions are right, there are many more seedlings than the small physical space of the pot can accommodate. The plan was always to weed the least healthy appearing seedlings and achieve the correct ratio of seedlings to soil to give the remaining ones their optimal chance.

The Menstrual Cycle: A Primer

Primordial follicles are quiet until puberty, when complex signaling from the brain starts the process of ovulation. Incredibly, it's these tiny follicles that produce the large amounts of estrogen that drive puberty as well as each menstrual cycle. There are several developmental steps taken by the follicle along the way to ovulation, and at each step the follicle has a slightly different name (see figure 3). For simplicity's sake we'll use primordial follicle for the ones waiting in the wings and follicle for those active ones on the main stage producing hormones, even though they may be in varying stages of development.

The signaling for a primordial follicle to be recruited to start the path of ovulation and then development along that pathway is very complex and requires coordinated signaling from several hormones from both the brain and ovary. Two of the main hormones from the brain that are involved with ovulation are follicle stimulating hormone or FSH and luteinizing hormone or LH. As the follicles develop the cells that surround the egg (oocyte) make two kinds of estrogen, estradiol and estrone—es-

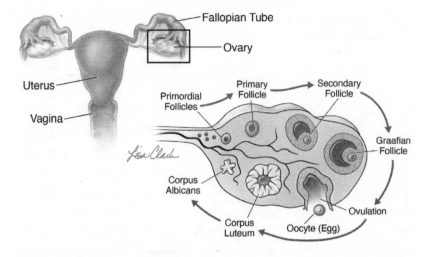

Figure 3: The Life Cycle of a Follicle

tradiol is a more potent estrogen. The amount of estradiol produced is significant as it has to travel through the bloodstream to affect multiple organs, including the brain as well as stimulating the lining of the uterus to develop. The follicle also makes small amounts of testosterone and other hormones.

The first half of the menstrual cycle is called the follicular phase. Via complex signaling one follicle dominates and the others disappear. This isn't waste; it's a group effort that leads to the follicle best suited for a healthy pregnancy. There is a constant stream of chemical communication between the follicle, the brain, and even the lining of the uterus. When estrogen levels are high enough, the brain sends messaging that triggers ovulation, which is the release of a mature egg now known as an ovum.

Ovulation marks the beginning of the luteal phase of the menstrual cycle. Some people have visions of the follicle bursting open, but it isn't under pressure. The follicle opens on the surface and the mature egg or ovum as it is now called makes its way to the fallopian tube. After ovulation the leftover tissue from the follicle organizes itself into a structure called the corpus luteum, which produces the hormone progesterone. This hormone stabilizes the uterine lining and makes other changes so implantation can be successful (progesterone is *pro-gest*-ation). The

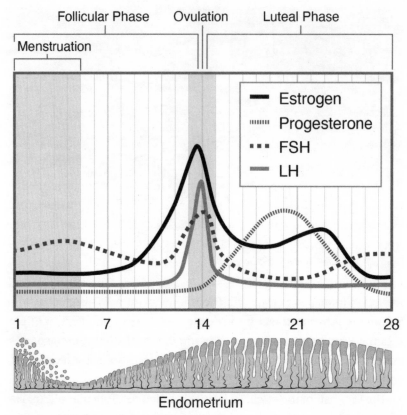

Figure 4: Hormone Levels and the Menstrual Cycle

trajectories or the four main hormones in the menstrual cycle are depicted in figure 4.

Imagine the cells that make up the lining of the uterus (the endometrium) as bricks. Estrogen builds and lays the bricks, but eventually a wall needs support. Progesterone acts like mortar stabilizing the lining. If implantation occurs, hormonal signaling from the embryo ensures the corpus luteum keeps producing progesterone until the placenta can take over. Without signaling from an embryo, a corpus luteum has a life span of fourteen days (range of twelve to sixteen), progesterone levels fall, and it shrinks becoming a small scar called the corpus albicans. It's the withdrawal of progesterone that destabilizes the lining of the uterus resulting in menstruation.

The cycle begins again when the brain signals the next wave of follicles.

The Menopause Transition

The menopause transition feels like the middle child of reproductive health. It has often been excluded or ignored under the false belief that it's not a big deal because it's not really menopause. Now we know it's a time of hormonal chaos and when many women have some of their worst symptoms. Almost twenty million American women are likely experiencing the menopause transition right now.

There are several key biological features of the menopause transition. There is an accelerated loss of follicles, alteration in hormone production by the remaining follicles, and changes in signaling from the brain. There are various potential reasons for these changes. At the level of the ovary, the primordial follicles themselves may be aging or the follicles that remain were never as healthy to begin with, hence why they never made it previously to recruitment. There are also age-related reductions in blood flow to the ovary, which may affect the ability to produce hormones. Some of the changes in brain signaling are in response to what is happening with hormone production in the follicles, but some are age related. Basically, it is a complicated process involving multiple mechanisms.

THE MENOPAUSE TRANSITION is of indeterminate length and can vary significantly woman to woman. African American women tend to have a longer menopause transition, although their age of menopause is the same. It's not possible to know the menopause transition is happening until it's happening. A skipped period or two could be stress or it could be the start. Some women may even have minor fluctuations in the amount of menstrual flow or the regularity of their cycles leading up to their menopause transition, but it's not possible to know while it's happening if that's a preamble to the menopause transition or not. That's often a source of frustration—you don't really know you're in the menopause transition until you're in deep.

Medically speaking the menopause transition is divided into two phases: early and late (see figure 5). The major differences between the two phases are changes in the length of the menstrual cycle, meaning the time between menstrual periods gets longer. During the early phase a woman is likely to see some of her cycles lengthen by seven or more days or she may even skip an occasional menstrual period. The late transition

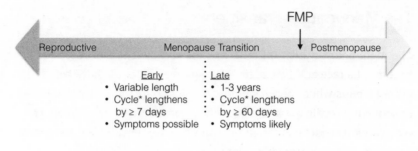

FMP

| Reproductive | Menopause Transition | Postmenopause |

Early
- Variable length
- Cycle* lengthens
  by ≥ 7 days
- Symptoms possible

Late
- 1-3 years
- Cycle* lengthens
  by ≥ 60 days
- Symptoms likely

*Cycle is from start of one menstrual period to the start of the next

Figure 5: The Menopause Transition—Early and Late

is characterized by more skipped periods—meaning sixty days between menstrual periods. When a woman starts skipping two menstrual periods in a row there is a 95 percent chance her final menstrual period will be within the next four years. Symptoms such as hot flushes or insomnia often start in the later menopause transition, but there is no hard rule here—some women have symptoms earlier than others and some may be skipping three or four periods in a row and be close to their final menstrual period and have no symptoms.

Every menstrual cycle during the menopause transition is dealer's choice, so it can really be menstrual mayhem. The closer to the final menstrual, however, the less responsive the primordial follicles, so skipped periods due to lack of ovulation become more common.

The only thing that is truly predictable about the menopause transition is that it's unpredictable.

Menopause and Postmenopause

The final menstrual period (FMP) marks menopause—at this point there are one hundred to one thousand primordial follicles remaining and they're incapable of ovulation. Women don't know their menopause birthday until twelve months after their final menstrual period, which can be annoying, but medically it only matters when evaluating abnormal bleeding or need for contraception. Postmenopause is the phase after the final menstrual period, but it's common to also say one is in menopause.

In describing menopause it's not uncommon for textbooks and articles to use the word "exhausted" when there are no more follicles capable of ovulating, but the ovaries aren't exhausted, tired, or used up. It's not as if they started a race and had to stop due to injury or inadequate training. Ovulation ends when it ends because that's the plan. If we applied that same tone to erectile dysfunction, we'd expect textbooks to declare that the penis is worn out. In medicine, men get to age with gentle euphemisms and women get exiled to Not Hotsville. Generations of medical professionals were trained with this language, and many have likely used these same words when talking with their patients—and that needs to change.

It was long believed that the ovaries were "nonfunctional" after menopause. Some of that was the inability to measure the very low levels of estradiol, testosterone, and other hormones in postmenopausal women. In the 1980s and early 1990s when I was in training, the technology we have now didn't exist. However, the false idea that the ovaries were dead after menopause also came from the long-standing belief that a woman's main value lay in her reproductive ability and so the end of fertility meant women were hanging around in the Grim Reaper's lounge waiting for their callout. So if the conventional "wisdom" is the ovaries have no value after menopause, there would be no need to study what you "know" to be true.

We now understand that the ovaries are involved in hormone production after menopause, albeit to a much lesser degree. This isn't because some of the follicles have gone rogue and are operating in stealth mode; rather, the ovarian stroma—the actual tissue of the ovary that contains the follicles—is able to make a hormone precursor called androstenedione that can be converted by other tissues into estrogens and testosterone. Therefore, removing the ovaries after menopause results in a small drop in levels of estradiol and testosterone, because it has a small effect on the ability of other tissues to make these hormones.

A Handbook on Hormones

To understand what's happening with hormones during the menopause transition and beyond, it's important to first step back for a primer. Hormones are chemical messengers; they're basically mini keys that roam the body looking for the right receptor (a lock) on cells. When the key fits the lock the message from the hormone is transmitted to the cell. Some hormones are produced in large amounts as they need to travel the body to impact other tissues, for example, the uterus and the brain, and some are produced in lower amounts for local use.

There are many important hormones involved in the menopause continuum, but some of the key players are as follows:

- **ESTRADIOL:** The technical term is 17-beta estradiol, but it is typically just called estradiol. This is the main estrogen before menopause. It's produced in large amounts in the developing follicle as it is meant to enter the bloodstream and have wide-ranging effects on many tissues. Estradiol is also made in smaller quantities in other tissues for local use, such as adipose (or fat) tissue, the endometrium (lining of the uterus), liver, brain, bone, and muscle. Estradiol levels vary significantly throughout the menstrual cycle; they may be as low as 30 pg/ml at the start of the follicular phase and be ten times that—typically 200–300 pg/ml—right before ovulation. During the menopause transition estradiol levels can even be higher than typical due to the erratic hormone signaling. After menopause estradiol levels drop significantly and generally they are 10–25 pg/ml, and the estradiol measured in the blood at this point represents hormone made in other tissues (such as fat or muscle) that has spilled over into the blood.
- **ESTRONE:** A weaker estrogen than estradiol. Like estradiol, it's also made in the developing follicle as well as other tissues. Estrone can be converted by tissues into estradiol and estradiol can be converted into estrone. This bidirectional flow happens inside cells, allowing for fine-tuning at a cellular level. After menopause the drop in estradiol production is more dramatic than the drop in estrone.
- **ESTRIOL:** Primarily made in the placenta. It isn't known to have any role in menopause.
- **TESTOSTERONE:** Produced in the developing follicle, the body of the ovary, and the adrenal glands. The main source of testosterone is the adrenal gland, so testosterone levels don't drop significantly with the final menstrual period; rather, there is gradual decline in levels over the life span that is primarily due to

age-related changes in the adrenal gland. The small amount of testosterone produced in the ovaries before menopause likely plays a role in ovulation.

- **PROGESTERONE:** Produced by the corpus luteum, which is the tissue that forms in the follicle after ovulation. Progesterone levels decline during the menopause transition because the corpus luteum can become less efficient at progesterone production or due to a longer time span between ovulations. By the time a woman is two years from her final menstrual period, only 50 percent of her menstrual cycles are producing appropriate levels of progesterone.

- **ANTI-MULLERIAN HORMONE OR AMH:** This hormone is produced by the follicles and is involved in signaling for ovulation—it's part of the communication system that acts as a gatekeeper on the pool of primordial follicles so the appropriate number are recruited into action each cycle. Without this kind of local control, tens of thousands of follicles or even more might vie for ovulation. AMH is valuable in the evaluation of infertility. There is ongoing work to see if AMH levels could be used as a predictor for menopause.

- **ANDROSTENEDIONE:** Made in a multistep process from cholesterol and is the precursor hormone made in the follicles that is converted into either estrone (and then estradiol) or testosterone (see figure 6; for the full process of converting cholesterol to hormones,

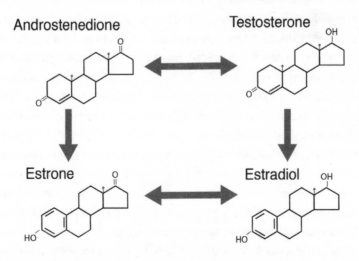

Figure 6: Production of Estradiol, Estrone, and Testosterone

see appendix A). It doesn't have any hormone functions itself per se. It's also made in the tissue (stroma) of the ovary and the adrenal glands, so with menopause there is a drop in levels but there is still plenty as it's no longer needed to make high levels of estradiol.

Estrogen and testosterone can be free in the blood or they can be bound to a carrier protein called sex hormone binding globulin or SHBG. Only the hormone that is free can interact with tissues. I remember SHBG with the following mnemonic—Seats Handy on the Bus, Girl? With less SHBG there are fewer seats on the bus, so more hormone out and ready to party, and with higher levels of SHBG there are more seats and so less hormone roaming the mean streets of the body. As testosterone binds more tightly to SHBG than estrogen (I think of it as aggressively pushing estrogen out of the way for the seats), lower levels of SHBG mean a bigger jump in the available testosterone versus estrogen.

How Hormones Change During the Menopause Transition

Basically, they're all over the place.

The thinking used to be that estradiol levels gradually dropped, triggering the brain to release more FSH in an attempt to rouse more primordial follicles to produce more estradiol. Basically, the idea was the brain is shouting at the ovaries because it hasn't received enough feedback in the form of estradiol. As we learn more about menopause, it turns out that there's more complexity here, and it's not always about estradiol. The high levels of FSH may not just be a by-product of the brain trying to trigger development of follicles, but they may also be responsible for some of the symptoms and conditions associated with the menopause continuum. For example, there is new evidence that rather convincingly suggests high levels of FSH may be a significant factor in osteoporosis. When we frame menopause as an estrogen deficiency, something that suits the patriarchal narratives of the loss of a "feminizing" hormone, we miss these other important hormonal changes.

Levels of estradiol, progesterone, and FSH can vary significantly cycle to cycle. Follicles can develop more slowly, resulting in a longer cycle. If the cycle is shorter than expected the first half is short-changed and proportionally more time is spent in the second half or luteal phase of the cycle, which is the time when women experience premenstrual symptoms (PMS). So multiple short cycles reduce the break a woman might otherwise have between PMS. Cycles with higher levels of estrogen can result in heavier periods, migraines, and breast pain, but swings in hormone levels cycle to cycle can also be the source of symptoms. Some women are more sensitive to changes in hormone levels—for example, only some women develop PMS or postpartum depression—and that same principle is at play here as the range of symptoms and their severity can range from distressing with a major impact on quality of life to minimal or none.

The Study of Women's Health Across the Nation, or SWAN, is an American study that enrolled a racially and ethnically diverse group of women in 1996 and has been following them since, and it has provided a lot of information about the trend of hormones over the menopause transition—consider the cycle to cycle changes we just discussed the trees, the trend is the forest. From SWAN four patterns of estradiol levels emerged:

- **RISE AND SHARP DROP:** A rise in estradiol levels during the menopause transition and then a sharp drop about one year before the FMP. This is the most common pattern among Caucasian women.
- **RISE AND SLOW DROP:** A rise in estradiol levels during the menopause transition and then a slow decline that continues for two years after the final menstrual period. This is the least common pattern with a similar distribution between races/ethnicity.
- **FLAT:** Estradiol levels start lower with less decrease. The most common pattern for African American women.
- **SLOW DECLINE:** Estradiol levels have a slow, gradual decline. This pattern is seen more commonly among Chinese American, Japanese American, and Hispanic women.

There are three patterns for FSH, a high, medium, and low rise—the latter is the least common. A lower rise in FSH is more likely to be seen when estradiol levels don't rise before the FMP, meaning there is a group of women who have less pronounced changes in both estradiol and FSH over their menopause transition.

Are There Hormone Tests for Menopause?

Short answer, no. It's the great period wait, Charlize Brown.

By the time a woman is postmenopausal, her estradiol levels are generally <25 pg/ml and her FSH >30 IU/ml, but this doesn't mean testing either hormone can make the diagnosis of menopause. First of all, hormone levels vary day to day. But as we've just discussed, the levels of these hormones can go up and down cycle to cycle so a random level with a low estradiol/high FSH could be menopause, but it could also be from a skipped period or two. Sometimes the very last ovulation can produce levels of estradiol and FSH that could be seen in a thirty-five-year-old.

Remember, we don't need hormone levels to know if a twelve-year-old girl who is growing in height and developing breasts is in puberty. Similarly, if a woman is in her forties and has irregular periods and/or hot flushes we know her hormone levels are changing and she is in her menopause transition. Testing hormones to "check" doesn't tell any woman about her progress in her menopause transition or when her final menstrual period is expected. Furthermore, it's unnecessary as hormone levels don't guide recommendations for menopausal hormone therapy (MHT), although these tests are valuable when periods stop before the age of forty (see chapter 6). Hormone testing is also valuable for research purposes and as part of an infertility evaluation, which isn't the scope of this book. For now, the diagnosis of menopause is based on age, a history of menstrual irregularity followed by twelve months of no menstrual periods (assuming no other medical explanation for the missed periods).

There are other causes of irregular periods, so a woman in her thirties or forties may need bloodwork to determine the cause; for example, thyroid disorders can produce irregular periods so testing may be indicated.

In cases where hormone levels are needed, for example, testing for polycystic ovarian syndrome or PCOS (a condition of disordered ovulation that affects 6 percent to 12 percent of women of reproductive age) or when primary ovarian insufficiency is suspected (see chapter 6), they are done via a blood test. Some practitioners offer hormone tests from saliva (salivary hormone testing) and they are *never* indicated. Salivary hormone tests are unreliable and don't even reflect what is in the blood. In my opinion, any provider offering salivary hormone testing for menopause-related concerns shouldn't be managing anyone's menopause.

What about determining the menopause transition for women who typically have irregular periods, such as those with PCOS or who have irregular periods for other reasons? For these women, it may not be possible to use the onset of menstrual irregularity as a sign the menopause transition is starting. A change in bleeding patterns from what is typical for that woman may be seen, but other symptoms may also develop as a sign of the menopause transition, such as hot flushes or difficulties sleeping and they can be treated regardless of the menstrual cycle. More research on the menopause transition and PCOS is needed.

Women who have had a hysterectomy, and endometrial ablation (a procedure that removes the lining of the uterus), or those with a hormonal IUD (intrauterine device) and are not having menstrual periods, won't have their period to mark their menopause transition or determine their date of menopause. If therapy is needed it can be started based on symptoms or risk factors.

BOTTOM LINE

- At the start of puberty there are approximately three hundred thousand immature follicles with oocytes (eggs) in the ovary, and by menopause one thousand or less remain, but they're no longer capable of ovulating.
- The menopause transition is a stage of variable length before the final menstrual period—characterized by erratic levels of hormones.
- The hallmark of the menopause transition is menstrual irregularities, and women who go more than sixty days between periods are in the late phase of their menopause transition—meaning their final menstrual period is three years or less away.
- There are many hormonal changes with the menopause transition—menopause is more than just changes in estradiol.
- Hormone levels should not be used to predict the timing of the final menstrual period, diagnose menopause, or to guide therapy for women over the age of forty.

Chapter 4

The Evolutionary Advantage of Menopause:

A Sign of Strength, Not Weakness

THERE'S A COMMON FALLACY THAT women were never "meant" to experience menopause. This assertion claims that menopause is an accidental state that resulted from longer life expectancies from modern sanitation and medicine, allowing women to live beyond their ovarian function. A benevolent patriarchal society allowed the failings of women—menopause—to be uncovered.

The tenacity of this myth is testament to the impact of patriarchal dogma. Erasing menopausal women from history is literally reducing women to the functioning of their uterus and ovaries. When something feels off balance I replace the word "women" with "men" to see how it sounds. If it sounds reasonable I'm more likely to consider the hypothesis worthy of further evaluation, but if we would never speak about men that way, then there's going to be a lot of side eye on my part.

Has anyone ever in the history of medicine ever uttered these words? "Through good sanitation and health care, men are now living long enough to develop erectile dysfunction?" Doubtful.

The Myth of Life Expectancy

Life expectancy is the average amount of time a person in a given community is expected to live from birth, and it isn't applicable for discussions about menopause. For example, a life expectancy of thirty doesn't mean everyone died after the age of thirty; it means 50 percent of people lived beyond the age of thirty and 50 percent died before the age of thirty. Consider identical twin girls, one dies two days after birth from an infection and the other lives for seventy-two years. They have an average life expectancy of thirty-six years, but that provides no useful information about the life of either twin.

Life expectancy has increased significantly over the years for both women and men. This is primarily due to more children surviving the first year of life as the result of sanitation, basic medical care, and vaccines. Until relatively recently in human history, the death rate in the first year of life was very high—at times 50 percent. Looking back at my own family tree, my great-great-grandparents John and Elizabeth Gunter had six children between 1846 and 1862; two of the boys—both named Thomas—died before their first birthday.

Historically, if you made it past your first birthday your odds at living a long life jumped dramatically.

Records from some of our earliest civilizations indicate if a man survived infancy, he had the *potential* to live to sixty to seventy years of age. One study looking at records of ancient kings, philosophers, and poets living before 100 B.C.E. (excluding violent deaths as the goal was natural life span) found those who enjoyed the privilege of this kind of station lived an average of seventy-two years. Those who experienced poverty likely had shorter lives due to malnutrition and accumulated injuries and the wear and tear of hard labor.

What about women? There isn't as much data, because women were less likely to have their births and deaths recorded. For example, in ancient Rome if a woman died before her husband, she was more likely to have her name inscribed on a tombstone than if he died first. As husbands were typically slightly older than their wives, they were more likely to die first, so deaths of younger women were over-represented on tombstones, making it appear as if more women died young or shortly after delivering a baby, when really there was what we in medicine call a sampling error.

The idea that women died so often in childbirth that most didn't live to see menopause has been advanced to support the concept of menopause as a modern experience, but for much of our recorded history maternal mortality wasn't likely higher than 1 percent or 2 percent. I blame much of this incorrect thinking on modern obstetrics, because what better way to stake a claim for your need than to insinuate most women will die without your interventions? While the plethora of orphans in popular eighteenth- and nineteenth-century English literature undoubtedly supported this supposed childbed culling of women, it's clearly counterbalanced with the crone archetype in ancient mythology and literature. But if your goal is to erase older women, only the stories without them are likely to be remembered.

We know women lived beyond the age of fifty, otherwise ancient Greek and Roman physicians wouldn't have been able to accurately record the average age of menopause. Pliny the Elder (Roman author circa 23–79 C.E.) mentions several women ninety years or older in his work.

Before the advent of modern sanitation and medicine, women who lived to the age of forty-five likely had a life expectancy of sixty-five to seventy years, much like men. This correlates well with observations from present-day cultures of hunter-gatherers who maintain a traditional way of life and have not accessed modern medicine. Among the Hadza, a society in Tanzania that has resisted settlement and was studied by anthropologists in the the 1980s when they were living in traditional ways, if a woman survived to the age of forty-five years she could expect to live a total of sixty-five to sixty-seven years.

Menopause is clearly not an artifact of industrialization or modern medicine. What sanitation, improved nutrition, and medicine appear to have given women *as well as men* are more years beyond seventy. Today in the United States a forty-five-year-old-woman can expect to live to almost eighty-three years, three years longer than a forty-five-year-old man.

Menopause and the Burden of Reproduction

When most people think of evolution and survival of the fittest they only consider the individual and their offspring. This can't apply to menopause, as postmenopausal women don't reproduce so they're no longer passing their genetics directly to the next generation. But after menopause, women can still protect their genetic legacy by contributing to the survival of their grandchildren.

The evolutionary advantage of menopause is grandmothers. It's known as the grandmother hypothesis, and there is plenty of science to back it up.

While it's true that most mammals—female and male—die relatively soon after they lose their ability to reproduce, humans are not most mammals. Pregnancy is much more of a biological investment for humans. Not only does it divert calories and nutrients, but in the world of mammals humans have awful deliveries. I know individually many people consider birth beautiful or their own delivery at least, and this is totally fair, but from a biological perspective, it's more of a just-good-enough situation that depends on women bearing the physical carnage. I saw a deer deliver in my yard, and this was a drop-and-get-up-and-go situation. Fast. Minimal blood loss. No visible physical damage. Then again, a fawn doesn't have to go to school.

Humans have longer and more difficult labors than most mammals due to our large heads at birth and the relatively narrow pelvis that allows us to walk on two legs. Intelligence and being able to walk upright, freeing hands for other tasks, have both conferred huge evolutionary advantages. The problem? Fitting the large fetal head needed for intelligence through the small pelvis we require to be bipedal. It's painful, tissues get damaged, and there can be significant blood loss. There is also the risk of maternal mortality, especially devastating evolutionarily speaking, because if a mother died during pregnancy leaving one or more children motherless, those children were more likely to die.

After delivery there's the toll of raising a child until it can care for itself. Human infants are uniquely vulnerable compared with other mammals at birth, in part because our brains and nervous system are far from being fully developed. Breastfeeding and raising children require additional calories for the family unit, and young children make it harder to find food and shelter.

Who can help offload some of these resource-heavy tasks? A grandmother. But she can only be gathering food and water, sourcing shelter, and providing child care if she isn't burdened with those tasks herself.

The most helpful grandmother hasn't recently finished with her reproduction; she's enough years from childbearing that she can leave her own offspring unattended.

It's a great theory, but where's the proof?

Researchers looked at birth and death records from women in the 1700s–1800s in Canada and Finland. What they found was the longer a woman lived, the more grandchildren she had. The researchers controlled for the number of children the grandmothers themselves had as that's obviously an important variable in the number of grandchildren.

Grandmothers weren't passing on genetics for an easier childbirth, because the grandmother effect extended to both daughters and sons. While genetics may have played some role—grandmothers who live longer may have genetics that also favor survival in infancy—genetics wasn't a major driver, as the grandmother effect disappeared with distance. If a grandmother's daughter or son lived close by, they had almost two more grandchildren compared with those who moved away. It wasn't just having a grandmother who was healthy enough to survive, it was being close to one that really mattered. It really does take a village.

Sure, you say. A young grandmother would be helpful, but a sixty- or seventy-year-old? It's true that hundreds of years ago grandmothers may have been younger than many grandmothers of today. However, the value of a grandmother didn't drop with age. For each decade a grandmother lived beyond the age of fifty, she had two additional grandchildren. Postmenopausal grandmothers were added value to the family unit and were the gift that kept on giving.

Grandmothers likely enjoyed a symbiotic relationship with the family unit. Providing food and caring for grandchildren increased a grandmother's worth. If a significant percentage of the family's calories are coming from the grandmother, it seems intuitive they would have been protected by the group, increasing the grandmother's odds of survival.

This is exactly what observations of the Hadza women have shown. According to work done by Dr. Kristen Hawkes and her team, Hadza women with a grandmother have more children than those without, and postmenopausal Hadza women spend much of their day foraging for food—even more time acquiring food than adult men. When her daughter is breastfeeding, the amount of time a Hadza grandmother spends foraging for food increases.

There is a belief that throughout much of our history it was men who acquired food from big game hunting, but that is an incredibly labor-intensive task and an unreliable source of food. While it suits the patriarchal man as protector narrative, in hunter-gatherer societies most of the family nutrition was supplied by foraging, and grandmothers excelled at this task. Bringing in big game may have contributed in other ways, for example, social standing within the collective.

Psychologists talk about two different types of intelligence, fluid and crystalized. Fluid intelligence includes thinking quickly, rapid recall, and multitasking, and peaks in our twenties and thirties. As we approach middle age, crystallized intelligence develops, which is how we use what we have learned and the practical application of that knowledge. This type of intelligence would have been especially helpful for ancestral grandmothers who were contributing to the collective, perhaps by locating food during times of drought and or identifying plant species that were safe to eat.

The only other mammals known to have menopause are toothed whales, the most well studied are killer whales or orcas. Like humans, female killer whales stop reproducing around the age of forty and can live to be ninety, so they, too, live approximately half of their lives after menopause. (Technically menopause isn't the best word as whales don't menstruate, they have an estrus cycle, but we'll use menopause as a stand-in.) Male killer whales die around age fifty.

Clearly female killer whales are not living past their menopause due to benevolent patriarchy.

Researchers have studied decades of data from killer whales in the Pacific Northwest. Like humans they live in small groups, are social, and are intelligent. Their offspring stay in the same pod, so following grandmother–mother–grandcalf dynamics is possible. Just like the human data from Canada and Finland and the Hadza women, a grandmother killer whale increases the likelihood her grandcalf will survive. If a grandmother dies, her grandcalf has an increased risk of dying for two years. Researchers also found that when food was scarce grandmother killer whales were best able to locate salmon, leading their pod to food, and they shared their catch with their grandcalves.

How Did Menopause Evolve?

Many people—doctors included—address this question from the wrong perspective by thinking in terms of ovarian *failure*. This is a product of biases that consider women weaker and those that suggest that male physiology represents some kind of human standard. This false hypothesis that it's a biological failing that leads women to end reproduction before men hardly seems different from the ancient Greek physicians thinking women were overly moist because their tissue was defective as compared with men.

The answer to how menopause evolved may be found with chimpanzees, our closest relative in the animal kingdom. We split from a common ancestor several million years ago and share over 98 percent of our DNA. Among our shared similarities? Ovarian function. Humans and chimpanzees both have ovaries with primordial follicles and menstrual cycles. Around the age of thirty-seven, chimpanzees, like humans, have an accelerated loss of primordial follicles and fertility starts to decrease. The difference is chimpanzees die around the age of fifty, meaning they don't live long after their ovarian function ends. Besides longevity there are some other key differences between humans and chimpanzees—chimpanzees have easier births and their babies are independent sooner than human babies.

So the question should not be why does ovarian function and consequently fertility have a hard stop around fifty? Instead the question we should consider is how did women become so physically successful that they began to live beyond their reproductive capacity?

This brings us right back to grandmothers.

Interestingly, chimpanzee grandmothers aren't invested in their grand babies, but for humans, being invested in a grandchild is survival of the fittest—the long game. Family groups with an interested and helpful grandmother would have had a survival advantage, and those genetics would have over time become dominant. The longer a grandmother lived, the more grandchildren and so on. It's also possible that a grandmother was of some value as a birthing attendant, as continuous support during labor from a doula has been shown to shorten the duration of labor, improve birth outcomes, and increase success with breastfeeding. While studies looking at modern doulas can't be directly applied to ancestral women, having someone with basic knowledge who is able to provide care and support was unlikely to be a negative.

Male killer whales die much earlier than females—around the age of fifty—likely because their longevity negatively affects the survival of the pod. Perhaps by competition for food or some other reason. While the evolution of men isn't our concern here, it seems a reasonable hypothesis that long-living human men also conferred advantages, either directly by helping their children and their grandchildren, by supporting the grandmother, or indirectly by raising the social status of their family unit or assisting the group in general. Because women live on average several years longer than men, it does make one wonder if our longevity as a species was driven by long-living grandmothers. I also acknowledge I may be way off base, considering female killer whale longevity doesn't drive male longevity, but I do like the idea of the Universal Matriarch orchestrating human longevity.

As an aside, I sometimes wonder if the reasons stories of women appeal so much to other women isn't just a work-around of the collective public silencing that has happened for centuries. Perhaps we are wired for collective storytelling as this would facilitate passing on vital information about finding food and water. If women were the primary foragers the ability to gather information this way would have been of supreme importance.

The Worth of Women Today Is Not Tied to Being a Grandmother

Human intelligence has allowed us to grow in many ways beyond our evolutionary programming, so while the grandmother hypothesis explains how we developed menopause, it doesn't mean that women only have value as grandmothers. What the grandmother hypothesis should do is give society a kick in the ass about the worth of women in menopause. It makes the patriarchal idea that woman's worth diminishes when ovulation stops even more offensive, because women in menopause literally helped drive evolution. We must also acknowledge that by choice or sadly because of infertility or the death of her children or grandchildren, not all women are grandmothers. Also, not all grandmothers add value to their children's lives.

Why Is Menopause Linked with So Many Medical Concerns If Grandmothers Are Part of the Plan?

Hot flushes? Osteoporosis? Heart disease? Vaginal dryness? What kind of plan is that?

There's no way around aging. If deterioration of the body were an impediment to evolution, I'm not sure where we'd be or even how to imagine that alternate evolutionary timeline. If heart disease that develops after menopause is maladaptive, what does that say about being a man? While accelerated bone loss starts in the years around the final menstrual period, the risk of fractures doesn't start to rise until a woman is around sixty years of age, so that works with a natural life span of sixty-five to seventy years. It's also unknown if the increased risk of fractures with age was the same thousands and thousands of years ago. Diet, exercise, and exposure to sunlight were vastly different as were many other variables that contribute to bone health.

Menstruation and pregnancy are part of evolution's plan, and yet they're both associated with distressing symptoms and health problems, some serious. The unfortunate reality of having a uterus and ovaries is carrying on despite the burden of bothersome symptoms. If hot flushes or night sweats were as they are today, it's unlikely they would have stopped most women from gathering food. It's also possible that a life lived mostly outside and/or the diet and increased physical activity resulted in fewer or different symptoms than women experience today.

Whenever I am bothered by something menopause or age-related, I remind myself that without menopausal women our world would likely be vastly different and life spans much shorter. And that menopause isn't a sign of weakness; rather, it's proof of strength.

BOTTOM LINE

- Menopause played an essential role in human evolution.
- Grandmothers confer a survival advantage for their grandchildren, likely by gathering food and assisting with child care and shelter.
- Some toothed whales, most notably killer whales, experience menopause, and grandmother whales are essential for survival of their grandcalves.
- Chimpanzees, our closest relative, also stop ovulating around the same time as humans, but die soon after.
- Women evolved to live beyond their ovarian function because menopause benefits society.

Chapter 5

The Timing of Menopause:

Understanding the Clock

THE AVERAGE AGE OF MENOPAUSE in the United States is fifty-one years and is the same across the country for African American, Chinese American, Hispanic, Japanese American, and White women. Older studies suggested African American and Hispanic women in America had a lower age of menopause, but data from SWAN (Study of Women's Health Across the Nation) attempted to control many factors that contribute to racial disparities in health and the data suggests there is no difference. Whether the age of menopause has risen for African American and Hispanic women and is now the same as White women or previous data that showed a lower age was spurious due to racism in medical research isn't known.

Women in Canada, the UK, Australia, Norway, Netherlands, Greece, and parts of Asia have a similar average age of menopause as women in the United States—fifty to fifty-two years—whereas women in developing countries tend to have a slightly lower age of natural menopause. Women who live at high altitudes (e.g., in the Himalayas or the Andes) also tend to enter menopause earlier.

Medically the age of menopause matters as many health risks are greater for women who enter menopause earlier; for example, there is an increased risk of cardiovascular disease, osteoporosis, and dementia.

These health concerns are greatest for women with a final menstrual period between ages forty and forty-five. Women who experience menopause early can reduce some of this increased risk with MHT (menopausal hormone therapy) (see chapters 17 and 18). A later menopause, meaning age fifty-four and beyond, is associated with an increased risk of breast cancer and endometrial cancer. When ovulation stops before the age of forty the diagnosis is primary ovarian insufficiency, and that requires a separate discussion (see chapter 6 for more).

Weighing all these outcomes together, an earlier menopause has a greater association with an earlier death than a later menopause because cardiovascular disease is far more common than breast and endometrial cancer. For every year menopause is delayed after the age of thirty-nine the risk of death from cardiovascular disease decreases slightly.

Is the Age of the First Period Related to the Age of Your Last One?

If a woman starts menstruating earlier she will not enter menopause earlier—the average age of menopause is the same whether the period starts at age nine or age fourteen. The only exception is when the first period starts at age sixteen or later, then the average age of menopause is slightly later—fifty-two years.

It seems counterintuitive that the age of the final menstrual period is independent from the age of the first one—after all, if menopause occurs when the follicle count drops below one thousand, wouldn't someone who started menstruating at the age of nine have a head start on running through their follicles compared with someone who started at the age of twelve? It turns out the number of cycles isn't what contributes to the loss of follicles; rather, it's the number of follicles lost with each cycle that matters. Also, it's important to know that even though both puberty and menopause are related to menstruation, the biological events that trigger puberty and the first menstrual period are vastly different than those that result in the last menstrual period. For example, the number of follicles is very important regarding the last period but is unimportant with regards to the first period. Think of the first menstrual period as a hose that was turned on for a time to fill a bucket and the last menstrual period as the consequence of a small hole that drained the bucket. Emptying the bucket is not a reverse of the process used to fill it with water.

Women with shorter cycles tend to enter menopause slightly earlier. One hypothesis is the hormonal signaling the results in a shorter cycle may be related to the rate of lost follicles each cycle. More research is needed in this area.

Genetics

By far the biggest contributor—some studies suggest genetics controls anywhere from 30 percent to 85 percent of the age of menopause. That's a large swing, but even 30 percent is a big number medically speaking. The stability of the age of menopause for thousands of years also supports a strong genetic component.

It's important to separate the influence of genetics from shared family environment because mothers and daughters typically live together for extended periods of time; so understanding what is genetics and what is the food or another variable takes some work. To resolve this very question one group of researchers in the United Kingdom looked at thousands of mother and daughter dyads or pairs and they also looked at sister-sister combinations within the same family unit. Identical twins were the most likely to have similar ages of menopause, not unexpected, but two sisters were more likely to have a similar age of menopause than mother-daughter combinations. A fascinating finding as both sisters and a mother-daughter combinations share 50 percent of their genes. The researchers concluded that sisters were more likely to have similar ages of menopause than mother-daughter pairs due to the impact of genetics plus environment—in general sisters spend more time in the same shared environment than a mother and daughter.

The role of mother's or sister's age is more predictive at the extremes, so if a mother goes through menopause at the age of forty-five or younger than her daughter has a greater chance of experiencing menopause at that earlier age. The same holds true if a mother's age of menopause is fifty-four or older.

All the genes and their variants that affect the age of menopause haven't been identified although some are known. For example, a harmful mutation in the BRCA gene that increases a woman's risk of breast and ovarian cancer lowers the age of natural menopause.

Smoking and Other Harmful Chemicals

Smoking has the next biggest impact after genetics, lowering the age of menopause by approximately two years. Smoking also shortens the menopause transition. Toxins from cigarette smoke accumulate in the ovarian follicles causing irreversible damage, and there are likely other negative effects on blood flow to the ovaries and hormone signaling. Exposure as a fetus to maternal smoking may potentially affect the age of menopause for that daughter later in her life as follicles are developing during pregnancy. The data on exposure to secondhand smoke—meaning what you may breathe by sharing a home or space with smokers—is conflicting, but long-term exposure (over twenty years) may slightly lower the age of menopause. This was something that always weighed on my mind as my mother was a heavy smoker when she was pregnant with me and both my parents were heavy smokers for most of the years that I lived at home.

According to the World Health Organization (WHO) the highest prevalence of cigarette smoking is Europe, where 19 percent of adult women smoke. The next highest regions are North America and the United Kingdom, where approximately 13 percent of women are smokers. Rates are significantly lower in other regions of the world—in the Eastern Mediterranean 3 percent of women smoke and in South-East Asia and Africa that number is 2 percent. Quitting smoking remains the best health intervention a woman can do for her menopause.

Endocrine-disrupting chemicals in the environment can interfere with hormones. Some are naturally occurring, such as lavender, and others are man-made and found in pesticides, plastics, industrial chemicals, and pollution. Higher levels of endocrine-disrupting man-made chemicals are associated with a variety of reproductive health concerns such as earlier puberty, infertility, endometriosis, and breast cancer. Higher levels of the endocrine disrupting synthetic chemicals known as PFAS (per- and polyfluoroalkyl substances) are linked with an earlier menopause—as much as two years earlier for women with high levels of exposure.

PFAS are used in nonstick cookware, water-repellent clothing, microwave popping corn bags and other food wrapping, and even some cosmetics. The data has been a little tricky to sort out because women generally have lower levels of these chemicals than men. The reason for the lower levels is because menstruation helps women eliminate PFAS, so women who go through menopause at the age of forty-five would be expected to have had higher levels than women whose final period is at the age of fifty-two. However, now we have data that measures levels before and after menopause, and higher levels of PFAS appear to be a contributing factor for earlier menopause.

Perfluorooctanoic acid (PFOA) and perfluorooctane sulfonic acid (PFOS)—the two PFAS linked most strongly with an earlier menopause—are no longer in production in the United States. They may be made in other countries and so may be found in some imported products. Even though PFAS themselves, or products that contain them, are no longer manufactured in the United States, they almost never degrade (they're often called forever chemicals) so more than 100 million Americans have PFAS in their drinking water—a legacy of environmental waste from manufacturing and products in landfill that degrade and release PFAS. Almost every American has measurable PFAS in their blood; however, levels have dropped since 2002 when manufacturing was phased out. There's no national drinking water standard for PFAS in the United States, so people don't know if their drinking water has concerning levels or not. How other endocrine-disrupting chemicals might affect age of menopause or the menopause transition isn't known.

Avoiding endocrine-disrupting chemicals is difficult as they are in the air, our water, and the soil. Some practical recommendations are to avoid microwaving food in plastic and to take shoes off outside the house and wash hands on coming inside to limit exposure to residue picked up outside due to contact with pollution, dust, and soil. Organic fruits and vegetables tend to have lower pesticide residues compared with conventionally farmed foods and this may appeal to some, but it's important to note that organic doesn't mean pesticide free as organically-certified pesticides are allowed. Switching to organic foods may be safer for farmworkers by reducing their exposure to endocrine-disrupting chemicals given they have the highest rates of exposure to pesticides and some may be exposed in unsafe work conditions, however, organic farming is more physically labor intensive and without regulation this could lead to exploitation of these essential workers in other ways. A full discussion of farmworker safety is beyond our scope here.

Cannabis is a naturally occurring endocrine disruptor, and one study suggested those who smoked heavily had fewer follicles stimulated during infertility therapy. This doesn't mean cannabis affects menopause; rather, given we know the endocannabinoid system (the receptors on which cannabis acts) has a role in reproduction and other studies have shown that cannabis may affect hormones, it's biologically plausible there could be an impact on menopause and so this needs to be studied. Many people are eager to believe a net positive for cannabis on every body system, but it is naive to assume activating the endocannabinoid system is beneficial. We don't know what we don't know, and at this point cannabis and menopause should be in the unknown category.

Overall Health and Reproductive Health

Women who report they are in poorer health are more likely to have an earlier menopause, and some medical conditions—such as autoimmune conditions and HIV—are associated with an earlier age of menopause. The reasons are likely complex and may vary from medical condition to medical condition, so more research is needed.

Delivering more children is linked to a later menopause, but this is probably because fertility is a reflection of follicle health and overall health—so correlation and not causation. In other words, actively trying to have more children isn't going to delay your last period. Interestingly, having taken the oral contraceptive pill (OCP) also is associated with a later menopause, possibly because OCPs work by suppressing the hormones that trigger recruitment of follicles, thus possibly delaying the loss of ovarian follicles that occurs each month with ovulation.

Several researchers have tried to sort out weight and menopause. Overall, it seems that being underweight is associated with an earlier menopause. Whether this is cause and effect, meaning a lower fat mass has a direct effect on follicle aging or women who are underweight are more likely to be in poor health (some medical conditions can lead people to be underweight) isn't known. There doesn't appear to be a link between being overweight and age of menopause.

A possible link between greater physical activity and an earlier age of menopause has been identified, but this connection is far from robust. While exercise can suppress the hormones that trigger ovulation and some people who exercise a lot may be underweight—meaning there are potential biological mechanisms—it's also clear that exercise has a net health benefit and overall is associated not just with longevity, but a healthier longevity. For more on the beneficial effects of exercise and menopause see chapter 7.

Studies on diet and menopause are hard to digest. For example, diets high in fat, carbohydrates, fiber, and vegetarian diets have all been linked with an earlier age of menopause, but an increased intake of vegetables, legumes, and meat have also been associated with a lower age. Studying diet and menopause is challenging because it requires distinguishing correlation from causation and accounting for social determinants of health. Also, diets high in fiber and a vegetarian/vegan diet are linked with many positive health outcomes, most notably a lower risk of cardiovascular disease. Finally, many studies on diet don't address the quality of the diet. As of today, there is no evidence that a specific diet can protect the ovaries or benefit reproductive health beyond the benefits of an overall healthy diet. For more on what makes a healthy diet in menopause, see chapter 21.

Alcohol consumption is associated with a later age of menopause. In these studies alcohol use was quite low, typically a drink a day. The link between alcohol and menopause isn't understood, so this doesn't mean a woman should increase her alcohol intake to try to counteract other factors that may lower her age of menopause. Just saying. There are other potential ways that alcohol may affect menopause that will be addressed in respective chapters.

Social Determinants of Health

Studies have linked not graduating college, being unemployed, and a lower socioeconomic status as a child with an earlier age of menopause. The reasons are not known, and more research in understanding the biological reasons is needed. Some data suggests unmarried women are likely to have an earlier menopause, but there's also work that says the opposite. Untangling marriage from economic stability and stress is hard. For example, during the COVID-19 pandemic, married families were less likely to experience economic instability and hunger than unmarried people. In addition, women who have more children tend to have a later menopause, and number of children may play a role in staying married. Data from the SWAN study shows no link between age of menopause and marital status for heterosexual women. There is unfortunately no data for lesbian women.

Some researchers have postulated that the physical act of heterosexual sex delays menopause. The hypothesis boils down to the penis being so mighty that it can drive hormonal changes that influence ovarian aging. I don't find the data compelling. The hypothesis rests on the fact that some research has found a trend toward a later age of menopause for women who have heterosexual sex at least once a month. However, women who have later menopause are more likely to be able to continue having sex as they're less likely to have painful sex due to changes from menopause. The study that made this claim controlled for estrogen levels as a proxy for genitourinary syndrome of menopause (GUSM), but levels of estrogen don't predict the ability to engage in sexual activity.

It also makes little evolutionary sense considering reproductive outcomes are generally poor in the late forties (for example, a higher rate of miscarriage, stillbirth, and maternal mortality), so extending the ability to reproduce by a few months or even a year at this end of the reproductive spectrum hardly seems advantageous. In fact, it seems the opposite because the worst thing for survival of young children is death of their mother, and pregnancies in the late forties would increase that risk. Also, if sexual frequency improved ovarian function, we would likely also see improvement with more sex at younger ages, but we don't.

Surgery and Menopause

A hysterectomy (removing the uterus), ovarian surgery (such as removing ovarian cysts), and uterine artery embolization (a procedure used to treat fibroids, see chapter 10) are all associated with a lower age of menopause. This is likely due to the impact of the surgery on blood flow to the ovaries as well as the inflammation that happens as tissues heal. Surgery to remove an ovarian cyst also has an additional impact. When a cyst is pulled away from the normal ovarian tissue, some normal ovary—and the follicles it contains—are also removed.

Tubal ligation or removing the fallopian tubes (salpingectomy) doesn't affect the age of menopause, but the latter does reduce the risk of ovarian cancer by 50 percent because many of these cancers originate in the fallopian tube.

Removing the ovaries (bilateral oophorectomy) before the natural age of menopause is known as surgical menopause, and clearly this impacts the age at which one's period stops. Surgical menopause is associated with worse symptoms of menopause, as well as an increased risk of cardiovascular disease, osteoporosis, and dementia. These risks are the greatest when ovaries are removed before age forty-five. While some of these risks can be reduced with menopausal hormone therapy (MHT), not all women want to take hormones and it isn't clear whether hormones can completely compensate risk-wise. Since 2008 the American College of Obstetricians and Gynecologists (ACOG) has recommended against incidental removal of ovaries—meaning for no medical reason—before menopause.

What about removing the ovaries after menopause? The small amounts of hormones produced may be important, because removing the ovaries between menopause and age sixty-five increases the risk of death—primarily due to increases in heart attack and osteoporosis. The increased risk isn't large—in one study surgically removing ovaries between the ages of fifty and fifty-four resulted in a 9 percent increased risk of dying before the age of eighty, but the fact that this increased risk exists suggests the small amount of hormones produced in the postmenopausal ovary play some role. Studies also tell us that removing ovaries after menopause may have a negative impact on sexual functioning.

For women with ovarian cancer, an ovarian mass that is suspicious for cancer, and those with genetic mutations that increase their risk of ovarian cancer, the risks associated with surgical menopause are worth it. Without surgery, most types of ovarian cancer are fatal. Women with the BRCA1 mutation have a lifetime risk of ovarian cancer of approximately 40 percent and that risk is 17 percent for women with BRCA2 mutation. In comparison the risk of ovarian cancer in the general population is 1 percent. Testing for BRCA mutations is only recommended for women who have specific risk factors, such as women with a strong family history of

breast and ovarian cancer or those with a moderate risk who are of Ash-
kenazi Jewish or Eastern European ancestry. Women should speak with
a genetic counsellor before embarking on any such testing.

What about women who are having a hysterectomy who have no sign
or history of ovarian cancer concerns? Given ovarian cancer is so hard to
diagnose early is it worth being liberal with removing the ovaries to prevent ovarian cancer or the need for another surgery down the road as a
sort of insurance policy? Can you imagine a world where we suggested
men who need testicular surgery for noncancerous reasons were advised
to just have their testicles removed to prevent further surgery down the
road? Everything sounds different when you translate it into men.

Ovarian cancer is scary. It's a horrible disease—the surgery and the
chemotherapy are brutal. There's no good screening and symptoms in
the early stages are vague, and women who have them are frequently
dismissed, so it's true we rarely pick up the disease before it's spread.
The five-year survival rate is just under 50 percent, so fear of ovarian
cancer is completely understandable. It's also important not to let that
fear distract us from the complications we could cause by removing
ovaries unnecessarily.

Like most gynecologists, I've seen many women die from ovarian
cancer, but what I don't see are when my patients die from cardiovascular
disease or osteoporosis or see their cognitive decline—my cardiology, or-
thopedic surgery, and neurology colleagues treat those outcomes. So I
and my fellow gynecologists have a disproportionate and biased fear of
ovarian cancers.

The impact of celebrity here—for both doctors and patients—is also
possible. In 1989 the comedienne Gilda Radner died at age forty-two from
ovarian cancer, and her death received widespread media coverage and
still comes up today. What is often left out was the fact that she had symptoms for months and her doctors never considered ovarian cancer. She
also had a higher than average risk due to her family history. Gilda Radner's story is a tragedy, but it isn't applicable to a woman at average risk
of ovarian cancer.

Approximately fifteen thousand women die each year in the United
States from ovarian cancer and three hundred thousand from heart disease, so a woman at average risk of cardiovascular disease and ovarian
cancer has a greater risk of dying from cardiovascular disease than ovar-

ian cancer, and removing her ovaries before the age of fifty-one only further increases her risk.

After a hysterectomy, there is approximately a 5 percent risk of needing another surgery to remove the ovaries at a later date. In some situations, the risk of needing another surgery may be higher, for example with endometriosis, a condition where tissue similar to the lining of the uterus grows in the pelvic cavity leading to pain and recurrent cysts on the ovaries. A woman with severe endometriosis who has endured several previous surgeries may desperately wish to avoid further surgeries down the road, so this is a situation where an in-depth discussion of risks and benefits is needed, and shared decision making about conserving or removing the ovaries should be considered.

It's clear that American women have historically received different counseling about removing their ovaries compared with women in other countries. In the early 2000s, 54 percent of premenopausal American women having a hysterectomy for noncancerous reasons had their ovaries removed versus 30 percent of Australian women and 12 percent of German women. That's atrocious and unacceptable. Women in Australia and Germany have a longer life expectancy than American women, so keeping their ovaries isn't exactly holding them back. In fact, it is almost certainly helping.

What's even worse is in America rates of surgical menopause are higher for African American women and the only explanation is racism—either individual doctors not bothering to explain surgeries to women, misperceptions about age of menopause for African American women, socioeconomic factors that lead African American women to get care from providers who are less invested in evidence-based medicine, or simply caring less about Black lives.

There are likely many factors that contributed to this American oophorectomy epidemic at the time of hysterectomy including out-of-date practices, a patriarchal "doctors know best" attitude, a cavalier approach regarding MHT fixing everything, racism, and fear of litigation regarding missed ovarian cancer. It appears guidelines are finally being adopted, so hopefully we'll see a reduction in this surgery. At one point money likely played a role, but OB/GYNs are reimbursed very poorly compared with other surgical specialties (after all, we're only operating on women). In the United States and Canada it seems the most money that a surgeon can make from billing an American insurance company or the provincial healthcare system in Canada for removing the ovaries at the time of hysterectomy is an additional $200, but often there is no difference in the payment between a hysterectomy with and without removal of the ovaries. Many American doctors are on salary and for them there is no financial incentive to removing the ovaries.

Medical Menopause

Some women are faced with an abrupt onset of menopause due to medications that dramatically reduce levels of estrogen. The three types of medications that have this effect are:

- **AROMATASE INHIBITORS:** Blocks the enzyme aromatase that converts androstenedione and testosterone into estrone and estradiol (see chapter 3), so they stop the production of estrogen in every tissue, not just the follicles. Symptoms of menopause can be severe because there is no local production of estradiol or estrone in tissues like the brain and the muscles. Women on aromatase inhibitors may experience widespread body pain and bone pain. They are used primarily for women with hormonally responsive breast cancers.
- **TAMOXIFEN:** A selective estrogen receptor modulator or SERM. It binds with estrogen receptors, blocking estrogen's path. In the breast this prevents estrogen from stimulating cancer cells. However, in some tissues SERMs themselves can act like estrogen— hence the term "selective." For this reason, menopause symptoms can sometimes be less severe with tamoxifen compared with other medications, because the estrogen-blocking effect varies tissue to tissue. Tamoxifen can act like estrogen on the uterus, thus increasing the risk of endometrial cancer (cancer of the uterine lining) and any abnormal bleeding while taking this medication should be evaluated.
- **GNRH AGONISTS:** Gonadotropin-releasing hormone agonists prevent the release of the hormone FSH from the brain, stopping ovulation and production of most of the body's estradiol. These

medications are used for women with hormonally responsive breast cancer and for women with fibroids, benign tumors of the uterus, and endometriosis—two gynecological conditions influenced by estrogen. Estrogen production in other tissues, such as the brain and the muscles, aren't impacted.

When taken before natural menopause, these medications produce the same symptoms of menopause as well as increase the risk of the health conditions associated with menopause, so women need to be vigilant about screening for cardiovascular disease and osteoporosis. Technically these effects are reversible if the medication is stopped, so it's not a true menopause, but for many women stopping them may not be feasible due to the risk of a cancer recurrence. When prescribed after menopause, aromatase inhibitors and tamoxifen can sometimes worsen menopause-related symptoms. GnRH agonists will have no effect after menopause as there are no follicles that can ovulate.

When GnRH agonists are prescribed for fibroids or endometriosis before menopause, a small amount of estrogen in the form of MHT can be used to reduce the symptoms and to mitigate the risk to the heart and the bones, but this option is not available for women taking these medications for a hormonally responsive breast cancer. There are often nonhormonal-based therapies to consider that will be discussed throughout the book. Preventing complications from these medications and reducing menopausal side effects is an important part of cancer survivorship.

BOTTOM LINE

- Timing of the final menstrual period (FMP) is a complex interplay of genetics, environment, and social factors that are intertwined in a way that's difficult to separate.
- Menopause between the ages of forty and forty-five is associated with an increased risk of medical conditions such as cardiovascular disease and osteoporosis as well as an increased risk of mortality.

- A sister's age is more predictive of age of menopause than the mother's age.
- Smoking reduces the age of menopause by approximately two years.
- Surgical removal of the ovaries under the age of sixty-five is associated with an increased risk of mortality, and the younger the age the greater the risk.

Chapter 6

When Periods and Ovulation
Stop Before Age Forty:

Why It Happens and the
Recommended Medical Care

PRIMARY OVARIAN INSUFFICIENCY OR POI is the term used when periods stop before the age of forty. At one point in the not too distant past this condition was called premature ovarian failure or premature menopause, but the name was changed for several reasons. Menopause isn't an appropriate term as it is permanent, but up to 50 percent of women with POI can expect some return in ovarian function (meaning they may ovulate again, albeit sporadically, and have occasional menstrual cycles). With menopause pregnancy is impossible, but it isn't with POI—some studies report pregnancy rates of 5 percent to 10 percent. Also, the word "failure" is pejorative.

Devoting a chapter to a condition that impacts 1 percent of women may seem like an odd decision, but unfortunately and inexcusably many women with POI don't get the right medical care—only about half are getting the recommended hormone therapy. Some have their concerns about missed menstrual periods or hot flushes dismissed because they're erroneously told they couldn't possibly be menopausal at this young age. Other women are given the correct diagnosis, but if they're not interested in assisted reproduction (fertility therapy) they aren't offered the appropriate treatment for POI. This focus on fertility while ignoring the increased risk of death associated with POI is a consequence of medical professionals and society viewing women's health in terms of reproductive function instead of ovarian function. Some women are offered therapy and decline because the importance of estrogen is never stressed—I've personally seen this situation several times with patients who have been referred to me for other reasons. Once I explain what MHT offers, they are very interested in the therapy.

POI matters outside of fertility because it increases a woman's risk of mortality due to higher rates of cardiovascular disease (primarily heart attack and stroke) and osteoporosis. It is also associated with a decline in cognitive function, and women who are diagnosed with POI are more likely to develop anxiety and depression and struggle with self-esteem issues. Bothersome symptoms such as hot flushes, night sweats, insomnia, and vaginal dryness can occur, but not with the same frequency as the menopause transition. POI is also a cause of infertility, which many women find devastating.

Whatever the reason, women with POI unfortunately have to strongly advocate for themselves, so if this chapter helps one woman it will have been worth it.

Surgical removal of both ovaries before the age of forty is often included in the POI category, even though it's clearly not reversible. While the treatment recommendations are the same for POI, there are some important distinctions—no testing is needed as there is no diagnostic dilemma or need to determine why the change in hormones has occurred.

What Causes POI?

No clear cause for POI is identified in approximately 90 percent of cases, which is frustrating. It's important that women know this when they start testing so they can be prepared to not find a specific answer. In this situation the diagnosis of POI is said to be idiopathic (medical jargon for unknown). The medical conditions or factors that raise the risk of POI include:

- **GENETIC:** Approximately 10 percent of women with POI will have a genetic cause identified, most commonly an abnormality involving the X chromosome. For some women the diagnosis will be caused by a single gene—the FMR1 (fragile X mental retardation 1) gene—on the X chromosome. Women with abnormalities in the FMR1 gene are also at higher risk for a neurological condition called ataxia (a problem with balance), and male family members who share this gene may have fragile X syndrome, a condition that involves mental disability and autism.

- **AUTOIMMUNE CONDITIONS:** This is a diverse group of conditions where the immune system attacks the body's own cells. There are more than eighty and they include hypothyroidism, type 1 diabetes, rheumatoid arthritis, and systemic lupus erythematosus. POI might be its own unique autoimmune condition and so the reason it's associated with other autoimmune conditions is that having one increases the risk of another. Or it's possible that POI could be a consequence of another autoimmune condition. POI can also be an early sign of a rare and potentially fatal disorder of the adrenal gland called auto-immune adrenal insufficiency.

- **CANCER THERAPY:** Certain kinds of radiation and chemotherapy are toxic to the primordial follicles in the ovary. When this happens it usually isn't a surprise—hopefully most women are informed in advance of this risk. But even then many women aren't offered the appropriate therapy. There may be ways to protect ovarian function for some women.

- **SURGERY:** Hysterectomy, ovarian surgery, and a procedure called uterine artery embolization (a treatment for fibroids) are all associated with POI.

- **POLYCYSTIC OVARIAN SYNDROME (PCOS):** A condition of disordered ovulation. Most studies link PCOS with a later age of menopause; however, one large study indicates the risk of POI may be 3 percent to 4 percent. More work here is needed.

- **INFECTIONS:** As many as 13 percent of women with HIV will experience POI. The exact reasons are not known. It may be the infection itself, the medications, other medical conditions associated with HIV, an increased risk of social determinants of health related to an early age of menopause, or higher rates of hysterectomy and other gynecological surgery. Mumps, a childhood infection, can rarely cause POI due to inflammation of the ovary.

Vaccination against the human papilloma virus (HPV) is *not* a cause of POI.

When and How to Test for POI

POI should be suspected when any woman younger than forty has missed three or four periods in a row, especially if she has symptoms such as hot flushes or vaginal dryness or has risk factors for POI. For women who are no longer having periods, either due to a hysterectomy or an endometrial ablation (a procedure that removes the lining of the uterus and is used to treat heavy periods), POI should be suspected when there are symptoms typically associated with the menopause transition.

Many women will skip three or four periods due to other medical conditions that are not POI, so the initial evaluation is testing to screen for POI and also to look for other explanations for the missed periods, such as thyroid abnormalities, weight loss, polycystic ovarian syndrome (PCOS), and pregnancy. It's also important to remember that symptoms similar to POI and the menopause transition can be due to other causes. For example, antidepressants can cause excessive sweating and a vaginal yeast infection can cause dryness.

The initial test for POI is to check the level of follicle stimulating hormone (FSH) in the blood (the hormone that stimulates the follicles, see chapter 3) as well as blood levels of luteinizing hormone (LH is also involved in ovulation), prolactin (a hormone produced by the pituitary gland in the brain), estradiol, and TSH (thyroid stimulating hormone) as well as a pregnancy test for anyone at risk of pregnancy. POI should be considered if the FSH is elevated, typically >25 IU/ml. All other causes of missed periods will have a lower FSH. The level of estradiol will be low with POI (<25 pg/mL, but it can be low in other non-POI causes of missed periods, so by itself it's not diagnostic of POI). A high FSH combined with a low estradiol is concerning for POI.

If the FSH is elevated, the test should be repeated no sooner than four weeks. If the FSH is >25 IU/ml on the second test, the diagnosis of POI is confirmed. At this point more testing is indicated:

- **TESTING FOR DIABETES:** Given the association of POI with autoimmune conditions.
- **HIV TESTING:** POI is more common among women with HIV.
- **ADRENAL ANTIBODIES:** A blood test that screens for autoimmune adrenal insufficiency, a condition associated with POI.
- **CALCIUM AND PHOSPHORUS LEVELS:** Blood testing that screens for hypoparathyroidism, a condition associated with POI.
- **ULTRASOUND OF THE OVARIES:** To identify any ovarian cysts. In some cases of POI the ovaries may be enlarged with cysts and there is a risk the ovary may twist on itself, affecting blood flow and leading to potentially serious complications (this is called ovarian torsion).
- **BONE MINERAL DENSITY TESTING:** A scan to diagnose osteoporosis as women with POI are at higher risk (see chapter 11). A baseline scan and then repeat testing every five years is indicated.
- **TESTING FOR GENETIC CONDITIONS ASSOCIATED WITH POI:** Most important for women hoping to get pregnant, but those who simply wish to know more about why they have POI may find the testing helpful. A genetic counselor is invaluable here because deciding on the best tests and interpreting the results can be complex. The basic genetic tests include a karyotype (looks at the number and structure of all the chromosomes) and testing for the FMR1 gene.

Treatment of POI

The risk of cardiovascular disease increases the longer a woman has POI, and studies have shown that estrogen can almost completely mitigate that risk and also help prevent osteoporosis. There are two ways women with

POI can replace their estrogen—with standard menopausal hormone therapy or MHT (see chapter 18) or with estrogen-containing contraceptives (see chapter 23).

Estrogen-containing contraceptives include the birth control pill, the patch, and the ring. The main reason to use one of these methods is need for contraception and cost—the generic birth control pill may be less expensive than some MHT. Some younger women with POI may also prefer to take an estrogen-containing oral contraceptive as they may be bothered with the association of MHT with menopause. Estrogen-containing contraceptives have three weeks of active medication and one week of placebo. The recommendation for women with POI is to skip the placebo week and take the active medication continuously, because some women with POI can experience hot flushes during a week without hormones as levels fall quickly. In addition, only using the estrogen three out of four weeks means 25 percent of the time there is insufficient estrogen to protect the heart and bones, so taking the medication continuously solves that problem. Women at high risk of blood clots shouldn't use these contraceptives, and traditional MHT may be their best option.

If a woman chooses MHT, a higher dose than is typically recommended for menopause is typically indicated to approximate the average estrogen production of the ovary in the thirties and early forties. Women with a uterus will need to take progestogen (a progesterone or a progesterone-like medication; see chapter 17) as estrogen given by itself can cause endometrial cancer (cancer of the lining of the uterus). MHT should not be relied upon for contraception. One option for women who wish to use MHT yet are at risk for pregnancy is a progestin-containing intrauterine device (IUD; see chapter 23), which will protect the uterus while also providing contraception.

The current recommendation is to take estrogen until fifty to fifty-two, the average age of natural menopause. Whether MHT should be continued after that will depend on symptoms and risk factors for medical conditions associated with menopause.

Women at high risk for breast cancer will need a more individualized discussion about their options. Women with POI who are hoping to get pregnant should be referred to an infertility specialist.

BOTTOM LINE

- Primary ovarian insufficiency or POI is a condition when ovulation stops before age forty, and it affects 1 percent of women.
- Some women with POI may still ovulate sporadically and a small percentage will get pregnant.
- POI can be genetic, related to autoimmune conditions, caused by previous cancer therapy or surgery on the uterus or ovaries, or related to other medical conditions, but often no cause is identified.
- POI is diagnosed by an elevated level of the hormone FSH measured at least four weeks apart.
- Women with POI should be offered estrogen therapy at least until the average age of menopause to reduce their risk of cardiovascular disease and osteoporosis.

Part 2

Understanding the Change:

What to Expect When You're Expecting Menopause

Chapter 7

Metamorphoses of Menopause:
Changes in Strength, Size, and Shape

MANY WOMEN START THEIR MENOPAUSE transition with one body, and end up on the other side with one that feels very different. This metamorphosis occurs because strength, size, and shape are all affected by both menopause and aging. There are already many unwelcome physical experiences with menopause, for example, random bleeding and hot flushes, so the addition of a physically changing body can add to the feeling of being overwhelmed or disoriented. Sometimes it can seem as if your body is a car with a new and completely different warning light that appears each day. An unwelcome exercise in, *"Oh what now?"*

Discussions about women's bodies are challenging. By the time a woman enters her menopause transition she has likely absorbed a lifetime of toxic messaging about her size and shape. Too fat or too thin. Too big or too small. At times it feels like the essence of being a woman is to be in a constant state of apologizing for your body. As female bodies change with both age and menopause, they may become even less like the impossible ideal set for them by a patriarchal society. The few women who do show their bodies in their forties and (gasp) beyond are praised as being age-defying if they are thin and look much younger, and they're labeled brave if they've visibly aged or have a roll of flesh yet are still willing to be seen in public. Most women in menopause don't even get a tryout for the *Sorry, Not Hot Enough World Championships.*

It fascinates me that we don't think less of ourselves because we can't play soccer like Megan Rapinoe or perform gravity-defying gymnastics like Simone Biles. I suspect many women are like me and marvel at what these women have accomplished with hard work and probably genetics. And yet if our bodies don't look like Jennifer Lopez at fifty—who also looks the way she does because of hard work and genetics—we feel judged by society.

Many of us are harsh on ourselves because of the ongoing toxic culture of bodies and beauty. It's worth noting that many of our beauty ideals are based on Western Art, and whether it was a sculpture from ancient Greece or a painting from the Renaissance, a woman's body was almost always created by a male artist for a male audience. The shape and size of an "ideal" woman's body has historically been at the whim of societal beliefs and sexual mores. There have been many cycles of female beauty being fleshier and leaner. Our modern obsession with thinness and its coconspirator fat shaming has persisted since the early 1800s, when a combination of Victorian beliefs and religious ideals linked what was believed to be excesses of the flesh with hedonism and sexual impropriety. Racism is also a significant contributor as race scientists advanced the lie that Black people were prone to dietary and sexual excesses. I recommend *Fearing the Black Body: The Racial Origins of Fat Phobia* by Dr. Sabrina Strings for anyone interested in learning more about the role of racism and religion in fat phobia.

Many women have had their health concerns dismissed because they were overweight. Not only is that cruel, it leads to substandard and inadequate medical care and disenfranchisement with the health care system, which turns women away from medical care.

There are no value judgments here—all bodies are worthy and beautiful. The goal is to provide information to understand how a body might change during menopause and beyond, the health implications, and ways to mitigate these changes.

Strength

One of the sentinel physical changes of aging is loss of muscle mass, which occurs at a rate of about 0.7 percent a year starting in the thirties and forties (there is some individual variation). This accelerates during the menopause transition, then levels back to age-related loss after menopause. There is some data that suggests estrogen in menopausal hormone therapy (MHT) may help slow the menopause-related loss of muscle mass, but this hasn't been proven definitively and isn't currently a reason to start MHT.

This progressive loss of muscle mass is responsible for what many call the slowing of the metabolism with age. Muscles are a major source of energy consumption, so the calories in/out equation becomes imbalanced when muscle mass decreases if the same amount of calories are consumed. Loss of muscle mass is also associated with insulin resistance, a condition where the body doesn't respond appropriately to insulin. This causes the body to produce more insulin to compensate, increasing hunger and also leading to weight gain. The combination of insulin resistance and weight gain due to loss of muscle mass is one of the reasons menopause increases a woman's risk of type 2 diabetes.

Muscles give us strength and the ability to move. They help with balance, and they strengthen bone—so another consequence of loss of muscle mass is an increased risk of falls and osteoporosis, both of which increase the risk of fractures and other injuries. When enough muscle mass is lost that there are health-related concerns, such as limitations in movement, the diagnosis is sarcopenia. Women develop sarcopenia earlier than men and often suffer more because women generally start with less muscle mass, have an accelerated loss of muscle during the menopause transition, and women live longer than men so they have more years over which to lose muscle.

The best way to slow the decline of muscle mass, and even reverse some of the loss, is through physical activity. Exercise is one of the main triggers to repair or replace muscle cells. It can't prevent age-related loss of muscle mass—even elite athletes lose muscle over time—but exercise is protective. Those with more muscle mass in their thirties are starting at a higher point muscle-wise, and those who continue exercising have a slower decline.

Physical activity doesn't just preserve muscle mass, it's linked with a myriad of other positive health outcomes, such as lower rates of heart disease and stroke, reduced rates of type 2 diabetes, improvement of glucose control for people with diabetes, reduction in many cancers, a lower risk of dementia, as well as benefits to the immune system. It's hard to find a part of the body that doesn't benefit from exercise. If exercise were a medication, every health care provider would be prescribing it and almost every patient would want it. After quitting smoking, exercise is the single greatest health intervention.

Think back to the grandmother hypothesis discussed in chapter 4. Historically, grandmothers were helpful because they were physically active gathering food and helping to care for grandchildren. One study of postmenopausal Hadza women revealed they spent almost thirty-seven hours a week foraging for food (moderate exercise according to the World Health Organization or WHO), so being physically active not only allowed grandmothers to contribute, but also helped them remain healthy so they could continue to contribute. Consider the imagery society often presents about women as we age. Frail, delicate, standing on the side lines cheering, and yet humanity has long depended on physically fit grandmothers.

The good news regarding exercise is that it's never too late to reap the rewards. In one study, adults aged sixty-five to eighty were 59 percent weaker than younger controls in their twenties, giving you an idea of the significance of the age-related difference in strength. After six months of strength training the older group made a significant dent in the gap and were now just 38 percent weaker than the younger adults. Even exercise in eighty- and ninety-year-olds can help build muscle mass and strength, while also improving balance and mobility and reducing falls.

Exercise goals for health maintenance include:

- **AEROBIC EXERCISE:** This is what gets your heart rate going. The minimum for good health is 150 minutes of moderate or 75 minutes of vigorous activity a week. Moderate activity means you can talk, but not sing while exercising. With vigorous activity, talking is a challenge. These are the lower limits of what is needed. Working toward 300 minutes of moderate exercise or 150 minutes of vigorous exercise a week is a good goal. Overall, only 40 percent of Americans are exercising to this extent, and it's much lower for women in the menopause continuum. Over a ten-year period, only 7 percent of women in the Study of Womens Health Across the Nation (SWAN) met these minimum requirements for physical activity.

- **MUSCLE-STRENGTHENING EXERCISES:** Think lifting weights, machines at the gym, or resistance bands. The goal is to target all major muscle groups on two or more days a week. Eccentric exercises, meaning working the muscle as it extends or lengthens—like the half of a bicep curl as the weight is lowered—are particularly stimulating for muscle repair and replacement. A review of resistance training is beyond the scope of this book, but a sports medicine physician, physical therapist, or trainer can make recommendations. The American College of Sports Medicine has good resources online. Some general recommendations to consider are eight to ten exercises per session that work the major muscle groups, two to three sets of eight to twelve repetitions (the last repetition should be difficult to complete), and over time the amount of weight should increase.
- **BALANCE TRAINING:** For women ages sixty-five and older, exercise programs with emphasis on balance can help prevent falls. While most exercise improves balance, specific attention to balance may provide additional benefit as women age. One evidence-based program is Tai Ji Quan: Moving for Better Balance® (TJQMBB), specifically designed for older adults at risk of falling and for people with balance disorders. The University of North Carolina Center for Aging and Health also has excellent videos for balance and strength training that can be accessed at med.unc.edu/aging/cgwep/exercise-program/videos/balance-exercises. A physical therapist may also be able to make specific recommendations about balance training programs.

Getting motivated to exercise is hard. If it were easy everyone would be doing it. I strive for about 150 minutes of exercise a week, a combination of running, biking, and weight training, but I'm trying to increase it based on the studies I read for this chapter and it's not easy. For the first few years of my menopause transition I was exercising about 250 minutes a week and was the strongest I'd been. And then, because of life—an arm injury, the stress of kids in middle school, increased travel, and writing *The Vagina Bible*—I somehow found myself exercising less and less until I was basically not exercising at all. I'd get back into it one day soon, I'd tell myself.

Fast-forward a couple of years and both my parents died in fairly short succession, in large part due to sarcopenia. Then one day I was sitting on the toilet and I couldn't get up without holding the wall. Three years before I had run a half-marathon.

So I got back into it. I was shocked at the difference just a few years made, and devastated after my first few runs. But I did what I tell my own patients—start with a ridiculously little amount of exercise, just keep at it every other day. Each time I tried to talk myself out of exercising—because there are always reasons to put it off—I reminded myself that exercise is like free money. Even a little is good. This attitude also still helps me today when my workout isn't what I had hoped. Look, would I prefer a $1,000 gift over $100? Yes. Am I turning down $100? Nope. After six months of what felt like plodding, I am running three miles (slowly) and I'm back into cycling. And my partner is an avid cyclist, and the idea of cycling vacations together is very appealing. I could focus on the fact that ten years ago my trajectory back into exercise would have been quicker, but instead I'm celebrating my perseverance.

If you're just starting, then whatever exercise you can and will do (and are likely to keep doing) is the right one. If you have heart disease, peripheral vascular disease, or osteoporosis, check with your health care provider before starting any new exercise program. People with mobility limitations or concerns about injury can consider exercises that focus more on gentle movements and balance like Tai Chi or Tai Ji Quan (discussed earlier). Tai Chi can even be performed in a chair.

It's important to pace yourself with any new exercise program. Many of us have the tendency to overdo it at the beginning, and you want to avoid weekend warrior injuries or the negative reinforcement of muscle pain that may limit your activities for several days, which is psychologically difficult and often leads people to give up.

How physically active a woman is during the day outside of any exercise program is also important healthwise. Being sedentary (e.g., watching TV, sitting at a desk, traveling in a car or on public transportation, sitting at a computer or using a smart phone, and reading) for eight or more hours a day increases the risk of premature death, and in America, 25 percent of adults are sedentary for more than eight hours a day. Sitting is not, however, the new smoking. The risk of mortality associated with smoking twenty to thirty-nine cigarettes a day is four times greater than that associated with a sedentary lifestyle.

Many of us in America have no choice but to sit for prolonged periods at a time—the irony that I sat for hours researching the negative health effects of sitting and writing about it isn't lost on me. Exercise doesn't reverse the negative health effects of prolonged sitting, so when possible consider what you can do to limit sitting. Some ideas include standing on public transportation if you are able instead of sitting, a standing work station, and limiting sitting outside of work hours when possible. I'm trying to move away from the video conferencing that became popular—and largely necessary—with COVID and replacing it with talking on the phone so I can stand and walk around the house.

Weight Gain and Menopause

Many women are bothered by weight gain during their menopause transition and/or find that losing weight after menopause is harder than it was previously. Several studies have tackled the weight-gain menopause issue, so this is a case of researchers listening to what women report and then investigating. The average age-related weight gain is approximately 0.3 kg (0.8 lb) per year and is primarily due to the loss of muscle mass that in turn reduces calories burned and raises insulin levels. Given the duration of the menopause transition, it's not uncommon for women to experience an age-related gain of 1.5–3 kg. Most of the gained weight is fat, so the percentage of body fat also increases with age. Menopause does have an effect here—more on that shortly.

Weight gain is complex. It's related not just to more calories/energy coming into the body than are being consumed and muscle mass, but also other factors, such as genetics, medical conditions, poor sleep, stress, depression, medications, as well as many social determinants of health. Medications may also drive weight gain. In one study that followed women over three years, researchers found women who were taking at least one weight-promoting medication gained more weight than women not taking any of these medications. While the actual amount was low, over many years this could add up. The medications identified as weight-promoting include antidepressants, beta-blockers, insulin, and steroids.

It's not possible to directly blame the medication based on this study as all of the background information on medical conditions and physical activity weren't known. In addition, there are complex interactions between social determinants of health and the conditions for which these medications are prescribed, such as high blood pressure or diabetes. But if a woman is experiencing unexpected weight gain, looking at medications and finding alternatives that may be more weight neutral are things to consider where possible.

There are also many things about weight gain that we don't understand. For example, researchers compared food and exercise diaries from Americans in 1988 and 2006 and found with the same calorie intake (and with the same general proportion of calories between protein and fat) and exercise, people in 2006 were approximately 10 percent heavier than they would have been in 1988. How we live our lives now is contributing to weight gain. Some potential causes are exposure to endocrine-disrupting chemicals, changes in gut microbiome, increases in problems sleeping, an increasing sedentary lifestyle, and rising rates of depression. Taking age-related or menopause-related changes out of the mix, weight gain over time—at least in America—is common.

Obesity, Abdominal Fat, and Menopause

Obesity puts people at greater risk for several medical conditions that are also linked with menopause, such as cardiovascular disease, diabetes, and dementia. Obesity also increases the risk of endometrial cancer and breast cancer after menopause. This doesn't mean all women with obesity will develop these problems. Like almost everything in medicine it's about increased risk. Being aware of these risks allows a woman to advocate for the right screening and treatment. Weight loss—even a small amount—may also help reduce or even eliminate these risks.

Weight is traditionally discussed in terms of BMI or body mass index, overweight being a BMI between 25.0 and 29.9 kg/m² and obese a BMI ≥30 kg/m² BMI. In America, approximately 35 percent of postmenopausal women have a BMI of 30 or higher. While obesity as defined by BMI is a cofactor in many health issues related to menopause, it isn't the best tool for assessing health risks. For some women BMI can overestimate risk and underestimate for others. BMI is a reflection of body size, and more data is emerging that tell us what matters isn't fat per se, but the location of the fat. So when we focus on the size of a woman, we ignore a major risk factor for her health—the fat we can't see.

There are two types of body fat. Subcutaneous fat, which is just beneath the skin and is the fat that can be grabbed with your hands (see figure 7). Typically it makes up about 90 percent to 95 percent of body fat. Visceral fat is inside the belly—around the stomach, liver, and other organs—and makes up the rest. Subcutaneous fat often feels like it's the most annoying, probably because of society's obsession with thinness, but it's visceral fat that's the most concerning health wise. This is because visceral fat is metabolically active in harmful ways—some even refer to it as active fat. It's associated with cardiovascular disease (heart attack and

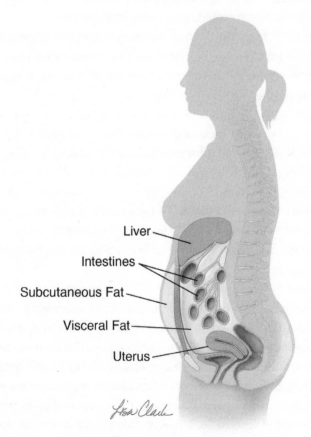

Figure 7: Visceral and Subcutaneous Fat

stroke), elevated lipid levels, fatty liver (a cause of liver failure), type 2 diabetes, arthritis, as well as other health risks.

During the menopause transition, women are more prone to gaining visceral fat. This may be why many think they're gaining more weight than they are, because their waistbands may be getting tighter. After menopause visceral fat makes up about 15 percent to 20 percent of body fat. There are several medical concerns associated with visceral fat, including:

- **REDUCED SENSITIVITY TO INSULIN:** A hormone that regulates the level of glucose (sugar) in the blood.
- **INCREASED INFLAMMATION:** May be a trigger or cofactor for many medical conditions.
- **RELEASE OF FATTY ACIDS INTO THE CIRCULATION:** Raises cholesterol and triglyceride levels. Interestingly, subcutaneous fat may help counteract this by absorbing circulating triglycerides.
- **NEGATIVE EFFECTS ON THE LIVER:** Blood from visceral fat drains to the liver before it reaches any other organ or tissue. This exposes the liver to high levels of inflammation and fatty acids, which can be damaging.
- **INCREASED ACTIVE LEVELS OF TESTOSTERONE:** Visceral fat lowers levels of sex hormone binding globulin (SHBG), the protein that carries testosterone and estrogens making more hormone available to interact with tissues (see chapter 3, remember Seats Handy on the Bus, Girl?).
- **INCREASED LEVELS OF ESTROGEN:** Adipose tissue makes estrogen and estrone from precursor hormones (see chapter 3), and visceral fat may be more effective at producing estrogens than subcutaneous fat.

The reasons women are prone to gaining visceral fat during the menopause transition aren't fully understood. One theory is the rising levels of follicle stimulating hormone (FSH; see chapter 3), but likely there are a combination of multiple hormonal changes acting in concert. Accelerated loss of muscle mass during the menopause transition may also play a role. One study suggests a link between surgically removing ovaries before natural menopause and visceral fat. Whether this is due to the earlier onset of low levels of estrogens, the rapid nature of the drop in estradiol and/or rise of FSH (removing the ovaries means the hormones immediately drop as opposed to a decline over several years), or the lack of hormones produced by the postmenopausal ovary isn't known.

Risk factors for visceral fat unrelated to menopause are smoking and lack of physical activity. During the menopause transition, 120 minutes of moderate physical exercise a week is enough to blunt the increase in visceral fat, but not to reverse any changes. Menopausal hormone therapy (MHT) may slow increases in visceral obesity during the menopause transition, although this is not currently a recommendation for prescribing MHT. While more work is needed here, it's clear MHT isn't associated with visceral weight gain.

The increase in visceral fat during the menopause transition and post-menopause matters because it may be one of the major reasons women have an increased risk of cardiovascular disease in menopause. But how do you know if you have visceral fat and are at increased risk?

Waist circumference, it turns out, is a good proxy for visceral fat. Yes, measuring with an old school measuring tape. I know, it feels positively retro given the technology of modern medicine. The measurement isn't taken at the narrowest part of the waist; instead, imagine a line dropped from the middle of the armpit down to the hip bone. The point where the lower edge of the tape meets the top of the hip bone is the measuring point. The tape shouldn't be pulled tight and the belly should be relaxed. According to the National Institutes of Health (NIH) a waist circumference of >88 centimeters (35 inches) for a woman is abdominal obesity. Each 1 cm (0.4 inch) increase in waist circumference over 88 cm (35 inches) increases the risk of cardiovascular disease by 2 percent. Between 1960 and 2000 the average waist circumference of Americans increased by approximately 15 cm (5.9 inches). For women with a waist circumference >88 cm (35 inches), a reduction of 5 cm (2 inches) lowers the risk of heart disease by 15 percent. Waist circumference may not be as reliable for Asian women and for women who are much shorter or taller than average, so more research is needed to help quantify risk of abdominal obesity for these groups.

It's important to note that not all health organizations use waist circumference to define abdominal obesity. The World Health Organization (WHO) uses waist-to-hip ratio, and to accommodate for height, researchers from the UK proposed a waist circumference-to-height ratio. It's frustrating that these don't always agree. Using BMI and the three methods for determining abdominal obesity there is a huge variation in whether or not I'm obese. I weigh 80.7 kg (178 lb) and am 179 cm tall (5 feet 10.5 inches) and wear a US size 10–12 for reference.

Knowing waist circumference can help a woman determine if she has a condition called metabolic syndrome, which is increased by menopause. Metabolic syndrome significantly raises the risk of heart disease, diabetes, and stroke. Metabolic syndrome is diagnosed when at least three of these five conditions are present:

- Waist circumference >88 cm (or >35 inches)
- High triglyceride level or taking medicine to lower triglycerides
- A low HDL or taking medicine to treat a low HDL (see chapter 8 for more)
- Hypertension (high blood pressure) or taking medication to treat high blood pressure)
- High blood sugar or taking medication to treat high blood sugar

Women with an increased waist circumference should make sure they have their blood pressure checked as well as a screen for diabetes and lipid tests (see chapter 7). The treatment for metabolic syndrome is exercise, weight loss, and medications to treat the abnormal lipids, diabetes, and/or the high blood pressure. While exercise doesn't specifically target visceral fat, it's beneficial overall and appears to reduce the risk of metabolic syndrome.

Weight Loss

Weight loss will reduce both visceral and subcutaneous fat. In one study, a weight loss of 6 percent to 7 percent (which was an average of 5 kg or 11 lbs lost) resulted in a 14 percent reduction in visceral fat. As weight loss can help prevent and treat metabolic syndrome, some women may have questions about how best to lose some weight, but I also appreciate for many women this can be a difficult and triggering conversation. If you are not interested in reading anything about weight loss, skip ahead to the next chapter. For any woman who wishes to learn more about weight loss, I hope to provide some general guidance.

I'm mindful about how I discuss weight. Many women have their valid medical concerns brushed off as being caused by obesity instead of being adequately investigated, and they've paid with their health and even their lives. I'm ashamed at the lack of welcoming spaces in medicine for women who are overweight. In addition, I've been on one long, continuous diet for thirty-one years and I wouldn't wish that curse on anyone. I can't think of one day where I haven't policed what I ate or felt guilt for not policing my food. For me it's a by-product of my mother telling me I was fat when I was a teen and growing up during the 1980s, which was a uniquely horrible intersection of thinness equating beauty as well as goodness and the nascent exercise culture. I was sixteen years old the first time I joined Weight Watchers and I weighed 70 kg (154 lbs). I was sixteen years old with a BMI of 21.8 and they let me join.

My coping strategy has been to lean into it, meaning I try to write down everything that I eat before I eat it, largely following a Mediterranean diet. This is called journaling. If I don't, I'm just going to silently count calories and judge myself, and so I have made not a peace, but a detente with this. When I journal it helps me decide if I am really hungry or not—for me hunger is an emotion, so I need to be mindful about whether I'm eating because I'm happy or sad or because my body needs fuel. Journaling also stops my food choices from living rent-free in my head and helps me lose the self-flagellation. Over time I've been able to shift my focus away from calories to the quality of my food choices. Admittedly it's a work in progress, and I'm not recommending this approach for anyone. But experts say that journaling is a low-risk intervention that can help with weight loss and weight maintenance.

It's important to acknowledge how hard it is to lose weight, but even more so to maintain that loss. Biologically our bodies are programmed to defend against weight loss, and in a Western society with ultra-processed foods readily available and often the least expensive option there's an added layer of difficulty. Also, how does one choose? High fat, low fat, low carb, paleo, keto, Mediterranean, vegan, Whole30, DASH, Atkins, flexitarian, and volumetrics to name a few. The number of weight loss plans is something else—the 2020 *US News & World Report* has a top 35 list! Yes, a top 35.

Many weight loss programs are fads, meaning they sound science-ish and fit with a trend, but when evaluated by experts they don't hold up. Given the inherent difficulty of nutritional science and the fact that it takes years of rigorous study to properly evaluate dietary interventions, the idea that a trend offers an answer that decades of research has yet to sort out would be laughable, except many people end up victimized by this predation.

Common themes with successful weight loss plans:

- **ATTENTION TO FOOD CONSUMPTION:** Whether it is avoiding animal-based products, eating at specific times (fasting), or counting carbs, fat grams, or calories. When there is attention to what is eaten there is usually a net calorie loss. This can be because calories were restricted on purpose or it may happen in a more indirect way, such as the feeling of fullness from the choice of food limits intake or the foods on the plan are lower in calories.
- **COOKING AT HOME:** Sticking to a plan is hard when other people are preparing food, so to truly follow a weight loss plan most people have to prepare the majority of their own meals. Multiple studies have linked meals away from home as a risk factor for obesity.
- **LITTLE TO NO ULTRA-PROCESSED FOODS:** Calorie intake is lower when these foods are avoided. Switching from a diet high in ultra-processed foods to any plan that isn't is likely to result in health benefits.

My friend Dr. Yoni Freedhoff, an expert in obesity medicine and author of the book *The Diet Fix*, has what I think is the most insightful advice for weight loss—the best plan is the one that works for you *and* is sustainable over the long term. Meaning can you follow this plan, when you adhere to it do you lose weight, and do you think you can eat this way for the rest of your life? If you feel as if you're missing out or it feels like a chore, it's only a matter of time before that plan stops working. That's why programs with so-called never foods don't work for me—for example, being a vegan or following a ketogenic diet. That approach makes me assign bad and good terms to food, and of course if I have trouble following the plan then I'm bad. Know thyself is very important.

Other methods for weight loss are medications and surgery. Medications can help people lose 5 percent to 10 percent of their weight, which can have significant health benefits. Some people don't lose much weight and others can lose a lot more than 10 percent. Medications aren't something to jump-start weight loss and then stop; to keep the weight off women have to continue taking them. There are several options, and an expert in obesity medicine is the person who can help a woman balance the potential risks against the potential benefits. Another method that can have significant and long-lasting effects on weight loss is bariatric surgery—women can lose 25 percent to 30 percent of their body weight. There is a small risk with the surgery itself, but given the health benefits from the weight loss, longevity is increased.

Obesity is a medical condition, but it's one of the few in which we assign or imply blame to the patient. It's also one of the conditions where medicine generally provides the least amount of guidance and support. What if we treated people with cancer or high blood pressure the same way? Can you imagine a world where a provider would give the diagnosis of breast cancer, imply it was the person's fault, and then send her out into the ether to find help? Fortunately, there are wonderful and kind experts in obesity medicine, and any woman interested in exploring weight loss should hopefully find a more patient-centric, evidence-based, and kind approach with them.

BOTTOM LINE

- Loss of muscle mass with age begins in the thirties and accelerates during the menopause transition.
- Exercise is good medicine—especially when it comes to menopause.
- Weight gain during menopause is more age related than hormone related, but hormonal changes contribute to redistribution of fat, so the age-related weight gain is preferentially deposited around the internal organs, increasing abdominal obesity.
- Abdominal obesity is a waist circumference of ≥88 cm (>35 inches).
- Abdominal fat is metabolically active and associated with a variety of medical conditions from cardiovascular disease to diabetes to dementia.

Chapter 8

The Heart of the Matter:

Cardiovascular Disease

ONE WOMAN DIES EVERY MINUTE from cardiovascular disease.

Do I have your attention? Good.

When most people think of cardiovascular disease (CVD) they think of a heart attack (myocardial infarction) or stroke, but cardiovascular disease is a broad category of medical conditions that impact flow of blood and consequently oxygen to tissues. CVD impacts circulation by affecting the heart (the pump), the blood vessels (the pipes), or both.

CVD is the number one cause of death for women—one in three women will die from CVD, and yet only 8 percent of women identify CVD as the greatest threat to their health. That's why it's so important that women and their providers expand their concept of menopause beyond the symptoms that get the most attention in the media and on social media, such as hot flushes, mood changes, and difficulties with sex. It's unfortunately still common for people to think of CVD as something that happens to men—men have crushing chest pain and heart attacks on television and in movies, but women seem to almost always die of cancer or tragic accidents. If we do think about women and CVD, it is something that happens at the end of their lives. And in one terrible sense, yes, CVD is something that does strike women at the end of their lives—it's just not happening at ninety-three years of age. Women die or have their lives seriously impacted by CVD in their fifties and sixties, and sometimes even in their forties.

Table 2. Common Cardiovascular Diseases

ANGINA	Chest pain due to reduced blood flow to the heart
ARRHYTHMIAS	Abnormal heart rhythm, can affect how the heart delivers oxygen to the tissues, and some types of arrhythmia can lead to blood clots that cause stroke.
ATHEROSCLEROSIS	Buildup of fat, cholesterol, inflammatory cells, and other substances in arteries (known as plaques). The plaques reduce blood flow and can burst, causing a blood clot that can block the artery. Atherosclerosis is a risk factor for heart attack and stroke.
HEART ATTACK	Reduced blood flow to the heart that is significant enough to damage the heart
HEART FAILURE	Damaged heart muscle that affects the ability of the heart to pump blood to the tissues
HYPERTENSION	Complex changes involving blood vessels, the heart, and chemical signals. It's not a disease per se; rather, it damages organs such as the heart, brain, and kidneys. It's a risk factor for heart attack and stroke.
PERIPHERAL ARTERY DISEASE	Reduced blood flow to the legs due to narrowed arteries; it causes pain and can damage tissues.
STROKE (ISCHEMIC)	A clot that critically reduces blood flow to part of the brain. Atherosclerosis increases the risk. Any condition that increases the ability of the blood to clot also increases the risk.

When women understand cardiovascular health and how that might change during the menopause transition, they may be able to take action to prevent CVD or to minimize the impact. Being proactive regarding therapy for CVD is literally life-saving.

What Is Atherosclerosis?

Atherosclerosis is a disease of the arteries and it's a major risk factor for CVD. It's the buildup of pockets of fats, cholesterol, inflammatory cells, and other substances in the walls of arteries—the areas of buildup are known medically as plaques. The plaques narrow blood vessels, restricting the flow of blood to tissues. A plaque can also burst, triggering a blood clot that can partially or completely block a blood vessel. Without sufficient flow of blood, the tissue starts to die.

Atherosclerosis is often thought of only with regards to the heart, and although it does cause angina (chest pain) and heart attacks, it can affect any artery. For example, a ruptured atherosclerotic plaque in an artery supplying part of the brain can cause a stroke, and the narrowing from atherosclerosis can lead to chronically reduced blood flow and damage to the kidneys. Peripheral artery disease is the reduced flow of blood to the legs due to atherosclerosis. It can cause pain in the legs and buttocks when exercising and even lead to gangrene (tissue death due to lack of oxygen). Diseases related to atherosclerosis are called atherosclerotic cardiovascular disease or ASCVD.

Risk Factors for CVD

Although rates of CVD are significantly higher for men than women before menopause, that gap narrows after menopause. CVD develops 7-10 years later for women than for men. There are likely many factors involved in the delayed onset of CVD for women versus men. One reason appears to be the increase in metabolically active fat (discussed in chapter 7) that occurs with the menopause transition. Men are more likely to deposit visceral or metabolically active fat, hence their higher rates of CVD, whereas before menopause women are more likely to develop subcutaneous fat (the fat you can grab). After menopause women begin accumulating metabolically active fat at a rate similar to men, increasing the risk of CVD through a variety of mechanisms including inflammation and higher levels of cholesterol and triglycerides. Before menopause estrogen may also be protective, possibly by making blood vessels more resistant to atherosclerosis and by regulating inflammation, so the loss of estrogen may directly play a role.

Besides menopause, there are traditional risk factors that impact CVD risk for both women and men, such as increasing age, smoking, lack of physical activity, being sedentary, being overweight, high blood pressure, and type 2 diabetes—although many of these disproportionately affect women.

Physical activity is the amount of exercise, such as running, walking, or riding a bike. Someone who is physically inactive is getting less than the recommended 150 minutes moderate activity/75 minutes of intense activity a week. Being sedentary is what happens when you aren't exercising and refers to prolonged periods of sitting or lying down (see chapter 7). Women are more likely to be physically inactive and are also more likely to live sedentary lives compared with men, especially as they age, further increasing their risk of cardiovascular disease. The reasons here are complex. Women have traditionally been excluded from sports due to gender discrimination and body shaming. Exercise is often promoted to women as a way to be thin, rather than a tool for health, and for many women there are limited or no safe spaces for exercise. It took me a lot of courage to join a gym when I was forty-five; I found the generally younger bodies intimidating, and it wasn't until I had achieved a certain level of competence—courtesy of a personal trainer—that I felt comfortable muscling my way into the free weights and onto the machines and ignoring the looks from the men who seemed angered or bewildered that I was taking up what they had erroneously believed to be their space.

Many women also had horrible experiences regarding exercise as a child, which can have lasting effects. When I was in elementary school, there was a national program in Canada called the Canada Fitness Award Program. Each year we were required to do six fitness tests, and then students were awarded gold, silver, and bronze badges based on their scoring. Those of us who didn't make the cut sat and watched as our classmates were called up one by one to receive their awards in front of the whole school. It was deeply humiliating, and I spent junior high and high school developing creative ways to avoid physical education class. It took years to overcome that trauma—it wasn't until I was twenty-seven years old that I even considered exercising for my health.

Type 2 diabetes is a significant risk factor for cardiovascular disease, so much so that before menopause type 2 diabetes cancels out the protective effect of estrogen, putting a woman at a greater risk for CVD than a man of the same age. This is why it's essential women get screened for type 2 diabetes, not only to prevent diabetes-related complications, but also so they can start screening for CVD earlier and receive preventative treatment for CVD as needed.

There are other factors that increase a woman's chance of CVD that aren't well understood. For example, both endometriosis and polycystic ovarian syndrome (PCOS) increase the risk of CVD as well as the odds of developing CVD at an earlier age. Women who developed diabetes during pregnancy (gestational diabetes), or high blood pressure during pregnancy, are also at increased risk for CVD. This association with reproductive tract disorders and CVD may be because these conditions share a root cause with CVD, but more research is needed.

Knowing if she is at higher risk for CVD may help a woman advocate for screening or consider making changes that may lower her risk, for example, increasing physical activity or quitting smoking. Unfortunately women typically receive less counseling than men about risk factors for CVD and what they can do preventative-health wise, only further compounding CVD risks for women.

Screening for CVD

Screening for CVD should be done every two to three years starting at age forty for women at average risk, but women at higher risk may need screening sooner and/or more often. Examples of risk factors that may warrant earlier screening include smoking, increased waist circumference, type 2 diabetes, or a personal history of endometriosis, PCOS, or diabetes during pregnancy.

Formal screening for CVD is a standard blood pressure check—normal is 120/80 mmHg or less. High blood pressure is diagnosed when the top number is >130 mmHg or the bottom is >80 mmHg. High blood pressure is a significant risk factor for atherosclerosis, and treating it lowers the risk of heart attack and stroke.

The other screening test evaluates the levels of lipids in the blood. Lipids are a group of molecules that cannot dissolve in water and are essential for the body to function. Every cell in the human body is constructed with lipids; they're also the building blocks for many important molecules, and they're a source of energy. However, lipids also play a role in atherosclerosis.

Cholesterol is perhaps the most well-known lipid. It helps keep the membrane around each cell water-tight; is used to make hormones, such as estrogen and progesterone (see chapter 3); and is a component of bile (a substance released by the liver that helps with digestion, especially absorption of fat). Most of the cholesterol in the body is made by cells (primarily in the liver), and the remaining approximately 20 percent comes from food. Cholesterol is only found in animal products, such as eggs, red meat, and dairy. High levels of cholesterol in the blood are linked with ASCVD. There is controversy about whether dietary cholesterol has as much of an impact on blood levels of cholesterol as once believed. Cholesterol is often found in foods that are high in saturated fat (see chapter 21), and it may be the saturated fat that poses the greatest harm, not the cholesterol.

As cholesterol is a fat and can't dissolve in water (it would float on top like oil on vinegar), it has to be packaged to travel in the blood. To do this the liver makes carrier proteins called lipoproteins: HDL (high density lipoproteins) and LDL (low density lipoproteins). HDL transports cholesterol from the tissues to the liver, where the cholesterol is broken down and emptied from the body via bile—low levels of HDL are a marker of an increased risk for CVD. LDL transports cholesterol to the tissues, and high levels are associated with an increased risk for CVD. The way I remember is H is also the first letter of HDL and higher and L for LDL and less—we want higher HDL and less LDL.

Triglycerides are storage fat and are transported throughout the body to be deposited in fatty tissue. The body makes triglycerides when there are additional calories in the diet that aren't needed, but triglycerides also come from food—most of the saturated fat that we eat are triglycerides. High levels of triglycerides are a risk factor for atherosclerosis.

Normal results for lipid screening tests are as follows:

- Cholesterol 125–200 mg/dL
- HDL ≥40 mg/dL
- LDL <100 mg/dL
- Triglycerides: <150 mg/dL (normal), 150–199 mg/dL (borderline high)

There are many factors that determine what kind of preventative therapy an individual woman might need, and a discussion about who needs to start medications is beyond the scope of this book. What women should know is if they have one or more major risk factors for CVD (such as an abnormal lipid profile, diabetes, high blood pressure, or smoking), and their ten-year risk of a heart attack or stroke is >10 percent (this can be calculated at tools.acc.org/ASCVD-Risk-Estimator-Plus/#!/calculate/estimate), then medication to prevent heart or stroke is likely indicated.

Women and Heart Disease: An Epidemic of Misdiagnosis and Undertreatment

There are tragic differences between the management of CVD for women versus men—42 percent of women die within one year of a heart attack versus 24 percent of men. Women under fifty-five who have a heart attack while in the hospital have two to three times the risk of dying compared with men of the same age. Some of this difference may be due to the biology of heart disease in women; for example, how the atherosclerotic plaque is disrupted causing a heart attack may be different in women versus men. But often it's death by misogyny. Sometimes this happens because studies have excluded women, so when women are getting what is referred to as the "best therapy" what they're really receiving is the best therapy for men. Another issue is the incorrect belief that women—especially young women—don't develop CVD. Other times it's women receiving less counseling about heart disease versus men or the fact that women are less likely to be prescribed statins, cholesterol-lowering medications, that can significantly lower the risk of heart attack and stroke, than men. Black women are especially less likely to receive statins.

Another very important point is women often have different symptoms of a heart attack compared with men. Most people are aware of chest pain or tightness—the classic elephant-sitting-on-my-chest sensation, but 42 percent of women having a heart attack don't have chest pain. Other so-called common symptoms of a heart attack—jaw pain, or sweating—are common for men. Women are more likely to have milder symptoms that may not seem related to the heart at all, such as a sudden onset of any of the following: shortness of breath, fatigue, body aches, cold sweats, palpitations, weakness, and unusual sensations (that they are hard to describe is part of the problem) in the back or arms. Sleep disturbances and severe fatigue with no explanation for several days or even weeks in the days and weeks before the heart attack can also occur. Almost two of every three physicians don't recognize these symptoms that are more typically experienced by women as a potential sign of a heart attack. In fact, women often have their symptoms brushed off as anxiety or hot flushes. As there is significant overlap in symptoms of anxiety, hot flushes, and a heart attack, it takes a dedicated health care professional to make sure all three are being considered, not just the two that aren't fatal.

Women themselves may ignore their pain as "not that bad," because for them the pain may really not be that bad. For example, for many women the pain of menstrual cramps is worse than the pain of a heart attack—after all, the force generated by the uterus during menstrual cramps is the same as the force generated during the second stage of labor. Yet, women with menstrual cramps are somehow viewed as weak and complainers. It's systemic gaslighting and it makes me want to scream.

I get that it's hard to wrap your brain around the idea that pain from a heart attack can be less severe than menstrual cramps; after all the heart muscle is literally dying during a heart attack while the uterus isn't dying during a period (although it may feel like that). The menstrual cramp–heart attack pain discrepancy underscores the biological complexities of pain. Pain from organs, like the heart and the uterus, is called visceral pain and it's processed differently than pain from, for example, a broken leg or a burn. It seems intuitive that women will have differences in how they express visceral pain as compared with men given all of the connections in the nervous system required for the menstrual cycle and childbirth, but when women are excluded from studies we don't learn about these difference and we miss crucial and potentially life-saving information. Consequently, much of the messaging women receive about heart attacks is that they should be clutching their chests because public education about heart attacks has really been about publicly educating men about heart attacks.

When a heart attack is suspected a person may need an angiogram, a test where dye is injected and travels through the arteries to identify a critical narrowing from atherosclerosis or a clot. There are two types of arteries in the heart that can become blocked—large and small. The standard angiogram is better suited to evaluating large arteries, but for women the smaller arteries are a frequent cause of heart attacks (this is called microvascular heart disease). So a woman with chest pain may erroneously get the all-clear because her larger arteries checked out when really there is a major concern with her small arteries that has been missed. Women with persistent chest pain or other symptoms of a heart attack and a negative angiogram may wish to make sure their cardiologist has expertise treating women so microvascular disease of the heart hasn't been overlooked.

BOTTOM LINE

- Cardiovascular disease is the number one cause of death for women.
- A woman's risk for cardiovascular disease rises after menopause and appears to be driven in large part by the accumulation of metabolically active visceral fat.
- Reproductive tract—related factors that increase a woman's risk of cardiovascular disease include a personal history of endometriosis, polycystic ovarian syndrome, gestational diabetes, and high blood pressure during pregnancy.
- Symptoms of a heart attack are often different in women versus men.
- Women without risk factors for cardiovascular disease should be screened with a blood pressure check and lipid profile every two to three years starting at age forty, but women with risk factors may need to start screening sooner or be screened more often.

Chapter 9

Is It Hot in Here or Is It Just Me?

Vasomotor Symptoms and How to Quench the Fire

WHEN MANY PEOPLE THINK OF menopause they think heat. This is because hot flushes and night sweats—collectively known as vasomotor symptoms or VMS—affect 80 percent of women at some point during their menopause continuum, and they affect almost 100 percent of women who take aromatase inhibitors (medications for a specific type of breast cancer).

Hot flushes are also known as hot flashes, although I prefer the word "flush" as for me flash evokes an instantaneous event, while flush feels like something that lingers for a few minutes, which is typical for this experience. My absolute favorite term is "hot bloom," which as we discussed in chapter 2 dates back to at least the 1700s—to me it really feels as if the heat is welling up inside my body and blooming out of my head. Some women like to call their hot flushes power surges, and whatever term works for you is just fine. After all, it *is* your experience.

Medically speaking, a hot flush is a wave of heat that envelops the head, neck, upper chest, and arms. It isn't just a feeling of heat; the body is warm to the touch. Hot flushes may be accompanied by sweating, redness in the face, nausea, agitation, and anxiety. The hot flush experience can vary woman to woman, but there's one constant—heat. Night sweats are hot flushes during the night that result in excessive sweating, and they're a source of sleep disturbance. They are also unpleasant, as waking up in soaked bedsheets is gross.

What Exactly Is a Hot Flush?

A hot flush happens when a wonky inner thermostat informs your brain that you're hot when you are not. Thermoregulation—the control of body temperature—happens deep in the brain in a region called the hypothalamus. Various hormones and neurotransmitters work together, receiving signals from the body and the environment, to keep body temperature in a relatively narrow zone. Reproduction and temperature control are closely related. For example, body temperature is highest midway between ovulation and menstruation due to elevated levels of progesterone. The theory is the slightly higher temperature during this time is favorable to implantation. Consequently there are neurons (nerve cells) involved in regulating both temperature and the menstrual cycle. A good analogy is thermoregulation and reproduction share the same motherboard.

The mechanisms behind vasomotor symptoms are very complex and not completely understood. It's not the estrogen levels that matter, otherwise girls would have hot flushes before puberty. A hot flush depends on a brain that had estrogen and then that estrogen is taken away. The faster the drop, the more profound the effect, which is why removing the ovaries before menopause leads to more hot flushes and more severe symptoms than the more meandering drop in hormones typical of menopause.

Estrogen has an interesting role in temperature regulation—it appears to suppress messages from a group of neurons that communicate about heat. With menopause, these neurons no longer have estrogen as a gatekeeper so the area of the brain with these heat-promoting neurons gets larger. Some research suggests that the elevated level of follicle stimulating hormones (FSH) with menopause may have a role in hot flushes.

Without the influence of estrogen, the thermoregulatory system becomes extremely sensitive to minor increases in temperature and responds in an exaggerated manner—so one flight of stairs feels like a long run in heavy clothes on a hot day. Think of it as part of your brain randomly yelling, "Fire in the hole" when all systems are operating just fine and there isn't estrogen around to say, "Don't be so shouty and honestly, let's gather all the facts first."

In an effort to cool off, blood vessels dilate and blood is shunted to the skin where it loses some of its heat. This is the wave of heat (and often redness) in the face, neck, upper chest, and arms. Sweat glands are also triggered to perspire. The heart rate goes up (this can contribute to a feeling of anxiety for some women) and there is reduced blood flow to the brain. This heat episode lasts an average of two to four minutes, stopping when the body temperature eventually drops from the cooling efforts. Because you were never hot to begin with, the body temperature is now lower than needed so there may be accompanying chills and some women are more bothered by the chills than the heat. Shivering may even occur to bring the now lowered body temperature back to normal.

Were you exhausted just reading about it? For some women these episodes happen twenty or thirty times a day. The intensity of vasomotor symptoms vary from woman to woman and are associated with difficulties sleeping, depression, and they negatively affect the quality of life. Some women are very bothered, and others not so much. It can be draining, stressful, and hot flushes make many women feel awful. Hot flushes are also unpredictable, meaning one day an activity triggers what seems like an endless wave of heat throughout the day and on another day that same activity may have no effect. The unpredictability just makes it worse because it can feel as if your body is out of control and that's unsettling.

Women with more moderate to severe vasomotor symptoms also have an increased risk for cardiovascular disease and stroke. Vasomotor symptoms don't directly cause heart disease by affecting the heart or blood vessels; rather, it's believed that the factor that predisposes some women to hot flushes also appears to predispose them to heart disease. One theory is hot flushes are more likely to occur when there is miscommunication between the nervous system and blood vessels, and this may also be a factor in heart disease and stroke. Women with moderate to severe vasomotor symptoms should be especially careful about being current on their screening for heart health, such as regular blood pressure checks and testing for high cholesterol and diabetes. Exercise is an intervention that can help lower these risks.

When Do Vasomotor Symptoms Start and How Long Do They Last?

The old thinking was vasomotor symptoms started at menopause (meaning the final menstrual period) and lasted for approximately two years. Now we know they can start during the menopause transition—even many years before the final menstrual period—and the hot flush experience lasts on average just over seven years. Data from the Study of Women's Health Across the Nation (SWAN) informs us that there are four distinct patterns of vasomotor symptoms among women in North America, and each pattern is experienced by approximately 25 percent of women:

- Starting earlier in the menopause transition and reducing after the final menstrual period.
- A later onset during the menopause transition, the most severe symptoms around the final menstrual period then slowly declining postmenopause, with an average duration four years.
- Few or none. Yes, it happens!
- "Super flashers" (a term coined by SWAN researchers) who start flushing early in their menopause transition and keep flushing long into their postmenopause, ten to eleven years total, or even longer.

This means there's approximately a 25 percent chance hot flushes will be minimal or nonexistent, a 25 percent chance of being a super flusher, and a 50 percent chance of falling somewhere in between. Some women may think they are super flashers when they are not as when women are asked to recall their hot flush experience, they report them more often than when that data is tracked prospectively day to day. This kind of recall bias is common with everything, not just in medicine, so it is vital to follow women in real time to find what they report. While hot flushes may be severe when they happen, only 6 percent of women have them daily and most women experience them on 30 percent or fewer days. This doesn't mean they don't suck; rather, even when hot flushes are common women are more likely to have days without hot flushes than with.

A variety of factors increase or decrease the risk of vasomotor symptoms:

- **ETHNICITY:** African American women report the longest duration of hot flushes—an average of eleven years or more, Japanese American and Chinese American women five to six years, and White and Hispanic women are in between.
- **SOCIAL DETERMINANTS OF HEALTH:** Poverty, lower level of education, and adverse childhood experiences (ACEs, see chapter 1) are all linked with an increased risk. Adverse childhood experiences can cause permanent structural changes to the brain that could make the brain more vulnerable to the process that triggers hot flushes.
- **SMOKING:** Current or former smokers have a longer duration of hot flushes.
- **MENTAL HEALTH:** Stress, depression, and anxiety increase the risk.
- **ALCOHOL:** Light drinking may reduce hot flushes, but heavier drinking has the opposite effect—more support for the Mediterranean diet and its one glass of red wine a day!
- **CAFFEINE:** Coffee, tea, and other drinks or food containing caffeine can trigger hot flushes for some women.
- **ANXIETY:** Women with high levels of anxiety are more likely to experience hot flushes. Anxiety can also mimic hot flushes—many of the symptoms are identical, for example, palpitations and sweating, and to make things more complex, women can feel anxious during hot flushes.

Hot flushes are typically worse in the afternoon and they can have seasonal fluctuations—worse in the summer months because heat and humidity can be a trigger. Keep this in mind when considering the need to start or change therapy—I recently had a bad run of hot flushes, and as of this writing I'm four years past my final menstrual period and four years on MHT. And then I realized my recent hot flush extravaganza started with a terrible, prolonged heat wave and so decided to do my best to cope and reassess my needs in winter. A week or so after the cooler weather came, my hot flushes disappeared.

Missed and False Hot Flushes

In studies where women wear monitors that physically detect hot flushes, the subjective—meaning what a woman experiences—doesn't always match up with what is recorded. In one such study, slightly more than half of the hot flushes went completely unnoticed by the woman—meaning physiologically a hot flush was happening, but it passed silently. This challenges the notion that hot flushes themselves are universally distressing. Interestingly, in this study positive emotions were more likely to trigger a hot flush than a negative one.

This same study also informs us of false—or what I call ghost—hot flushes, meaning a woman reports that she's experiencing a hot flush but it is not occurring physically—up to 88 percent of women experienced false hot flushes. (I prefer ghost flushes, as "false" sounds pejorative, and women are already often accused of fabricating symptoms.) Ghost hot flushes were likely to be triggered by frustration and reduced feelings of control, as well as exercise and cigarette smoking.

What does this mean?

It's important to remember that nothing is experienced until your brain tells you it's experienced. Emotions, mood, and probably even expectations affect levels of neurotransmitters, and these changes may heighten, dampen, create, or abolish many sensations including hot flushes. This is the mind-body connection. More work is needed to understand what's occurring when a woman is experiencing the sensation of a hot flush and one isn't happening physically. Possibilities include other emotional experiences being interpreted as hot flushes due to expectations (meaning twenty years ago before menopause that same experience would have been interpreted differently as hot flushes were not expected), or the brain signaling for hot flushes is actually occurring but there is simply no physical response (remember, a hot flush is the result of wonky signaling), or other reasons.

It's clear that studies that only report hot flushes that women record in diaries may not be providing the whole picture, because women may be recording ghost flushes or they may not be aware when a hot flush is physiologically present. We also don't know all the implications of these other hot flush experiences; for example, we don't know if ghost hot flushes or undetected hot flushes increase the risk of cardiovascular disease. More work here is needed.

I am often asked about FemTech, new technology such as devices, apps, or online services for women's health, and many products I've been shown to date appear worthless to me. It is either a more expensive solution to interventions currently available, the service or product is based on hypothesis alone and there is no backing data, or it seems downright stupid. However, I wonder about a portable, inexpensive hot flush monitor? Might the ability to accurately detect what is happening physically be useful in studies to understand the implications of the range of the hot flush experience and cardiac health or to determine response to menopausal hormone therapy (MHT)? I think back to my summer heat wave–provoked run of hot flushes and had I access to an app that had accurately tracked my flushes might I have seen this was an annual August occurrence and instead of worrying that my MHT was no longer working, I could have been reassured that this was a temporary, albeit annoying, phenomenon. I'm also open to the possibility that the app might have informed me there was no difference in the frequency of my hot flushes, suggesting I was just more bothered because the weather was unusually hot. As worry may exacerbate hot flushes, might this knowledge have even reduced my bother factor from my hot flushes even sooner?

Cultural and Genetic Factors

The vasomotor experience varies around the world. Women who live in countries where menopause is viewed as a life change and aging isn't considered a negative are generally less bothered by symptoms. Perhaps a lack of gloomy connotations and attitudes makes it easier to get educated as well as normalizes symptoms—when women know what to expect they may be less bothered by their symptoms. Also, when aging women are looked down upon by society that can make the first hot flush seem like an expiration date. Not feeling that you're headed for society's trash heap is likely helpful given the complex interplay between emotions and neurotransmitters. Other factors that may play a role are regional diets, physical activity, climate, and access to quality, affordable health care.

Genetics may also play a role in the diversity of the vasomotor experience. There is some data that suggests variations in a gene on chromosome 4 could be associated with an increased risk of hot flushes—this gene is part of the code for those motherboard neurons discussed earlier that have a dual role in both reproduction and temperature control. Perhaps it's possible one day we may have a genetic test that could predict if a woman is more or less likely to be a super flusher, and that may affect how some women feel about starting MHT or affect how we screen for heart disease.

The incidence of hot flushes is lower in some Asian countries, most notably Japan. In the 1980s the anthropologist Dr. Margaret Lock and her group found only 20 percent or so of Japanese women experienced hot flushes. The main theories that evolved from this finding were diet—specifically phytoestrogens—and societal expectations. Since then phytoestrogens as an intervention have proven to be largely ineffective for hot flushes—both in food and supplements—although it's possible a lifetime of eating a high phytoestrogen diet primes the body in a way to make these foods more useful. Genetic differences offers another possibility as Japanese women are more likely to be capable of converting the phytoestrogen daidzein into equol, a more active substance. However, Japanese women who eat more soy don't have a lower rate of hot flushes, so it seems there's either science we don't yet know about phytoestrogens—especially those in soy—or they have minimal effect.

At the time of Dr. Lock's study there was no Japanese word for hot flushes, so her group decided upon three phrases that seemed to best describe the experience. A follow-up study by other researchers twenty years later used an expanded list of terms to try to capture the hot flush experience, and at this point in time there was an increased number of Japanese women reporting vasomotor symptoms. It isn't known if this is because the Western concept of menopause had permeated Japanese culture—the word "hotto furasshu," a loan word from English for hot flushes, was now in use—or these newer phrases better captured the experience. Interestingly, chilliness was a common vasomotor symptom among women in Japan.

The anthropologist Jan Morgan Zeserson raises an important point about the lack of a Japanese word for hot flushes—shouldn't an experience felt by almost 20 percent of women have a word? He offers the possibility that perhaps the lack of a word or other cultural reasons didn't leave room to discuss the experience of hot flushes, even when asked directly by researchers. Researchers have since addressed that very question, comparing the hot flush experience from women of Japanese descent and those of European descent living in Hawaii. First the women completed questionnaires by mail about their vasomotor experiences and then had their hot flushes recorded for twenty-four hours via portable monitoring equipment so there was objective data. By survey 26 percent of Japanese American women reported hot flushes compared with 47 percent of European Americans. However, when the women were monitored the number of hot flushes was the same between the two groups. So cultural factors may affect what some women are either willing to report or what they feel, meaning a hot flush is happening but based on a variety of factors is not as bothersome.

It's important to distinguish whether women in some cultures or countries truly have fewer vasomotor symptoms, whether they have the symptoms but aren't bothered by them, or whether they have hot flushes and night sweats and there are cultural barriers to reporting that experience—even in a medical study. My takeaway from this is without objective monitoring of symptoms, studies reporting different rates of hot flushes by culture or ethnicity may lead to under-reporting for some groups. In addition, we need to understand more about what is happening when women feel they are having a hot flush but physically are not, and when a hot flush is physically occurring but it passes unnoticed.

Weight and Hot Flushes

Fat-phobia among health care providers has caused many women with hot flushes and night sweats to be dismissed. *"If you'd just lose weight"* isn't appropriate medical therapy nor is it compassionate, and the horrible implication is some women deserve their symptoms.

The relationship between weight and vasomotor symptoms is complex. Some researchers have suggested the estrogen produced by fatty tissue may be protective, while others have postulated that fatty tissue could act like insulation, making it harder for the body to dispel heat. Thinking back to the four patterns of hot flushes that we discussed earlier, women who are overweight are more likely to be in the group that has earlier hot flushes and are less likely to continue to have them for long periods of time after the final menstrual period. But if excess insulation from fatty tissue were truly a mechanism, then there shouldn't be a pattern of fewer hot flushes after menopause.

Several studies have addressed weight loss, and while the findings are not robust, there may be some benefit to weight loss although women should be offered therapy for vasomotor symptoms regardless of weight or waist circumference. The Women's Health Initiative trial (a large study that looked at MHT, see chapter 17) had a dietary intervention arm and women who lost weight were more likely to see a reduction in hot flushes. Even a 4.5 kg (10 lb) weight loss had some benefit. It's unknown if this is because of a direct effect of weight loss, or if weight loss may improve other medical conditions indirectly benefiting hot flushes.

Is Something Else Causing My Hot Flushes and Night Sweats?

While hot flushes or night sweats in the late forties and beyond, especially if menstrual periods are irregular or have stopped, are likely due to menopause there could be other causes. Women can have two medical events that have converged at once. The younger a woman is when hot flushes and night sweats occur, the more attention should be paid to ruling out other causes. Also, if therapy for vasomotor symptoms is ineffective, these other causes should be considered or reconsidered.

Some of the more common conditions that also cause hot flushes and/or night sweats are as follows:

- Thyroid conditions
- Diabetes
- Sleep apnea, mostly night sweats (see chapter 16)
- Anxiety
- Excessive alcohol
- Medication side effects, including supplements
- Cancer
- Tuberculosis

Treatment of Hot Flushes and Night Sweats

Treatment of hot flushes is often neglected, which isn't acceptable. While they're not directly dangerous, they can dramatically affect quality of life for many women. When hot flushes and night sweats are untreated, health care expenditures are higher and women are more likely to miss work. Many women are also brushed off during their menopause transition with the mistaken belief that hot flushes don't start until menopause. For others the medical options are presented in a way that falsely amplifies their side effects and risks.

Many menopause guides start with advice for women to dress in layers and have access to a fan (like a courtesan, I guess!?) before embarking on any therapy for hot flushes. These therapies have never been tested, but most people know that if they're hot, removing a layer or two of clothing helps. Also, with layers women can do things such as taking off their jacket or sweater before climbing the stairs (or other heat-causing activities), potentially reducing events that trigger hot flushes.

I spend a significant amount of time considering the temperature forecast and if there will be air-conditioning before I get dressed, because getting mildly overheated can trigger a hot flush. I find it helpful to wear short-sleeved shirts and dresses and in the summer I often have my hair in a bun or a ponytail so I don't feel as if I have a fur coat around my neck. Truthfully, I don't know if this results in fewer flushes or if when the heat hits I'm less annoyed because there are fewer things touching my skin to irritate me. I'm a little nervous about a certain beautiful velvet long-sleeved dress, because when I get a hot flush the desire to take something off is pretty overwhelming. I often find myself taking off my top layer before I've really registered the heat. Clothing designers really need to consider vasomotor symptoms. As one of the goals with treating hot flushes and night sweats is to reduce their bother factor, if dressing differently makes you feel less bothered, then that's great. If not, that's also okay.

It seems as if I'm bombarded daily with Instagram ads about clothing made from fabric with special cooling technology. Unsurprising given my Internet search history, but there's no data to say a woman will have fewer hot flushes or night sweats if she wears certain pajamas or underwear. If a woman thinks a fabric feels cool against her skin then it may help her, and feeling prepared clothing-wise may reduce stress. I bought a pair of silk pajamas from the company Lunya to try them out. Their data didn't sway me, but the idea of washable silk did. Also, the top has a large vent in the back, and that design element seemed thoughtful for a woman with vasomotor symptoms. I'm unsure if they've made any difference, but they feel cool against my skin and are cute and comfortable, and I like wearing them.

Nonmedication Options

Cognitive behavioral therapy or CBT involves harnessing the mind-body connection. This doesn't mean hot flushes are made up or "all in our head"; rather, hot flushes can have an impact on how we feel, and the reverse is true because the same neurotransmitters that direct thoughts and behaviors can also impact hot flushes. CBT for hot flushes involves education about what's happening medically as well as about developing skills that help replace any negative beliefs with those that are more positive or at least more objectively accurate. For example, in response to a hot flush I might think, "My brain feels like the antechamber of hell," and "This is never going to end." Those negative thoughts are cognitive distortions, meaning they feel accurate (like, they *really* feel accurate) and maybe even rational, but they overemphasize the negative. These thoughts ultimately leave people feeling worse, which may make the hot flush more bothersome. These negative thoughts may also strengthen parts of the brain involved in messaging about hot flushes actually increasing the risk or severity of hot flushes.

With CBT one goal is to learn to replace cognitive distortions with something more accurate. For example, "This is only going to last two to four minutes; that's the time it takes to brush my teeth." It takes practice to do this. CBT is typically combined with slow, deep breaths to slow the heart rate and lower blood pressure, decreasing some of the physical changes of the stress response. Whether CBT is physically stopping the heat or affecting the brain's perception isn't known. Regardless, studies on CBT show that it can lead to changes in the brain that are visible on imaging. When taught by a clinical psychologist or when self-guided at home, CBT can help many women suffering with hot flushes. When I feel a hot flush coming, I do my best to pause, take three slow, deep breaths, and tell myself, "Humans couldn't have evolved to this point without the strength of women in menopause."

Another mind-body therapy that has been shown to be effective at reducing hot flushes is clinical hypnosis, which involves achieving a very deep state of relaxation by working with a hypnosis practitioner supplemented with at-home practice.

Nonmedication options that have not proven effective are exercise (still good for you though!), changing diet to increase phytoestrogens (see chapter 19), wearing a magnet against the skin, and paced respiration. Paced respiration means aiming for fifteen minutes twice a day of slowing breathing down to five to seven breaths per minute (a typical respiration rate is twelve to sixteen breaths/minute) as well as at the start of each hot flush. Even if the data was good for paced respiration, it's simply not practical to take a fifteen-minute breathing break at the start of each hot flush—for women with ten hot flushes a day that would be three hours of paced respiration!

Acupuncture hasn't shown to be effective in clinical trials where a sham or placebo comparison group was used. While some women report feeling better, this may be because acupuncture isn't just the needles, it's also being with a practitioner who is being attentive, and studies tell us that kind of companionship can make people feel better. As long as women are informed of the science, if this option makes them feel better it's their body and their choice.

Pharmaceutical Hormones

The gold standard treatment for vasomotor symptoms is menopausal hormone therapy or MHT, and it's the estrogen that has the bulk of the effect (women with a uterus will also need a progestogen). MHT and the different types of progestogens are converted in depth in chapters 17 and 18. In general, the recommendations are to start with the lowest dose therapy that can relieve the symptoms. Doses as low as a 0.014 mcg estradiol patch have been shown to be helpful for some women, but the majority of women need the equivalent of a 0.025 mcg daily dose. For women who cannot use transdermal therapy, this is the equivalent of 0.5 mg of oral estradiol and 0.3–0.45 mg of conjugated equine estrogens (CEE). Estradiol and CEE are equally effective (see chapter 17 for more on these two hormones). It typically takes at least six weeks to see a substantive improvement, which is more evidence it's not the estrogen levels per se as those are elevated within twenty-four hours of starting therapy.

Progestogens, especially the progestins, in the typical dose used in MHT can augment the effects of a low-dose estrogen. These hormones may be an option for some women when estrogen isn't an option, for example, when estrogen even in very low doses triggers migraines or other side effects, or for women with a history of endometrial cancer where their oncologist advises against estrogen. Oral progesterone 300 mg a day (a dose higher than typically used in MHT) can also help hot flushes as well as with sleep disturbances. Both estrogen and progestogens are unfortunately contraindicated for women with a history of breast cancer.

Nonhormonal Prescriptions

When people think of medical therapy for vasomotor symptoms they often think only of hormones, but there are a wide range of effective nonhormonal prescription medications. Some women and their providers can get hung up on potential side effects without giving these therapies a try, but overall studies tell us these options are generally well-tolerated. Remember, this isn't a marriage; a medication can easily be stopped if it's not providing a net benefit for quality of life. Nonhormonal prescriptions include the following:

- **ANTIDEPRESSANTS:** Using an antidepressant for hot flushes doesn't mean a woman is depressed or her hot flushes are imaginary; rather, the chemical changes that result in hot flushes appear to involve many of the same neurotransmitters as depression. Paroxetine mesylate (Brisdelle) 7.5 mg and paroxetine hydrochloride (Paxil) 10–20 mg (higher than 12.5 mg may add more side effects without much additional benefit) can be very helpful for hot flushes and also reduce nighttime awakenings from night sweats—a definite bonus. It's unclear if there is a meaningful difference, besides cost, between paroxetine mesylate and hydrochloride. Other antidepressants helpful for hot flushes are citalopram (Celexa) 10–20 mg/day, escitalopram (Lexapro) 10–20 mg/day, and venlafaxine (Effexor) 75 mg/day. Starting with a generic when available for any of these medications is the most cost-effective approach. It's generally worth starting with the lowest dose and waiting six to twelve weeks before increasing the dose if needed. Some of these medications can affect libido, make orgasm more difficult, or inhibit it completely (it's reversible), so something to watch out for. See chapter 15 for more.

- **ANTIEPILEPTIC DRUGS:** Some medications that prevent seizures are also useful for vasomotor symptoms. There is a large amount of data on the drug gabapentin, which is a generic and has been around for decades. The dose is typically 300 mg at night, and can be increased if needed to 300 mg three times a day. This is still a low dose for this medication, and the dose can be increased if necessary up to 2,400 mg a day. Gabapentin is especially helpful for women with sleep disturbances related to night sweats. Side effects (including sexual) of gabapentin are uncommon in the 300–900 mg a day range and it can be quite effective at this dose—I have personally had a lot of success with low-dose gabapentin in my practice. At higher doses sedation, headache, dizziness, and swelling in the legs can occur. The other option is pregablin (Lyrica), which has some similarities to gabapentin, although it is more expensive and in the United States it's a scheduled substance—meaning special prescribing as we do for opioids is needed. Pregablin can sometimes be helpful when anxiety is a concern. Women who can't tolerate gabapentin due to dizziness or other side effects may do better side-effect-wise with pregablin.
- **CLONIDINE:** A blood pressure medication that can help some women with hot flushes, but is less effective than estrogen and other prescription nonhormonal therapies. It may take up to three months of use to see an effect. Side effects are light-headedness, dizziness, dry mouth, and constipation.

Botanical Options

In general, these products are poorly studied if they have been formally evaluated at all. Many of the existing studies suffer from what we in medicine call methodological flaws—meaning the study design is poor and conclusions aren't possible. Often the number of women enrolled is too few to be meaningful or vasomotor symptoms aren't recorded using standardized techniques, or there is no control group so distinguishing between true effect and placebo isn't possible. Many people wonder why not recommend a placebo, what's the harm? It's not ethical for physicians to recommend placebos and duplicity aside, they're less effective than people think and the placebo effect is usually temporary.

Another issue with these products is contamination with hormones and antidepressants—meaning medications that *do* treat hot flushes. Women are then unknowingly exposed to medications that could have risks for them. Supplements are also a rapidly increasing cause of liver failure and other serious medical complications, either due to the actual substance in the product or contaminants (see chapter 22 for more). Here are some of the most common botanical therapies often used for vasomotor symptoms and what we know about them:

- **BLACK COHOSH:** Also known as *Actaea racemosa,* black cohosh is a plant native to Eastern North America. Indigenous North Americans originally used the roots and stems to help with labor and a variety of illnesses, although it was never a traditional therapy for hot flushes. It made its way into the American folk remedy lexicon in the 1800s. Studies show no benefit with black cohosh versus placebo and there are reports of liver damage. One study found 25 percent of thirty-five black cohosh supplements in America didn't contain any black cohosh at all! Imagine the outcry if 25 percent of antibiotic prescriptions didn't contain any antibiotics? The investigators undertook the study as they wondered if some of the reports of harm from black cohosh were related to accidental contamination during harvesting with the roots and stems of similar-looking plants with known toxicity to humans. The adulterated black cohosh contained plants native to Asia, meaning they weren't accidentally harvested along with North American black cohosh but likely a purposeful switch. With the bulk of the data showing no benefit and 25 percent of supplements not even containing black cohosh, I recommend giving it a pass.

- **CANNABIS:** There isn't much data, except for one yet to be published study that tells us 27 percent of women have tried cannabis for their symptoms versus 19 percent having tried MHT. It's a small study and only included female veterans, so it's unclear if it reflects the general population or not. As of 2020 there's no reliable data on the effectiveness of cannabis for vasomotor symptoms. Cannabis is an endocrine disruptor, so the potential for effect is there, but the assumption shouldn't be that it's beneficial. More research is needed before recommending. Cannabis has become a part of medical folklore. For example, there is the myth that Queen Victoria used cannabis for painful periods. She didn't; that myth emerged in the 1990s. Hashish was recommended by Dr. Tilt in his book on menopause from the 1800s (we met him in chapter 2), not to treat hot flushes rather to quiet menopausal women "driven to the verge of insanity by ovario-uterine excitement." (As an aside, I always wonder if these women who were supposedly oversexed were the ones who still wanted to have sex and now didn't have to worry about getting pregnant, but their husbands had lost their sex drive or had erectile dysfunction. After all, lack of sex in a heterosexual couple-ship can often be because of the man.) Dr. Tilt believed cannabis was an anaphrodisiac (antiaphrodisiac or reduced sex drive) based on his observation that it caused impotence in men (cannabis is associated with an increased risk of erectile dysfunction).
- **FLOWER POLLEN EXTRACT:** This is a product called relizen, sold under several brand names, that is purported to have antioxidant and anti-inflammatory properties. There's only one small study comparing relizen with placebo, and at three months there was a significant improvement in vasomotor symptoms. There was no long-term follow-up. One short-term study is not a lot to go on, but some women may wish to give it a try.
- **HOMEOPATHY:** The guiding principle is that a very dilute amount of a substance similar in some way to the underlying condition is effective therapy. Homeopaths claim the original substance is diluted so much that the water retains memory, and it is the memory of the original substance that supposedly makes the remedy effective. For example, tiny amounts of *Candida* for

yeast infections or lachesis for menopause. What is lachesis? Diluted venom from a pit viper. I'm not entirely sure how to approach the idea of poisonous snake venom being *like* menopause. There are all kinds of terrible jokes here, all at the expense of women. Homeopathy is a pseudoscience, and the dilution principle isn't consistent with the known scientific laws of the universe. Hard pass.

- **PHYTOESTROGEN SUPPLEMENTS:** These products contain a variety of isoflavones or other phytoestrogens. Products that contain soy, red clover, flaxseed, and hops fall in this category. The more popular products claim to contain high levels of genistein and/or daidzein or the metabolite equol. Of all the botanical therapies, soy supplements are the most tested. One product, S-equol, may be slightly effective for some women; otherwise there's no conclusive evidence that any of these products are effective, although they appear safe.

- **VITAMIN E:** Doses of 400–800 IU (international units) a day have mixed results for vasomotor symptoms. If there is benefit it's mild at best. Doses of 400 IU a day or more are also associated with an increased risk of mortality, so that's a "no" for vitamin E.

- **DONG QUAI:** This is the dried root of the plant *Angelica sinensis* and is commonly found in traditional Chinese medicine. Dong quai isn't effective for hot flushes or night sweats, and there are concerns about potentially dangerous interactions with blood thinners as well as unresolved issues concerning an increased risk of cancer.

- **EVENING PRIMROSE OIL:** This oil is extracted from seeds from the evening primrose plant or *Oenothera biennis*. It has been used in many remedies for gynecological symptoms, from premenstrual syndrome, to breast pain, to hot flushes. Despite its widespread use there is essentially no data to support its efficacy.

New Research

There is research looking at a medication called fezolinetant, which has the ability to quiet the nerves that are overactive temperature-wise without the influence of estrogen. Preliminary studies show a lot of promise—an 80 percent reduction in hot flushes. Expect more data on this therapy soon.

BOTTOM LINE:

- Vasomotor symptoms affect 80 percent of women and often start years before menopause, the average length is seven years, and for many women they can persist long into menopause.
- Estrogen is the most effective therapy for vasomotor symptoms.
- The most effective nonmedication options are CBT and hypnosis; acupuncture is ineffective.
- There are several nonhormonal therapies: paroxetine mesylate and hydrochloride, escitalopram, and low-dose gabapentin seem to be the most effective and have the most favorable side-effect profiles.
- Phytoestrogen supplements and black cohosh, two of the most popular botanical therapies, have not proven to be effective in studies.

Chapter 10

Menstrual Mayhem:

Abnormal Bleeding and What to Do About It

CHANGES IN BLEEDING—BOTH IN amount and regularity—are a universal experience leading up to the final menstrual period. It may not feel normal, especially for women who have had regular menstrual periods until this point in their lives, but it's typical. So typical that menstrual irregularity is one of the medical signs that the final menstrual period is approaching (see chapter 3).

From a medical perspective, abnormal bleeding matters for several reasons. It can be a warning sign for other medical concerns, such as endometrial cancer (cancer of the lining of the uterus) and thyroid conditions. The volume of blood lost because of abnormal bleeding may be medically concerning. There's also the impact on quality of life, which should never be underestimated. One can only ruin so many pairs of underwear before one is so done. Every person who downplays the ongoing mental wear and tear of irregular bleeding should be required to wear a contraption attached to their pelvis for a couple of *years* that intermittently leaks blood, and then they can get back with me about whether it's really *that* bad.

Some women may have only a few missed periods or one or two heavier periods. Others have a lot of irregular bleeding, yet don't find their bleeding problematic once they know their experience is typical and cancer/precancer has been ruled out as a cause. Many women want treatment because their bleeding is bothersome, and others may need treatment because the bleeding is medically concerning. The range of women's responses to their bleeding is as diverse as the bleeding patterns of the menopause transition.

It's not possible to diagnose the cause of any woman's abnormal bleeding without sitting down with her and listening to her medical history, doing a physical exam, and possibly ordering some tests. The goal of this chapter is to review the bleeding patterns and why they happen, what is concerning and why, and explain common tests and treatments so women can understand what is happening to their bodies and be empowered to advocate for themselves.

Abnormal Menstrual Bleeding—What *Exactly* Does That Mean?

Menstrual bleeding is considered abnormal when it doesn't follow a regular pattern or it's too heavy. A typical bleeding pattern is a menstrual period every twenty-four to thirty-eight days from start of one menstrual period to the first day of bleeding in the following cycle. An abnormal bleeding pattern can be an irregular cycle, meaning more than a seven-day difference in length from cycle to cycle; for example, twenty-five days between the first day of the period for one cycle is followed by thirty-seven days for the next. Other abnormal bleeding patterns include frequent periods (every twenty-three days or less), long interval between periods (more than thirty-eight days), skipped cycles, spotting between periods (intermenstrual bleeding), and bleeding after sex (post-coital bleeding).

Volume-wise a normal menstrual period is 30–80 ml of blood (1–3 ounces)—I know, it often seems like a lot more. Accurately measuring menstrual blood loss isn't practical for obvious reasons, so blood loss is considered heavy in the following situations:

- Leaking through menstrual products enough to soak clothes or bedsheets
- Needing to change a soaked menstrual product every hour for several hours

- Clots larger than a quarter
- Bleeding for longer than seven days

Many times I've asked a woman if her periods are heavy only to hear "no" in response, but when I ask that same woman is she's leaking onto her clothes or "flooding" she replies that she does. This doesn't mean she's unaware of her own body; rather, this heavy bleeding is typical for her and/or her concerns about the amount of bleeding have previously been wrongly dismissed by a medical professional or parent. Personally, I prefer the word "flooding" to describe heavy periods because it seems most women understand that means soaking their clothes or narrowly avoiding a CMI—a critical menstrual incident.

The amount of blood lost with each menstrual period often increases during the menopause transition, which comes as a surprise to some women. The cultural shame women are made to feel about their menstrual cycles often prevents them from discussing their experiences with other women, and too often medical professionals fail to inform women about what to expect or they dismiss women's experiences. Making women feel as if their bodies are broken and they are the only ones having flooding, when it's a common experience, is a form of oppression.

I remember asking for a tampon in a nightclub bathroom when I unexpectedly got my period in my late forties, and a very kind woman about twenty years younger handed me a regular-size tampon. I struggled not to laugh at its puny size, what was that against my mighty mature menstruation? But I also smiled, because it's the menstrual equivalent of someone thinking you're much younger than you are. At forty-seven my motto was *Go super-plus or go home!* I did take the opportunity to explain the heavier periods in your forties to this young woman and her friends who were wide-eyed in horror.

There should be no uterine bleeding after menopause, so all bleeding that happens after the final menstrual period is considered abnormal. When menstrual periods are very irregular—as is common in the menopause transition—it can be easy to mistake bleeding after menopause for just another wonky, late period. This is especially true for women with medical conditions that affect ovulation, such as polycystic ovarian syndrome or PCOS, some of whom may typically go eight months or more between periods. Also, not every woman tracks her periods during the menopause transition, including gynecologists! Was the last period seven months ago, thirteen months ago, or nineteen months ago? Um, maybe? In these situations where timing of the last menstrual period is unclear, it's always best to err on the side of caution and treat the bleeding as abnormal because missing a precancer or cancer would be devastating.

Endometrial Cancer

This is cancer of the lining of the uterus. While it is more common after menopause, it should always be considered as a potential cause of abnormal uterine bleeding during the menopause transition. There are several types of endometrial cancer, the most common is called endometrioid. When caught early, this cancer has a survival rate of 90 percent. Some factors that increase a woman's risk of endometrial cancer are related to increased exposure to estrogen with insufficient progestogen (progesterone or progestin) to counterbalance that effect. This is why taking estrogen in MHT without adequate progestogen (see chapter 17) and obesity (a body mass index or BMI of 30 or more) are associated with this cancer. Other risk factors include type 2 diabetes, the medication tamoxifen (see chapter 5), and genetic factors. Hormonal contraception—including the levonorgestrel IUD—lowers the risk.

This connection with obesity and endometrial cancer exists because fatty tissue makes estrogen via the enzyme aromatase (see chapter 3), so the greater the BMI the more estrogen produced. For every 5 unit increase in BMI the risk of endometrial cancer increases approximately 50 percent. It's important women know about this connection with endometrial cancer in the same way that women with a family history of osteoporosis should know about their increased risk—knowledge allows women to make informed choices. Unfortunately, only approximately 50 percent of women are aware of the connection between obesity and endometrial cancer, so they may not know to advocate for testing if they have abnormal bleeding or for therapy (progestogens) to lower their risk. With this knowledge some women may try to lose weight, which can also be helpful. It appears many doctors are hesitant to discuss the connection, in one study of women with endometrial cancer only 30 percent had been told by their provider about the link with obesity. Conversations about weight can be hard, but it seems that women either get no information or they are fat-shamed and neither are acceptable.

An ultrasound can be useful in ruling out endometrial cancer for women who have bleeding after their final menstrual period, but it is not useful for this reason before menopause. This is because the thickness of the lining of the uterus is what is used on ultrasound to determine risk for cancer, but before menopause the lining is normally thick because of the menstrual cycle. After menopause the lining should be thin, so ultrasound is much more useful.

When an ultrasound can't be used to screen for endometrial cancer (before menopause) or a thickness in the lining is detected in an ultrasound after menopause a sample of tissue from the lining of the uterus is needed for diagnosis.

Abnormal Bleeding Between Age Forty and Menopause: How to Think Like a Gynecologist

Remember back to our bricks-and-mortar analogy for the menstrual cycle (chapter 3). Estrogen builds up the lining (lays the bricks) and progesterone released with ovulation stabilizes the lining (the mortar). Progesterone production stops when there is no pregnancy, the lining is destabilized and comes out, exposing blood vessels that bleed. Menstrual blood is a combination of the endometrium (the lining) and this blood from the vessels. The uterus stops the bleeding with powerful contractions that squeeze the blood vessels, essentially applying pressure just as you might do when you pinch a bleeding nose. The pressure slows the bleeding giving the blood's clotting mechanisms (coagulation system) a chance to work and the bleeding stops.

With this in mind, the root causes of abnormal bleeding include the following:

- **ENDOMETRIUM:** The lining of the uterus, either too thick or too thin. Hormonal changes are the most common cause. Polyps (see figure 8) are localized overgrowths of the lining of the uterus that hang from a stalk (their risk of being cancerous is about 1 percent). Hormonal contraception and menopausal hormonal

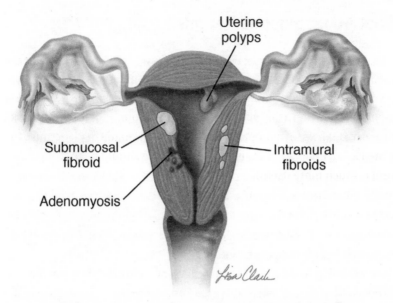

Figure 8: The sources of abnormal menstrual bleeding: fibroids and polyps

therapy or MHT can also affect the endometrium (lining), as can supplements that have been adulterated with hormones. Cancer and precancerous changes are always a consideration and less commonly infection.

- **MYOMETRIUM OF THE UTERINE MUSCLE:** Fibroids, known medically as leiomyomas, which are benign tumors of the uterine muscle; and adenomyosis, a condition where the lining of the uterus grows into the muscle (see figure 8). More on these two conditions shortly.

- **ISSUES WITH THE BLOOD'S ABILITY TO CLOT:** For women ages forty and older this is almost always due to anticoagulant medications (also known as blood thinners), such as rivaroxaban, warfarin, and apixaban. Aspirin can also affect bleeding as can many supplements, either because the botanical ingredients affect the clotting system or interact with anticoagulant medications or because they've been adulterated with prescription medications.

The color of the blood doesn't indicate the cause of the bleeding, but the pattern or volume may help point your provider in one direction or another. (See supplemental table 1, p. 337.)

What About Skipped Periods?

Skipped periods, two, three, even five in a row, are a normal part of the menopause transition. If every woman with skipped periods were evaluated then every woman would need multiple evaluations over her transition. So the answer as to who needs an evaluation is *it depends,* on the risk of cancer and the likelihood that another medical condition not related to menopause is the cause.

Is the bleeding otherwise a normal flow with no bleeding in between? This is likely the menopause transition, but changes in bleeding are worth reporting to your provider because women with risk factors for cancer/precancer may need to be evaluated, especially if the periods are heavier or lighter than expected.

Hypothalamic amenorrhea is a medical condition that may be mistaken as menopause. This is a condition where the signaling from the brain to the ovary is affected so there's no trigger to start the development of a follicle each month. The result is low levels of estrogen and no periods or infrequent periods. Hypothalamic amenorrhea is most often caused by stress, sleep disturbances, weight loss, excessive physical exercise, but can be triggered by any illnesses. Estrogen levels are low, just as with menopause, but unlike with menopause levels of follicle stimulating hormone (FSH) are also low. Diagnosing hypothalamic amenorrhea is important as the low estrogen levels increase the risk of osteoporosis.

What About a Super Soaker Event?

Some women may have an episode of massive bleeding during the menopause transition, so much so that urgent or emergency care is needed. This can happen out of the blue or it may occur superimposed on a background pattern of irregular and/or heavy bleeding. Either way, it's frightening to see so much blood and it's medically concerning. If you are soaking through one pad an hour for two hours or you are concerned about the bleeding, it's time to urgently speak with a medical provider or seek medical help.

Menstrual Mayhem—Understanding the Evaluation

How each individual woman is evaluated will depend on many factors including, but not limited to, her age, whether she takes hormones or other medications including supplements, her previous bleeding patterns, other medical conditions, and her family history. For example, polyps are not a common cause of bleeding, but a woman taking tamoxifen should be evaluated for a polyp regardless of her bleeding pattern as that medication significantly increases the risk of polyps. It's also important to consider the cervix as a cause of bleeding and to ensure that cervical cancer screening is up to date.

A physical exam can typically rule out the cervix as a likely cause of the bleeding and also ensure the blood isn't coming from the vagina, or vulva. A pelvic exam will determine whether the uterus is enlarged, raising suspicion for fibroids or adenomyosis. If cervical cancer screening isn't up to date, it should be performed. Blood tests may be indicated to make sure the blood loss isn't medically concerning and to evaluate thyroid function and the level of a hormone called prolactin (high levels can signal a medical condition that affects menstrual bleeding). It's also *always* important to rule out pregnancy. Other testing, for example, screening for thyroid problems, may be indicated based on individual factors.

An ultrasound of the uterus may be needed to evaluate the size and shape of the uterus, potentially identifying causes of bleeding, such as fibroids, polyps, and adenomyosis, but many times it's appropriate to proceed with some therapies without an ultrasound. A tissue sample from the lining of the uterus may also be needed to rule out cancer or precancer. The sample may be obtained in the office using a small straw-like device passed through the cervix into the uterus, called an endometrial biopsy, or in the operating room with a procedure called dilation and curettage or D & C. There are advantages and disadvantages with each procedure, and the best one for a given woman will depend on many individual factors.

An endometrial biopsy involves being awake in the office and is similar in many ways to an IUD insertion. Some women find it mildly uncomfortable and others find it very painful. Unfortunately, many options to reduce the pain from this procedure have been investigated and none are particularly helpful. Techniques discussed for pain control with IUD insertion in chapter 23 may be applicable here. Many women unfortunately are given no option to stop when an endometrial biopsy is painful, and this can lead to some avoiding the test in the future when indicated, potentially putting them at risk for missing a cancer.

How these tests will play out—which ones a woman may need and in what order—are dependent on many factors and beyond the scope of this book.

Tell Me More About Hormonal Bleeding

The hormonal chaos of the menopause transition can lead to high levels of estrogen, low levels of progesterone, or both. This can cause a sort of Goldilocks situation with the endometrium—too thick, too thin, or disorganized (think of the instability of a haphazardly constructed brick wall or shoddy brick work). Basically, never quite right. A thick or a disorganized lining can result in heavy and/or longer bleeding, and when bits of the lining break off intermittently (think of sections of a brick wall being unstable), the result is irregular bleeding. Irregular bleeding can also be the result of irregular ovulation. And if the lining is too thin due to low levels of estrogen from prolonged periods without ovulation, then the lining of the uterus becomes raw, leading to bleeding.

Whether a woman needs to have an ultrasound or not depends on many factors, but with a normal-size uterus and a low concern for cancer/precancer, it may be fine to start therapy and then if it's ineffective, proceed with an ultrasound. Even if women do have fibroids or adenomyosis—other causes of heavy periods that may be identified on ultrasound—the initial medical treatments are typically the same as hormonal bleeding.

The first line of treatment options for hormonal bleeding include the following:

- **LEVONORGESTREL IUD:** The most effective medical therapy for heavy periods—it reduces blood loss by 70 percent to 80 percent per cycle and can help with irregular periods by stopping them altogether. It may also help period pain. See chapter 23 for more.

- **TRANEXAMIC ACID:** This medication helps the blood clot and is taken for five days of the menstrual cycle during bleeding. It reduces blood loss by up to 50 percent per cycle. Many women like the idea of a medication they only take when they are bleeding.
- **HORMONAL CONTRACEPTION:** This includes estrogen-containing birth control pills, the patch, the vaginal ring, progestin only pills, as well as depo medroxyprogesterone acetate. The implant is less effective at controlling irregular bleeding, so typically isn't recommended here. Blood loss may be reduced by 50 percent or more depending on the methods. Hormonal contraception with estrogen can treat both heavy and irregular periods and also reduce period cramps as well as treat hot flushes. See chapter 23 for more on these medications.
- **NONSTEROIDAL ANTI-INFLAMMATORY DRUGS:** Also known as NSAIDs, these are anti-inflammatory pain medications available over the counter (OTC) and in higher doses as a prescription. Ibuprofen and naproxen sodium are two common examples. When started one or two days before a period, they can reduce the amount of blood for up to 80 percent of women. The volume of decrease is not the same as with the other methods listed, but they can help many women and also reduce menstrual cramps.
- **PROGESTOGENS:** When periods are irregular and heavy, an oral progestogen for eleven to twenty-one days a month and in the right dose can often regulate cycles and reduce the flow. The progestins are more effective here than progesterone. See chapters 17 and 18 for more on progestogens.
- **STANDARD MHT:** Tends to be less effective at controlling this kind of bleeding. See chapters 17 and 18 for more information.

There are surgical options when medical therapy isn't effective. Most providers strongly recommend at least three to six months with a medical therapy, and preferably trying at least two of them before opting for a surgical procedure. While complication rates from surgery are low, they happen, and I encourage women to consider how they might feel if they were to have a surgical complication and hadn't previously tried a medical therapy. Ultimately, it's a woman's body and it's her choice.

An endometrial ablation is a procedure where the lining of the uterus is destroyed. It can be done in the operating room or in the office, depending on the method chosen and patient preference. This procedure is only indicated when cancer/precancer has been ruled out. Though some women have no periods after this procedure, many will continue to have bleeding; it just won't be heavy. Success rates vary depending on the procedure selected. Women younger than forty-five years and those with painful periods are more likely to be dissatisfied with the outcome.

The definitive procedure is a hysterectomy, which can usually be accomplished vaginally or via the operating telescope, meaning two or three small incisions in the abdomen. Hysterectomy rates are higher in the United States versus other industrialized countries. While some of this is driven by some gynecologists who recommend surgery over medical therapies and even racism, some women simply want a hysterectomy because they want to be "done with it" bleeding-wise. While some of these women may be swayed to trying medical therapy by emphasizing the effectiveness of nonsurgical therapy, it's important to remember that American women have to pay far more for their medical care compared with their British and European counterparts to whom they are often compared in studies on the rate of hysterectomies.

In the United States, women without insurance may pay more than $1,000 for a Mirena IUD and $150 a month for tranexamic acid. Even with what is considered good insurance, these options can still cost a lot in copayments. Now add in the cost of office visits, ultrasounds, and other tests that may be needed, and that could be hundreds or possibly thousands of dollars depending on the insurance. This could even be for several years. And what if you pay all that money and you are still having bleeding? Given the bizarre American system, the copayments to treat the bleeding with medication could be higher than the copayment for a hysterectomy, so some women are financially incentivized for surgery. One of the many sad truths about American health care is women can't always afford what we providers may recommend as the first-line option, or they can't take the risk that the nonsurgical therapy may not be effective. In the United Kingdom every therapy listed in this chapter has no out of pocket expense and in most European countries there is universal health care that covers some or all of these expenses.

And then there is sick leave—full-time employees in the United States have an average of eight days a year of sick leave. Almost 40 percent of working Americans have no sick leave, and in lower wage industries that number is almost double. The United Kingdom and most European countries have paid sick leave, and of course no one is worried about losing their health care if for some reason they are forced to leave their work because of illness. Many women can go back to work as soon as one week after a hysterectomy (depending on the type of hysterectomy), and most by two to three weeks. Again, when looking at the multiple office visits that may be needed to manage abnormal bleeding time off could be a factor in some women choosing surgery.

Women with bleeding concerns who are in their later forties may feel differently about trying medical options versus women in their early forties who may have to take these medications for a longer period of time. This might be one situation where developing an accurate blood test for predicting the time to the final menstrual period could be useful. For example, if a test existed that could accurately predict menopause was two years away versus five years away, it may affect how a woman in her later forties thinks about surgery. What we do know now is once a woman is going sixty or more days between periods, it's very likely her periods will stop within four years.

Tell Me More About Fibroids

Fibroids—medically known as leiomyomas—are benign (noncancerous) tumors of the muscle of the uterus or myometrium (see figure 8). They can cause heavy bleeding, painful periods, and when very large can put pressure on the bladder and cause discomfort or the need to go to the bathroom more often. Fibroid growth is influenced by estrogen, so they almost always get smaller after menopause when estrogen levels drop. The small amount of estrogen in MHT is not enough to trigger their growth.

By the age of fifty almost 70 percent of White women and 80 percent of Black women will have at least one fibroid. Why so many women get fibroids isn't known, but one theory is related to the ability of the uterus to self-repair after pregnancy—the stretching of the uterus to accommodate a growing fetus and placenta traumatizes the tissue, so a self-repair mechanism is essential to allow for repeat pregnancies. Possibly with fibroids the repair mechanisms may be triggered inappropriately, leading to the accumulation of excess muscle tissue. Fibroids often appear earlier and cause more symptoms for Black women. While the reasons for this difference aren't entirely known and social determinants of health may play a role, fibroids in Black women are more likely to have elevated levels of the enzyme aromatase, and this enzyme is essential in the local production of estrogen. With more estrogen produced locally, the fibroids can grow faster, producing more symptoms and cause problems earlier in life.

Fibroids are a bit of a conundrum. Size is not always a reliable indicator that the fibroid is causing symptoms, so it's hard to know why some are problematic while others are bystanders. Fibroids can lead to heavy bleeding by mechanically preventing the uterus from squeezing to reduce blood flow, but as they can affect the behavior of blood vessels it is likely there are other ways they interfere with bleeding. Fibroids that distort the lining of the uterus are called submucosal fibroids, and those embedded in the muscle of the uterus are known as myometrial; these are most likely to cause abnormal menstrual bleeding (see figure 8). Sometimes fibroids can outgrow their blood supply and the tissue starts to die, which is very painful.

Fibroids don't become cancerous, but there's a very rare cancer of the uterine muscle called sarcoma that can be mistaken for a fibroid. Far fewer than 1 percent of fibroids are sarcomas. The risk of sarcoma increases with age, and there may be findings on ultrasound that raise or lower the suspicion. A rapidly growing fibroid may be more concerning for cancer, although even then the absolute risk that this is a sarcoma is still low.

I often hear women ask why there are so few treatments for fibroids, but there really are a wide variety of options, including medications to control bleeding and even shrink fibroids, procedures to shrink fibroids, and surgery—either to remove the fibroids or a hysterectomy. If we compare fibroids to a similar type of condition in men, benign prostatic hypertrophy, which is a benign overgrowth of tissue in the prostate, the range of therapies are essentially identical. I wonder if some women are left with the impression there are few treatment options because they've had their bleeding dismissed as "not that bad," or the full range of treatment options was never discussed?

Treatment options for fibroids include all the medication options discussed previously for hormonal bleeding, although women who have a very distorted uterine cavity from fibroids may not be candidates for the hormonal IUD as it may not fit well. Another option is a medication called a GnRH analogue, which affects the signaling from the brain to the ovary, creating a reversible chemical menopause (discussed previously in chapter 5). This therapy was until recently only available as an injection, but now there is a pill. GnRH analogues are very effective at reducing bleeding from fibroids. This can be a short-term bridge to stop bleeding while tests are being performed or before surgery, but it may also be a longer-term option and MHT can be added to prevent bone loss and other symptoms of menopause.

Procedures and surgeries for fibroids include the following:

- **SURGICAL REMOVAL OF THE FIBROIDS:** Called a myomectomy. Sometimes this can be done with a telescope inserted into the uterine cavity via the vagina, but other times this requires abdominal surgery. This may not be a definitive procedure, because there may be tiny fibroids that are not visible that grow to replace those fibroids the surgeon removed.
- **UTERINE ARTERY EMBOLIZATION OR UAE:** A procedure where a radiologist identifies the major blood vessels that supply the fibroid and injects special material to block the flow of blood, causing the fibroid to die. This can cause significant pain that can last for several days. One study compared surgical removal of fibroids versus UAE and reported that quality of life was higher at two years with surgery, but many women are very satisfied with their results after UAE. The complication rates between the two procedures are similar.
- **FOCUSED ULTRASOUND SURGERY (FUS):** The fibroid is precisely identified with an MRI scan as well as the structures that need to be avoided, such as the bowel and bladder, and an ultrasound delivers sound waves that heat and destroy the fibroid.
- **HYSTERECTOMY:** Removing the uterus is the most effective and immediate therapy.

One consideration is procedures like these are associated with a lower age of natural menopause (see chapter 5 for a review). Surgical decision making is complex and involves previous therapies tried, desire to keep the uterus, what is available locally, other medical conditions that may make some procedures riskier than others, and estimated time to menopause, which is when bleeding from fibroids should stop.

Tell Me More About Adenomyosis

Adenomyosis is a condition where the lining of the uterus grows into the muscle (see figure 8). There are a variety of ways this can increase both the amount of bleeding with a period as well as pain, but adenomyosis doesn't cause bleeding between periods. Adenomyosis is rare for women who have never been pregnant; the main hypothesis is the damage to the wall of the uterus from the stretching during pregnancy leads to microscopic cracks that allow the lining to grow into the muscle.

Women with adenomyosis may have a slightly larger uterus, and sometimes there are findings on ultrasound or magnetic resonance imagining (MRI) that increase suspicion. Adenomyosis is what's known in medicine as a diagnosis of exclusion—meaning there are no definite tests that tell us whether it's adenomyosis, so other conditions are ruled out and if nothing else is found and the symptoms fit, then the conclusion is the heavy bleeding is due to adenomyosis.

There are no adenomyosis-specific therapies; the first-line therapies are those recommended for hormone-related bleeding, such as the levonorgestrel IUD, birth control pills, or Depo-Provera. While GnRH analogues (discussed earlier for fibroids) aren't approved for adenomyosis, they could be used. If bleeding is significant or hormonal medications aren't initially effective enough, a short course of GnRH analogues can be used to stop the bleeding and then a switch can be made to the levonorgestrel IUD or other hormones. It's not wrong to try an endometrial ablation when adenomyosis is suspected, but the failure rate may be higher. The definitive therapy is hysterectomy.

Bleeding After the Final Menstrual Period

Up to 11 percent of women will have bleeding after their final menstrual period (FMP), most of which occurs in the first few years. Once a woman is three or more years from her FMP her chance of this bleeding is <1 percent per year. Whether it's a heavy flow or a pinkish tinge, bleeding after menopause should never be brushed off as one last hurrah as there is a 6 percent to 10 percent chance the cause could be endometrial cancer. Bleeding after menopause is such a sensitive sign of endometrial cancer that up to 90 percent of women diagnosed with endometrial cancer had at least one episode of bleeding after menopause.

There are fewer non-cancer causes of bleeding after menopause because there is no ovulation to trigger irregular bleeding or to stimulate adenomyosis. Fibroids also shrink. The main causes include the following:

- **CANCER OR PRECANCER:** Endometrial cancer, but cervical cancer is also a consideration as one of the groups most affected by cervical cancer are women in their early sixties. The older a woman is when she has her bleeding after menopause, the more likely it is to be endometrial cancer or precancer. Factors that increase exposure to estrogen without a progestogen increase the risk of endometrial cancer, such as obesity (production of estrogen in fatty tissue) and taking estrogen in MHT without a progestogen.
- **A THIN UTERINE LINING:** Without estrogen the lining of the uterus can get so thin that it bleeds intermittently. This is the most common cause of bleeding after menopause.
- **A THICK UTERINE LINING:** Estrogen produced in fatty tissue or from MHT can cause the lining to thicken (lay bricks), and without the stability of a progestogen the lining breaks off intermittently. Supplements that have been adulterated with hormones are another cause.
- **GENITOURINARY SYNDROME OF MENOPAUSE OR GUSM:** Meaning the bleeding isn't from the uterus, but from the vagina. Looking at underwear there is no way to determine the source of the blood. This bleeding happens when the vaginal tissues get very thin without estrogen (see chapter 13 for more).
- **POLYP:** the risk of cancer in a polyp increases with age and for women after menopause.
- **CLOTTING ISSUES RELATED TO BLOOD THINNERS:** Even when a woman is taking these medications, cancer and precancer must always be considered.

• **MENOPAUSAL HORMONE THERAPY:** MHT can cause bleeding for some women after menopause (this doesn't include expected bleeding for women who take it in a cyclic fashion, see chapter 18). When this bleeding happens it can be due to too much progestogen versus estrogen, so the lining gets overly thin, or not enough progestogen so the lining gets thick. Unexpected bleeding on MHT needs an evaluation to make sure it isn't cancer, although depending on the circumstances, abnormal bleeding in the first six months of starting menopausal hormone therapy may sometimes be monitored. This is a shared decision made between a woman and her provider.

Tests to rule out cancer include an ultrasound to look at the thickness of the lining of the uterus; when it's ≤4 mm this can exclude more than 99 percent of cancers. This test is less effective to screen for cancer before the final menstrual period as the lining of the uterus can normally be thicker than 4 mm. The other option is either an endometrial biopsy, a D & C, or a hysteroscopy (all discussed previously). If the ultrasound shows a very thin lining but the bleeding continues, then more testing is needed.

Treatment for cancer and precancer is beyond the scope of this book. There are many treatment options for GUSM (see chapter 13). A polyp should be removed and MHT may be helpful for women with bleeding due to a thick or thin lining of the uterus.

BOTTOM LINE

- Bleeding abnormalities are characteristic of the menopause transition and can include heavy periods, longer periods, irregular cycles, and bleeding in between cycles.
- The most common cause of bleeding during the menopause transition is the hormonal chaos that's characteristic of that phase.
- Fibroids and adenomyosis are common causes of heavy periods; they may also cause painful periods but they don't cause irregular bleeding.

- Heavy bleeding can often be controlled with medications, and there are several options.
- All bleeding after menopause is abnormal and requires an evaluation.

Chapter 11

Bone Health:

The Basics of Bone Biology, Osteoporosis, and Preventing Fractures

"I AM HERE TO SCARE you about osteoporosis" was the opening line from a lecture I attended in 2019. I couldn't have put it better, so I, too, am here to scare you about your bone health and osteoporosis. The goal is to raise awareness about the significance of osteoporosis and its devastating impact for many women, as well as to explain the screening process and fracture prevention.

Osteoporosis is a condition where the bones become fragile, increasing their risk of fracture. It's characterized by a decrease in the amount of bone (bone mass) and microscopic alterations to the architecture (see figure 9). There are also other changes in bone quality that aren't well understood. The net result is the structural integrity of the bone is impaired. Bone health is on a continuum—while osteoporosis reflects one end of the scale and the highest risk of fracture, many more women have low bone mass, which also increases their risk of fracture. This used to be called osteopenia, but that term is no longer in use.

If you are in your late twenties, you're losing bone as you read this. Bone is constantly remodeled, meaning it's reabsorbed and new bone is produced—so much that the entire skeleton is replaced approximately every ten years. After a woman reaches her peak bone mass in her late twenties, the balance tips slightly in favor of bone loss and there is a small

Normal Bone   Osteoporosis

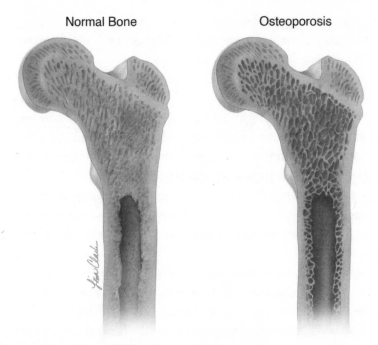

Figure 9: Normal bone (left) and bone with osteoporosis.

but steady decline in bone mass of <0.4 percent per year. Estrogen is a major player in bone formation, so the time of most rapid bone loss starts approximately one year before the final menstrual period, lasting about three years. On average a woman can lose 6 percent of her bone mass during these three years, but some women can lose a lot more—up to 3 percent to 5 percent a year. After this period of rapid loss, bone is lost at a higher rate than before menopause—0.5 percent to 1 percent a year. Aging also affects bone integrity in other ways.

In addition to menopause and age, other factors that affect bone mass and fracture risk including the following:

- **AGE OF MENOPAUSE:** An earlier menopause means more life lived after menopause, a period of increased bone loss. A woman whose menopause is age forty-five years or younger has a fracture risk 1.5–3 times higher than a woman who experiences menopause at age fifty or older.
- **ALCOHOL:** ≥3 units a day is associated with an increased risk—FYI 2 units is 175 ml (6 ounces) of wine.

- **ANOREXIA NERVOSA:** Low bone mass is common and when anorexia starts early this may affect a woman's peak bone mass. Extremely low body weight can stop ovulation for many women, resulting in very low levels of estrogen and there are other hormonal changes with anorexia that also affect bone. Calcium deficiency intake due to dietary restrictions may also be a factor.
- **GENETICS:** The greatest contributing factor to bone health.
- **MEDICAL CONDITIONS:** Such as rheumatoid arthritis, type 2 diabetes, Cushing's disease, and hyperparathyroidism.
- **MEDICATIONS:** Common examples are the contraceptive depot medroxyprogesterone acetate (DMPA), steroids, and aromatase inhibitors (medication for breast cancer), and heavy use of cannabis.
- **NUTRITION:** Especially calcium and vitamin D deficiency. Calcium is constantly flowing in and out of the bone, so when intake is insufficient there isn't enough calcium for remodeling and if intake is very low the body can even use the bone as a source of calcium reserves. Vitamin D helps with calcium absorption from the intestine and is important in muscle health, which has an indirect effect on bone remodeling. Also, weak muscles can contribute to falls, a major risk for fractures. It's not uncommon for people to hear that soda causes brittle bones, but there is no sound science backing up that assertion. Caffeine may slightly reduce the amount of calcium absorbed from food, but when a postmenopausal woman is getting enough calcium in her diet there's no effect on bone health. It takes a combination of low calcium intake and a daily caffeine consumption of the equivalent of three cups of coffee a day to increase bone loss.
- **PHYSICAL ACTIVITY:** Stress on bone from weight bearing and from muscles is important in maintaining bone health. Osteoblasts—the cells that build bone—are actually stimulated by mechanical signals from exercise.
- **RISK OF FALLS:** Falls to the side are especially risky. Activities that work on strengthening muscles and balance can help reduce falls.
- **SMOKING:** There are multiple ways smoking negatively affects bone health. Peak bone mass is lower and bone loss is accelerated throughout the lifetime, but especially after menopause.

Women who smoke lose an additional 2 percent of bone density for every ten years after menopause.

In the United States two-thirds of women ages fifty and older have either low bone mass (51 percent) or osteoporosis (15 percent) (see figure 10). White women have the highest risk, African American women the lowest, and Hispanic and Asian American women are in between risk-wise, although some data suggests Mexican American women (approximately 50 percent of Hispanic women in America) may be at higher risk than White women. The prevalence of osteoporosis varies around the world, with the highest in Norway and the lowest in Nigeria.

One of the first things you learn on your surgical rotation in medical school is the devastating impact of a hip fracture. If a woman aged sixty-five years or older is living independently and breaks her hip, one year later she has a 50 percent chance of being unable to live independently, a 40 percent risk of being unable to walk independently, and a 30 percent chance of no longer being able to get in and out of a bath. And the odds she will die by the time the year has passed are 17 percent.

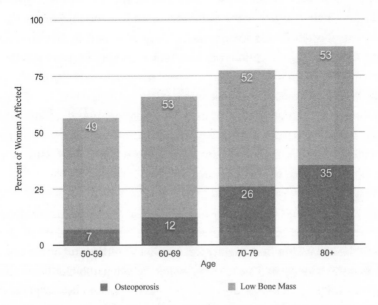

Figure 10: Osteoporosis and Low Bone Mass in American Women Ages 50+

And that's just hip fractures. There are vertebral (spine) and other fractures, kyphosis (a deformity of the spine that is a forward curvature, pejoratively called a dowager's hump), chronic pain from fractures, incontinence as women can't get to the bathroom in time due to pain and/or mobility issues, lung problems (related to healed rib fractures that now restrict the movement of chest muscles), and depression—never mind the emotional toll of losing one's independence.

Let's put osteoporosis and low bone mass in perspective with other major health conditions. The lifetime risk of breast cancer is 15 percent. The lifetime risk of a hip fracture is 17 percent. Fractures from osteoporosis and low bone mass lead to as many hospitalizations as strokes and heart attacks. And yet it seems as if we don't take bone health as seriously as these other health conditions. A woman is far more likely to get her screening mammogram than her screening for osteoporosis, and most women who have a hip fracture—an event that should trigger therapy for osteoporosis—don't get the right follow-up.

It feels as if there's a cultural acceptance of osteoporosis, which is tragic and fills me with rage. Perhaps society just expects women to get frail, so why be concerned about something that's "normal"? Maybe the needs of women as they age are irrelevant when society decides they're no longer hot enough so they should just be quiet and accept their dotage? There's also a false belief among some that prevention is ineffective or medications to treat osteoporosis are too risky. Osteoporosis isn't in the news like breast cancer or contraception concerns, which always makes me feel that women are reduced to boobs and babies, so many women may simply be unaware of their osteoporosis risk or that it is a significant health concern and there is preventative therapy as well as treatment. And finally, who wants to talk about a disease that we associate with crones, hags, and little old ladies? Even if women have concerns or are aware of their risks, they may not feel a space has been created for discussion.

Whatever the reason, it's women who suffer.

I'll admit my bias upfront. My mother died at age eighty-six from osteoporosis. Every single complication of osteoporosis that I've listed, she endured. She had her first fragility fracture in her fifties, and by the time she died she had lost at least 12 cm (5 inches) in height. She had so many hospitalizations due to fractures with extended stays in rehab that I lost count. It wasn't until she was critically ill from the disease that her osteoporosis was even treated. Before that her crumbling bones were just shrugged off as normal. When I pressed her to get screened for osteoporosis she was told it was unnecessary, the implication was that all these fractures were "normal" and when I had her ask about treatment she was told the potential side effects made the medications too risky.

There were challenges making her home safer from falls. I had a team come to the house to make safety recommendations, and they called in a panic about the number of throw rugs, which lead to falls and therefore are kryptonite for fragile bones. The physical therapist sounded frantic as he ran around the house scooping them up, as well as detailing the litany of other safety concerns—for example, a staircase with no hand rail that made my mother feel so unsteady that she walked down it *backward* so she could hold the wall with her hand that hadn't been recently fractured. When I visited a month later all the throw rugs were back in place and the handrail never materialized. Making changes in your seventies and eighties is hard—being stubborn is probably one reason many people live that long. That's why planning how you will live in your older years is important when you are younger. Making your home safer in your seventies and eighties can feel as if you're giving in to aging, while making these same changes in your fifties and sixties (or even earlier) can feel as if you are taking charge and being proactive.

In the end, my mother brushed her knee against a wall, fracturing her patella (knee cap)—as well as her tibia (a bone in her lower leg)—setting off a cascade of events that led to her leg being amputated. My father couldn't bring himself to give the consent, and so the task of explaining the surgery to my mother and providing consent to the surgeon fell to me. She never got over the amputation physically or mentally, and our rocky relationship ended with her blaming me for the loss of her leg. She died a few weeks later.

How Do I Know If I Have Osteoporosis?

Any woman who had a fragility fracture (meaning a fracture without an obvious reason, such as trauma) should automatically get the diagnosis of osteoporosis. For other women, the diagnosis of osteoporosis is made with a scan called a dual energy X-ray absorptiometry or DXA (pronounced dexa), and it evaluates the density of bone in a vertebra (part of the spine) and the top of the femur (the thigh bone, which is part of the hip). It's commonly referred to as the bone mineral density (BMD) test. It uses a very low dose of X-rays—about the same radiation one gets spending a day in San Francisco. There is more portable equipment that scans the wrist or ankle, but this testing is less accurate.

Screening for osteoporosis with a DXA is recommended at least once for all women at age sixty-five, when a follow-up evaluation is needed depends on several factors. If at sixty-five a woman has a normal bone density (a T score of -1 or higher) or mild bone loss (a T score of -1.01 to -1.49) her chance of developing osteoporosis in the next 15 years is less than 10 percent. However, women with moderate bone loss (T score of -1.50 to -1.99) or advanced bone loss (-2.00 to -2.4) are at risk for developing osteoporosis within a few years and may need repeat testing in 1–5 years (this depends on a variety of factors and is beyond our scope here).

Women should not wait until they are 65 to consider their bone health as those who are at increased risk for osteoporosis should be tested sooner. There is controversy on when screening should begin for these women. Some experts say a woman who is postmenopausal with one major risk factor for osteoporosis, such as smoking or a family history, should be tested.

There are also two tools to help determine if a woman under the age of 65 should have a DXA scan to determine her bone density. The first is the osteoporosis self-assessment tool or OST, which helps identify women more likely to have low bone density. The equation is (weight in kg - age in years) x 0.2, and a score of <2 is associated with an increased risk of low bone density.

The other is the Fracture Risk Assessment Tool or FRAX, designed by researchers at the University of Sheffield in the United Kingdom, a free tool to help women ages forty to ninety and their providers assess the risk of a major fracture (go to sheffield.ac.uk/FRAX/index.aspx or enter "FRAX tool" in the search engine—there is even a metric converter for those who don't know their weight and height in kilograms and centimeters). When the risk of a major fracture in the next ten years is >9.3 percent a woman should be formally tested for osteoporosis.

The FRAX tool doesn't incorporate every risk factor nor does it account for many nuances. For example, a woman who smokes two packs of cigarettes a day is at higher risk than a woman who smokes half a pack, or a parent with multiple fragility fractures likely confers a higher risk than a parent who had one fracture. So it's always important to individualize the approach to screening. There may be times when the FRAX score doesn't indicate a significant risk, but formal testing for osteoporosis is still indicated.

Understanding Bone Mineral Density

A BMD result is reported as a T score, which is unfamiliar terminology for many people (see figure 11). The T score compares a woman's bone density with a typical reading for a thirty-year-old and reports that result in standard deviations or SD. A standard deviation is a way of expressing what falls within the expected range and what does not. A T score of –1 SD and higher is the expected range, a T score between –1 and –2.5 is low bone mass and osteoporosis is a T score of –2.5 or lower.

My T score was –1.2 for my femur when it was tested a few years ago (given my family history I was tested at age fifty), meaning I have mild bone loss. This doesn't mean I've lost bone compared to when I was thirty or that I'm on a more accelerated bone loss trajectory. Think of a BMD

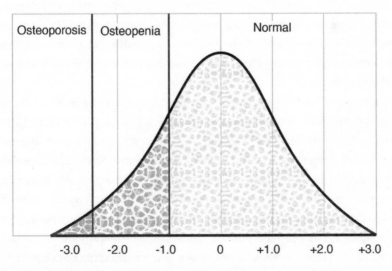

Figure 11: Bone Density and T Scores

like measuring weight—your weight today doesn't tell you what your weight was like five or ten years ago or what it will be in five to ten years from now; it only tells you about your weight on the day you were weighed. I do many things to maintain bone health, including never smoking, weight bearing exercises, and having adequate calcium and vitamin D. I also took the birth control pill for many years, which is good for bone density. Part of me was a little annoyed with my results, all that work and it's not normal? And then I reminded myself that considering my genetics, perhaps without all this work I'd be looking at a bone density of −1.5. If my bone density in five or so years is still −1.2, then perhaps this may be where I've been hovering BMD-wise for a while.

It's important to know that the T score is only one piece of the puzzle. Age, height, weight, family history, race, and a variety of other factors contribute to the risk of fracture. Once a woman knows her BMD she can go back to the FRAX and input her results. If her risk of a major fracture is ≥20 percent or risk of a hip fracture is ≥3 percent in the next ten years, then therapy for osteoporosis is recommended.

Fitness Prevents Frailty, and Fractures

Many people think of exercise as good for your heart, but it's also one of the best things you can do for your bones. Weight bearing activities as well as muscles pulling on bone stimulate production of new bone. Exercises that involve a component of balance also reduce falls, and exercises that work on posture can help prevent and treat the curvature in the spine called kyphosis.

Exercise is so helpful that it can help reverse bone loss, even for women who have lost a significant amount of bone mass. The Lifting Intervention for Training Muscle and Osteoporosis Rehabilitation (LIFTMOR—a great acronym) trial was an eight-month study of women, average age sixty-five, with low bone mass or osteoporosis who performed bone-targeted high-intensity resistance and impact training (HiRIT) thirty minutes twice a week compared with a matched group participating in a low-intensity exercise program. The intervention exercises involved deadlifts, squats, overhead presses, and jumping chin-ups with drop landings. The traditional thinking had been these exercises were too dangerous and could lead to more fractures, but in this study the weights and resistance were slowly introduced with close, expert supervision for posture and technique. Although it's a small study, the results showed a gain of bone mass and there were no fractures or serious complications from the exercises. We definitely need more studies like this, because proving these kinds of exercises are safe and effective for osteoporosis would be revolutionary. Women shouldn't embark on this kind of program without supervision, but finding a physical therapist or appropriate trainer who is experienced in working with women who have osteoporosis—after clearance from your doctor—is something to consider.

Women who are generally fit with no limiting health conditions should consider the exercise goals already discussed in previous chapters—at least 150 minutes of moderate-intensity aerobic activity (e.g., brisk walking) or 75 minutes of vigorous-intensity aerobic activity (e.g., jogging or running) every week and strength training two or more days a week. From an osteoporosis prevention standpoint, balance training and posture exercises are recommended at age sixty; starting them earlier as a preventative measure and so you have the skill set down is likely a good idea.

Women with low bone mass or osteoporosis should also learn spine-sparing strategies. Bending and twisting the spine with everyday activities can increase the load on the spine, causing fractures. For example, a woman with severe osteoporosis can fracture a vertebra just bending down to tie her shoes. It's important to bend at the hips not the back, and instead of twisting to grab something, taking a step to turn your whole body. Good information on a variety of exercises, including balance and posture, can be found at the following places:

- Osteoporosis Canada, osteoporosis.ca/bone-health-osteoporosis/exercises-for-healthy-bones
- StandTall® and other exercises for healthy posture, found at the International Osteoporosis Foundation, iofbonehealth.org/news/stand-tall-four-simple-exercises-healthy-posture
- National Osteoporosis Foundation, nof.org/preventing-fractures/exercise-to-stay-healthy

While this seems like a lot of time devoted to exercises (about forty-five to sixty minutes a day), it doesn't have to be all at once. Consider how much time it takes to go to the doctor for an appointment, never mind the time (and pain and cost) of treating fractures or the expense of being unable to live independently. Ultimately it's probably time neutral or even time saving to prevent all of that with exercise. Remember, exercise is money in the bank of your health.

Got Vitamins?

Milk is good for your bones, right?

Many people are surprised to learn that no study has linked milk with a reduction in osteoporosis. In fact, a group of researchers plotted the risk of a hip fracture and milk consumption by country and there was no correlation between lower odds of hip fracture and countries that drink more milk. The United States has one of the highest rates of milk consumption in the world and one of the highest rates of hip fracture. There is even data that links milk consumption with an increased risk of fractures, possibly due to the increase in height for milk drinkers because longer bones have a greater fracture risk. See chapter 19 for more on milk and health.

Calcium is a threshold mineral, meaning extra calcium above the daily requirements won't build more bone or be stored in bone for later use; rather, it's dumped in the urine. Insufficient calcium can lead to lower bone mass—because there isn't enough to support the constant replacement of bone—but high levels don't prevent or solve problems.

Women ages nineteen to fifty need 1,000 mg of calcium a day, and women fifty-one years and older should get 1,200 mg. For some women dairy may be that source, but fortified soy or almond milk, sardines, tofu, canned salmon with bones, turnip greens, chia seeds, kale, bok choi, and figs are also good sources. For women who can't get enough from their diet, a calcium supplement is recommended, and in this situation it is best to take a combined calcium and vitamin D supplement as vitamin D helps the body absorb the calcium. If you think you're getting 500 mg of calcium a day from your diet and your needs are 1,000 mg, then a 500–600 mg supplement will suffice. Remember, the idea of a supplement is to get you to the recommended intake, not to over shoot. Calcium supplements aren't benign; they increase the risk of kidney stones (all that extra calcium in the urine). There was a concern that calcium supplements could be a factor in increasing the risk of heart disease, but that appears to have been resolved and no longer a cause for worry. Approximately 33 percent of women in the United States take a calcium supplement.

Another important micronutrient for bone health is vitamin D. In addition to helping the body absorb calcium it helps with the flow of calcium in and out of bone, and has many other important functions, including muscle health and the healthy functioning of the immune and nervous systems. The recommended daily intake for vitamin D is 600 IU (international units) a day for women ages nineteen to seventy and 800 IU a day for ages seventy and over. Vitamin D includes both vitamin D2 (ergocalciferol) and vitamin D3 (cholecalciferol). Vitamin D3 is made in the skin in response to ultraviolet B (UVB) rays from the sun and we also get vitamin D3 from food, such as fatty fish, beef liver, butter, and egg yolks (if you hadn't guessed, it's a fat-soluble vitamin, and I remind myself every time I have butter that I'm getting my vitamin D). Vitamin D2 is only found naturally in a few foods, but many foods are fortified with vitamin D2. Both vitamin D2 and D3 are converted into the usable form of vitamin D, called calcitriol, by the liver.

Someone with light skin may get enough sunlight in the summer to make adequate vitamin D in five to ten minutes with only their face and hands exposed to the sun, but it may take thirty minutes or longer for someone with dark skin, because melanin (the pigment that results in darker skin) blocks ultraviolet light, so less gets through to the cells that produce vitamin D. It is also more challenging for many people to get enough sunlight during the winter compared with summer as the further you get from the equator the shorter the days and the sun is lower in the sky, reducing UVB exposure. Also, when it's cold people are covered up so less skin is exposed to the sun and/or people spend more time indoors. Air pollution may also affect the sun's rays, reducing UVB exposure. Another consideration is the ability to produce vitamin D decreases with age.

There's a lot about vitamin D that we don't yet know. For example, African American women tend to have lower levels of vitamin D but they also have a lower rate of osteoporosis, so levels may only tell part of the story. Furthermore, how your body uses the vitamin D you have may also matter.

In the 1990s there was a string of studies linking vitamin D deficiency to a litany of medical conditions, and measuring vitamin D levels became the rage. It seemed as if we were recommending vitamin D to almost everyone for everything. While it's true many studies linked a variety of illnesses to lower levels of vitamin D, what we don't know is if people who were unwell spent less time outdoors, meaning was low vitamin D the result of the illness, not a cause? Vitamin D has been extensively studied and there's no evidence linking low levels with cancer, heart disease, or type 2 diabetes. What we do know is that vitamin D hype led to a lot of unnecessary testing that added tens of millions of dollars to health care costs.

Approximately 35 percent of women twenty years and older take a vitamin D supplement, although there's no evidence that routine supplementation prevents osteoporosis or fractures for women with normal vitamin D levels. Moreover, 97 percent of Americans have vitamin D levels in the normal range (20 ng/ml or higher, although it's important to note that there is some controversy about the normal range with some experts stating 30 ng/ml should be the low end of normal). I suspect most of us in America have levels of 20 ng/ml or higher because many of us are so terrible with sunscreen and get at least thirty minutes of direct sunlight every other day. Because it's difficult to get enough vitamin D from diet, it's very reasonable for women who spend a lot of time indoors, women with darker skin, women who are fastidious with sunscreen, and those who cover most of their skin while outdoors (for religious reasons or sun avoidance) to consider a vitamin D supplement. As the ability to make vitamin D reduces with age, it is also reasonable for women ages fifty and older to take a supplement.

Vitamin D supplements in the recommended doses—800–1,000 IU a day—are very safe (400 IU a day appears to be ineffective at improving health, so don't bother with this lower dose). An 800 IU dose increases the blood levels by approximately 10 points. At this dose there is essentially no risk of toxicity, so most women are better off wearing sunscreen and taking a supplement. Supplements are either vitamin D3 (made from lanolin exposed to ultraviolet light) or vitamin D2 (made by yeast exposed to ultraviolet light)—both are converted in the liver equally to calcitriol— your liver doesn't care which one you take and you don't need to know your vitamin D farmer. Many providers recommend a daily vitamin D supplement for women at risk of osteoporosis. Testing for vitamin D is not recommended routinely; simply assess whether you are getting enough through sun exposure and diet and supplement as needed, although testing is indicated for women with osteoporosis.

Medications to Reduce Bone Loss

In the United States women who have had a fragility fracture, who have osteoporosis on BMD testing (a T score of −2.5), or a high fracture risk based on FRAX scoring are candidates for therapy. In Canada, medical therapy is recommended for women ages sixty-five years or older with a BMD of −2 or lower. There are many factors that go into the decision regarding medical therapy for osteoporosis and a full discussion of these is beyond the scope of this book. The goal here is to present the basics so women are in a position to better advocate for themselves. Before starting medical therapy it is important that women try to maximize non medications options discussed previously such as quitting smoking, cutting back on alcohol intake, ensuring there is adequate calcium and vitamin D intake, and balance and weight bearing exercises.

Estrogen in menopausal hormone therapy (MHT) is highly effective at preventing menopause-related bone loss. In the Women's Health Initiative (WHI) trial conjugated equine estrogens (CEE) plus the progestin medroxyprogesterone acetate reduced the risk of fractures of the hip and spine by 34 percent. We know that both oral and transdermal estrogens are equally effective. The CEE/bazedoxifene combination (estrogen plus a selective estrogen receptor modulator) is also effective at preventing osteoporosis. See chapters 17 and 18 for more on these medications. When estrogen is stopped women will experience that period of accelerated bone loss seen in the late menopause transition, so MHT just puts that on hold, and then bone loss continues at the more accelerated postmenopausal rate. There is no specific bone density where estrogen is recommended for osteoporosis prevention, but family history and other risk factors should be discussed to determine if MHT makes sense for osteoporosis prevention.

Raloxifene is a selective estrogen receptor modulator, meaning it acts like estrogen on some tissues but not on others, that reduces spine fractures, but not hip fractures. It also reduces the risk of breast cancer. Side effects include worsening of hot flushes and an increased risk of blood clots. There are more effective drugs for fracture prevention, so it's typically only considered for women with a low risk of blood clots for whom other options aren't appropriate or women with osteoporosis who also have an increased risk of breast cancer.

A class of medications called bisphosphonates are the mainstay of osteoporosis prevention and treatment. These drugs inhibit the action of cells called osteoclasts, which break down bone in the process of remodeling. They can be taken orally daily, weekly, monthly, and by intravenous injection every three months or even once a year, depending on the drug. Bisphosphonates are very effective for preventing hip and spine fractures for women with osteoporosis, and several are also approved for prevention of osteoporosis. There are a lot of nuances with these medications; they are typically given for up to five years and then the need to continue is evaluated.

Use of bisphosphonates rose after the Women's Health Initiative (WHI, see chapter 17) was published and women were frightened away from estrogen. Then information was published about the rare side effects including osteonecrosis of the jaw (basically exposed, dead bone in the jaw) and atypical fractures (fractures not due to osteoporosis) and then bisphosphonates had had their own WHI-like moment in the press and as expected their use plummeted. Osteonecrosis of the jaw is an awful complication, and the risk is 1/10,000 to 1/100,000 patients treated per year. However, the risk of blindness with drugs for erectile dysfunction (phosphodiesterase inhibitors) is 3 per 100,000 men per year, and I've yet to see a headline discussing that complication. The way society amplifies rare complications of life-saving therapies for women yet ignores complications when it's about amplifying the glory of the penis is exhausting and harms women. These rare complications from bisphosphonates are more common among women receiving high doses, especially when getting the medication intravenously, for those also on chemotherapy for cancer. Poor oral health and extensive dental work while on these medications is also a risk.

All Osteoporosis in Postmenopausal Women Isn't *Just* Menopause

It's important not to blame menopause for everything—almost 50 percent of women who are past menopause and have osteoporosis will have another diagnosis that could be contributing to their osteoporosis, such as vitamin D deficiency, inability to absorb macro and micronutrients from diet (such as after bariatric surgery or a condition called celiac disease, which is gluten intolerance), thyroid disorders, overactive parathyroid glands, and Cushing's disease.

BOTTOM LINE

- All women should be aware of their risk factors for osteoporosis, even women who are years away from their menopause transition.
- Women entering their menopause transition should evaluate their risk of osteoporosis; the OST and FRAX are two tools that may be used.
- All women age sixty-five and older should have a bone density scan, but many younger women need testing.
- Calcium supplements and vitamin D supplements are helpful when women are unable to get the recommended daily amount from diet and sun exposure.
- Estrogen and bisphosphonates are preventative medications for osteoporosis.

Chapter 12

This Is Your Brain on Menopause:

Brain Fog, Depression, and Dementia

MANY WOMEN REPORT BRAIN FOG or forgetfulness with their menopause transition, some develop depression, and for others some of the changes that could lead to dementia or Alzheimer's disease may be triggered during this time.

Though science matters in all things menopause, in discussing brain health we have perhaps the clearest example of the need for facts. This is because many harmful cultural narratives tie a woman's competence to her hormones. We're accused of being too hormonal before each period, during our period, during pregnancy, and after having a baby. And what happens when we finally rid ourselves of these supposedly toxic hormones? Our brains are now supposedly unable to function. Judging women by their hormones is the ultimate ad hominem attack, or perhaps a better term is an "ad feminem" attack, and it's this character assassination that is the core tenet of the patriarchy.

The insult of it all aside, there are many ways tropes about women and their so-called hormonal brains are destructive. When women are expected to be less competent with age there is no urgency to report troubling symptoms, so women may suffer in silence thinking what is happening is normal. Medical conditions that affect the brain are already unfairly stigmatized in many cultures and countries, so add in the shame of having a supposedly hormonal brain as well as the societal disdain toward women as they age, and it's a wonder any woman over forty reports any concerns with their brain health.

These biases also lead medical providers to reject the concerns of women who do self-advocate, and if it's supposedly common knowledge that women get less competent with age or that women are hysterical hypochondriacs, then there is less urgency to study their concerns.

Fortunately, in the past twenty years several excellent studies have examined women's brain health in menopause, and now we can be guided by facts as opposed to harmful stereotypes and clichés.

The Brain and Hormones—Some Basics

The brain is greatly influenced by estrogen—both by estrogen made in the ovary (mostly estradiol) and by estrogen manufactured locally in the brain. There are many complex ways estrogen is involved in brain function. For example, estrogen increases blood flow to the brain, enhances brain metabolism (meaning how the brain receives and uses chemicals and nutrients), and improves brain connectivity (how the different regions of the brain communicate and coordinate with each other). Estrogen even helps clear beta-amyloid deposits (proteins that contribute to the development of Alzheimer's).

Estrogen also boosts activity of serotonin, an important neurotransmitter involved in mood and in the signaling required for some aspects of memory and executive functioning. Executive functioning is a combination of memory, flexible thinking, and self-control to organize and use information to achieve goals. I think of executive functioning as the mind being able to prioritize and focus effectively on tasks. Estrogen is crucial to the brain's role with reproduction, for example, it's part of the hormonal signaling that tells the brain to trigger ovulation (chapter 3) as well as temperature regulation to optimize implantation (chapter 9).

This doesn't mean that women's brains are unable to function without estrogen. Girls have amazing, capable brains before they enter puberty and many women who never take estrogen continue to achieve great things after their final menstrual period. After all, our ancestors managed with their low-estrogen brains to find food and water when it was scarce, likely using their memories from previous famines or droughts or possibly even recalling what their own mothers may have told them about foraging during difficult times.

It's possible that the reduction of estrogen in a brain primed to have high levels through decades of exposure and/or the hormonal chaos of the menopause transition causes symptoms for some women either due to an underlying genetic risk or because of other biological vulnerabilities.

While estrogen matters, it's also only one piece of the puzzle. There are other changes with menopause that could potentially impact brain function. For example, the rise in levels of follicle stimulating hormone (FSH) or inflammation from the increase in visceral fat (see chapter 7).

Women's brains also have a unique plasticity—the ability to change or rewire in response to hormonal cues. This is what enhances bonding with a newborn and allows a mother to be so attentive to her baby's needs, such as recognizing subtle changes in crying or facial expressions and then to act accordingly. Hormonal changes with delivery repurpose many functions to this new, all-important task—infant survival. This is why many mothers feel they have baby brain, and they're not wrong. It's not that they are less capable but rather the brain has shifted resources to become hyper-focused on one specific and evolutionarily vital task—survival of their baby. Considering the vast resources pregnancy requires and the extreme vulnerability of the end product (the baby), this is a very logical use of brain function.

The responsiveness of a woman's brain to hormonal changes and the ability to rewire in response to hormone triggers are likely part of the reason that women are at higher risk for depression compared with men and may explain hormonally mediated depression and mood changes (for example, during their menstrual cycle—premenstrual mood dysphoric disorder or PMDD and postpartum depression). This ability to rewire in response to hormonal cues may also explain some of the changes experienced by some women during the menopause transition.

Brain Fog

Like many women, I have forgotten my car keys or missed a meeting and then worried I had menopause brain. Surely this was the beginning of a rapid decline into forgotten hankies stuffed up my sleeve and in my bra.

Approximately two-thirds of women report these same cognitive difficulties during their menopause transition, meaning some kind of memory problem or forgetfulness. It's often commonly referred to as "brain fog." Maybe it's a concern about misplaced keys, problems with word finding, or an inability to focus on a task. Several studies have looked at this phenomenon. For example, during the SWAN (Study of Women's Health Across the Nation) participants underwent tests of cognition and memory over several years, and these women were followed prospectively—an ideal way to follow changes as they occur. Women had a reduced speed at which they were able to process information as well as a decrease in something called verbal episodic memory, which is the ability to recall a list of words or remember a story. These were subtle changes that didn't leave the women forgetful or unable to function; rather, the researchers summed it up as an impact on the ability to take in new information.

Another group of researchers compared women ages forty-five to fifty-five with men of the same age and found the women performed better than the men with memory tasks before menopause, but during the menopause transition and afterward that advantage became less apparent. This point feels important enough to emphasize. Yes there is a temporary change, but even with that change women still out-performed men.

(There's another mantra for your hot flush cognitive behavioral therapy.)

These menopause transition changes in brain functioning are temporary and disappear once the menopause transition is over. This is an important point that I hope normalizes the experience and helps women feel reassured about what is happening. There can be a *pause* in learning, and in many ways the menopause transition does feel like a break in your stride—but this isn't an early sign of deterioration. Perhaps a good analogy for the hormonal chaos of the menopause transition is like a computer uploading a new program. During the upload (the menopause transition) things run a little slower. Once loaded, there may be a glitch or two before this new program is running smoothly and then things settle as the new program takes over. After all, both computer code and hormones are forms of language.

What about hot flushes and night sweats? Might those lead to memory issues? That sounds intuitive, but looking at the women in SWAN there was no link between those experiences and how the brain processed information or on memory. Depression, anxiety, and sleep disturbances can definitely influence how the brain works, and if a woman develops those conditions during her menopause transition they may impact her brain function, but it's not the transition per se but the depression or anxiety.

What about women who say they just don't feel as sharp after their menopause transition? To answer this question researchers looked at memory and cognition over time—before the menopause transition, during, and afterward. What they found was the cognitive function does change, but it's simply a function of aging. Remember, a woman who starts her menopause transition at the age of forty-seven and ends at fifty-three has also experienced six years of aging.

Some women feel that their brain is functioning worse than what it appears to be when evaluated, or perhaps their lived experience doesn't match up with what they're reading in this book right now—that menopause-related changes are typically minimal and temporary. Studies tell us that women who are under more stress, have depression or anxiety, have other health concerns, or who aren't sleeping well and/or who have more vasomotor symptoms are more likely to judge their cognitive performance more harshly. Vasomotor symptoms can even prime the brain to be more receptive to negative experiences. This is the mind-body connection in action.

Many women in midlife are under incredible amounts of stress as women bear more financial burdens because of gender inequalities. For example, women are paid less than men for the same work, they typically perform more unpaid caregiver functions, and during times of financial crisis are more likely to lose their job. As stress, especially financial stressors, may play a role in many health conditions, we must also step back and look at the stress that society uniquely imposes on women.

I asked my partner, who is eight months older, what he blamed when he lost his car keys? He laughed and said, "Well, age or stress of course." Why would anyone blame menopause, he wondered? It was interesting to see the liberty of never absorbing a lifetime of toxic messages about one's body. I also know I'm with a true feminist, because he immediately rejected the hypothesis that menopause could make women less competent.

The way we think about menopause feels like an exercise in confirmation bias about the supposed ineptitude of older women. So influenced by society to believe that menopause affected memory and brain function, even I failed to consider that I probably wasn't misplacing my car keys any more than usual—after all I've always been organizationally challenged. It wasn't until I read the studies about what is typical and compared my experiences with a similar aged man that my biases were revealed to me and I felt relieved.

What should a woman do who feels that she may be experiencing cognitive changes or having memory issues?

- **BE REASSURED:** Temporary changes with memory, attention, and the feeling of brain fog are typical symptoms of the menopause transition, and *while they feel alarming they aren't a cause for alarm.* This isn't a sign that there's a steep memory cliff ahead. Dementia in midlife is rare for women who aren't at genetic risk for early-onset Alzheimer's disease.
- **GET SCREENED FOR DEPRESSION, ANXIETY, AND SLEEP DISTURBANCE:** These affect cognitive performance and when treated memory may improve.
- **GET EVALUATED:** For other health conditions that may be associated with memory issues or a feeling of brain fog. Some medical conditions to consider are sleep apnea, thyroid disease, and diabetes. Medications may also leave some people feeling fuzzy or affect memory, so a review of those is in order.
- **EXERCISE:** At least 150 minutes a week of moderate activity is the goal. This comes up repeatedly, I know, but it's one of the best things a woman can do for her brain health.
- **CONSIDER STRESS:** There's no easy fix here, but a psychologist may be able to help reframe life stressors, give support, and provide strategies for coping. I find many women underestimate the amount of stress they're experiencing.
- **FORMAL MEMORY TESTING:** This is called neuropsychiatric testing and it's only indicated when memory or other cognitive concerns are worsening with no explanation or are interfering with how a woman lives her life. Women at genetic risk for early-

onset Alzheimer's disease should be referred when they have any concerns about their cognition.

What about menopausal hormone therapy (MHT)? There's no data to support that it will stop this *temporary* cognitive decline. If hot flushes or depression improve with hormones, then there may be an indirect impact on temporary memory concerns. Women should be reminded that if these temporary changes in cognition don't improve on MHT, increasing the dose of estrogen isn't likely to be the answer.

Depression and Menopause

Depression isn't just feeling sad, it's a medical condition associated with sadness that won't go away, hopelessness, low energy, and little interest in activities that once brought pleasure. Depression can affect emotions, thoughts, behavior, sleep, appetite, cognitive ability, and physical health. The menopause transition is associated with an increased risk of depression—depending on the study anywhere from 19 percent to 36 percent of women may experience depression during this phase. The reasons are complex, and it appears the hormonal chaos allows depression to emerge in women who are at risk. Typically, the brain is able to compensate for the myriad of hormonal changes that happen with the menopause transition, and the low levels of estrogen after the final menstrual period, but some women may have a reduced ability to adapt to the changes in the hormonal milieu.

That depression is associated with menopause isn't surprising—women have higher rates of depression versus men and depression can be triggered by hormonal changes, for example, premenstrual mood dysphoric disorder (the more extreme version of PMS) and postpartum depression. Women who enter menopause before age forty-five, and especially those with primary ovarian insufficiency (see chapter 6) have higher rates of depression than women whose final menstrual period is much later. It seems the longer a woman is exposed to estrogen from her ovaries, the lower her odds of menopause transition-associated depression. One estimate suggests a 5 percent decrease in risk of severe depression for each two-year delay in menopause. This shouldn't be taken as a cause and effect with estrogen levels—in fact studies don't link levels of estrogen with depression—although interestingly in one study higher levels of testosterone were associated with a greater risk of depression.

Depression that emerges during the menopause transition is likely due to a combination of the hormonal chaos, length of exposure to estrogen throughout the lifetime, genetics, medical health, and social determinants of health. And the more of these added, the greater the risk. Some specific factors that have been identified include the following:

- **ADVERSE CHILDHOOD EXPERIENCES OR ACES:** Negative childhood experiences such as emotional abuse, chaos in the family due to divorce, or food insecurity affects brain structure and function. The areas affected are the hippocampus and prefrontal cortex, which are also areas especially influenced by estrogen and are involved in memory. Women who have experienced two or more ACEs are more likely to experience menopause-related depression.
- **EMOTIONS:** Women who have negative attitudes towards aging and menopause and those who experience more negative emotions (such as worries or pessimism or anxious thoughts) are at greater risk of depression. This doesn't mean the emotions or thoughts cause the depression, but that an association has been identified in studies.
- **INSUFFICIENT SLEEP:** Difficulty sleeping is a symptom of depression, and lack of sleep can worsen depression.
- **LOWER SOCIAL SUPPORT:** Being unhappy in a marriage, being single, and having few close friends or family. Social relationships protect the brain just as estrogen does.
- **SMOKING:** The mechanism isn't known, but there is a definite association.
- **SOCIAL DETERMINANTS OF HEALTH:** Such as financial hardships and stress.
- **VISCERAL FAT:** It's unknown if this is cause or effect. Meaning, is the inflammation or hormone changes from the metabolically active fat contributing to depression or are the hormonal changes of depression, such as changes in cortisol, increasing the risk of visceral fat?

What depression doesn't appear to be linked with? Surprisingly, hot flushes.

One could look at this list and think, ugh. And it's true many aren't possible to change, but for women who haven't started their menopause transition there may be opportunities to shore up your brain's defense against depression, such as working on sleep, quitting smoking, or forging new friendships. Often women find their social circles getting smaller in their late thirties and early forties for a variety of reasons—moves, new relationships, breakups or divorces, kids, and life to name a few.

Women should be screened annually for depression. A good tool is the PHQ-2 (where PHQ stands for Patient Health Questionnaire), which is simply two questions: In the last two weeks how often on a 4-point scale where 0 = not at all, 1 = several days, 2 = more than half the days, and 3 = nearly every day have you been bothered by:

- Little interest or pleasure in doing things?
- Feeling down, depressed, or hopeless?

When the score is 3 or greater further evaluation for depression is indicated.

A full explanation of the treatment of depression is beyond the scope of this book. Many women with mild depression manage well with psychological therapy, such as counseling with a psychologist or other licensed therapist or cognitive behavioral therapy (CBT). Moderate to severe depression typically requires antidepressant medications in addition to psychological therapy. Estradiol in MHT can be effective in treating mild to moderate depression that emerges during the early menopause transition. It seems there is a window of opportunity here for estradiol to help, as toward the late menopause transition and after the final menstrual period estrogen no longer has an antidepressant effect.

Dementia and Alzheimer's

Women are at higher risk for developing dementia and Alzheimer's disease (a type of dementia) compared with men, and when women develop these conditions they often develop them earlier. Women with a later menopause (longer lifetime exposure to estrogen) have a lower risk of dementia, and women with menopause before age forty-five are at higher risk. With that in mind it's reasonable to ask how does this relate to menopause and can menopausal hormone therapy (MHT) help reduce that risk?

Many factors that are unrelated to estrogen can increase a woman's risk of dementia and Alzheimer's disease. For example, diet (see chapter 21), lack of exercise, smoking, and high blood pressure and diabetes (the latter two negatively affect blood vessels, reducing blood flow to the brain). Genetics also increase the risk of Alzheimer's disease, specifically a gene called APOE4, which appears to raise the risk for women even more than men. The APOE gene provides instructions for making a protein called apolipoprotein E. There are several versions of the APOE gene, and people who inherit the version called APOE4 are at higher risk of developing Alzheimer's, and there appears to be an interaction between APOE4 and estrogen that increases the vulnerability of younger women to Alzheimer's during the first few years of postmenopause.

Many women wonder about MHT for prevention of dementia or Alzheimer's disease. Data tells us that starting MHT after the age of sixty or more than ten years from the final menstrual period may increase the risk of these conditions. Women with lower cognitive function at baseline were especially vulnerable to the MHT-associated increased risk of dementia.

For younger women the data is a little more complex. Many researchers wonder if there is a critical window during the menopause transition or very early after the final menstrual period where the estrogen in menopausal hormone therapy (MHT) may be preventative therapy for dementia. Two studies—the KRONOS early prevention trial and the KEEPS trial—enrolled women within three years of their final menstrual period and followed them for four years to evaluate the impact of oral conjugated equine estrogens (CEE) or transdermal estradiol on cognitive function. Neither study showed any improvement over the short term, but as the changes of dementia and Alzheimer's start in the brain long before there are any measurable physical sign, researchers wondered if brain images might hold early clues.

Several years after the KEEPS trial finished, researchers brought the women back to reevaluate their brains. At this point the brain scans of women who had taken CEE had some negative changes in blood vessels compared with women taking placebo, while women using transdermal estradiol had less of an effect, but there was no change in performance of the cognitive function tests. Whether this effect on blood vessels might translate into an increased risk of dementia down the road or is a spurious finding isn't known.

In this same study, researchers scanned the women's brains for amyloid plaques, which are seen with Alzheimer's disease and show up on brain scan years before symptoms. What they found was women who carried the APOE4 gene and were using transdermal estradiol had a reduction in deposits of amyloid plaques, but this effect wasn't seen among women who weren't APOE4 carriers. It's not known if estrogen when given early might reduce the plaques for all women, if the women who were APOE4 carriers were uniquely sensitive to estrogen, or if there is another explanation.

Currently, there's no evidence to support starting MHT to reduce the risk of Alzheimer's disease or dementia for women at average risk. There is evidence that quitting smoking, a healthy diet, and regular exercise can help—in fact approximately 50 percent of the risk for Alzheimer's disease is related to these potentially modifiable factors. There are also some unanswered questions about potentially negative effects of estrogen on blood vessels in the brain over the long term, and the effect seen on brain scans was more pronounced with the oral CEE versus the transdermal estradiol, raising the possibility that this change may be related to increased clotting in the blood vessels (oral estrogens affect blood clotting while transdermal do not, see chapters 17 and 18). More work here is definitely needed. Whether women with APOE4 gene should consider estradiol for brain health at menopause is beyond what we can discuss here, and women at high genetic risk for early Alzheimer's should be under the care of physicians with experience in this area.

BOTTOM LINE

- Estrogen influences many aspects of brain health and functioning, but with menopause the brain appears to adapt to the new hormonal environment.

- The hormonal chaos of the menopause transition can lead to temporary cognitive changes; there are factors that may make these changes feel more concerning than they are with objective testing measures.
- Depression may emerge during the menopause transition, likely due to an underlying vulnerability combined with changing levels of hormones.
- Women with milder depression may benefit from estrogen in MHT.
- Dementia and Alzheimer's disease are more common in women than men; for most women starting MHT to protect the brain isn't indicated because of many still unanswered questions.

Chapter 13

The Vagina and Vulva:

Genitourinary Syndrome of Menopause and the Therapies

CHANGES TO THE VULVA AND vagina due to menopause used to be called vaginal atrophy, but now we use the term "genitourinary syndrome of menopause" (GUSM). While it's true the vaginal tissues do atrophy, meaning they become thinner and can shrink, this older terminology was problematic. First, the vagina is only one of the structures affected. The bladder, urethra, clitoris, and vulva also undergo changes related to the lower levels of estrogen. And then there's the point that atrophy is synonymous with shrinkage. Women are already diminished by society as we age, so a term that makes the vagina sound like a decrepit shrinking violet is unacceptable.

GUSM isn't a catchy acronym, but it's more encompassing and reminds everyone—women and their providers—of the potential scope of the problem. Here we'll discuss medical issues related to the vagina and vulva; for more on the bladder and urethra, head to chapter 14.

GUSM is common—as many as 15 percent of women report manifestations during their menopause transition, and eventually up to 80 percent of women will experience some symptoms. Many women with GUSM don't get the care they need. Some don't perceive their symptoms to be menopause-related, others think there are no safe treatment options, many women are dismissed by their providers, and some just don't feel comfortable enough to discuss sexual concerns.

Women who are the most bothered by symptoms of GUSM are forty-five to sixty-four years of age, but it isn't known if the symptoms truly reduce over time, if women give up seeking care for their symptoms because they have been dismissed or ignored too many times, or if the lack of a sexual partner or other health conditions leads to a shift in priorities.

Vulva and Vagina 101

Let's start with a brief introduction to the vulva and vagina (anyone wanting an in-depth review should pick up my book *The Vagina Bible*). The vagina is the inside; it's a fibromuscular tube lined with mucosa (specialized skin). It connects the uterus with the vulva, which is on the outside. In other words, where the clothes touch the skin is the vulva. The vulva includes everything from the mons (just below the pubic bone) to just before the anus (see figure 12). Where the vagina and the vulva overlap at the opening is known as the vestibule.

The labia minora, which are the inside lips, vary in size—for 50 percent of women they protrude beyond the labia majora and this is normal.

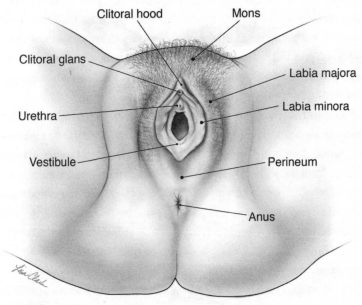

Figure 12: Vulva

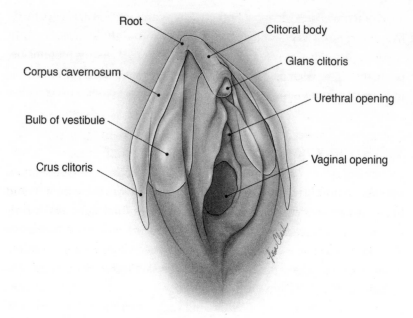

Root
Clitoral body
Corpus cavernosum
Glans clitoris
Bulb of vestibule
Urethral opening
Crus clitoris
Vaginal opening

Figure 13: Clitoris

The labia minora have a small amount of fat and may sometimes have erectile tissue. They are also filled with specialized nerve endings. The labia minora divide close to the glans, the visible part of the clitoris—the top joining the clitoral hood and the bottom turns into the frenulum (which is very sensitive) that merges with the lower aspect of the glans. Given the specialized nerve endings and these connections with the clitoral glans, tugging and pressure on the labia minora can be very stimulating for many women.

The external part of the glans is relatively small (it may look like a kidney bean or a small candy to some people) and is partially covered with skin called the hood. The entire clitoris itself is much larger—the glans is just the tip of the iceberg—and is shaped like an inverted Y with four arms instead of two. One set of arms is called the bulbs and the other the crura. The bulbs and crura come together at the body and then join with the glans (see figure 13). The clitoris is intimate with the urethra, so that's why many women have an area that is very sensitive in a good way around the urethra and/or just inside the vagina right beneath the bladder. This is often called the G-spot, but it's not one spot. In medicine we call it the clitorourethral complex, and the area that feels pleasurable often varies person to person. If this isn't a particularly pleasurable spot for you, that's okay. Everyone is built differently.

When women achieve orgasm via vaginal penetration it's because the penis or fingers or sex toy is bumping or tugging or otherwise stimulating the clitoris, but it's important to note that 1 out of every 3 don't orgasm with vaginal penetration alone, because the mechanics just don't do it for their clitoris. Fingers, tongues, and sex toys offer far more precision than a penis. Orgasms with penile penetration—Dr. Sigmund Freud's so-called vaginal or "mature" orgasm—aren't superior to orgasms brought about by direct clitoral stimulation with fingers or any other method. Freud likely had no concept that the clitoris was more than the glans, but regardless, the idea that there could be no real pleasure without the mighty girth of a penis has become a harmful, misogynistic trope that's simply untrue. After all, lesbians report more orgasms during sex than heterosexual women.

Changes with Menopause

The vulva and vagina undergo significant changes either directly from the lack of estrogen or indirectly because of the reduction in blood flow to the tissues. Collagen production also decreases with age. Collagen is a protein that, among other things, gives tissues their strength and stretch, so the loss of collagen with menopause and age leads to increased tissue fragility and decreased elasticity. Physically, the tissues appear pale, and when GUSM is severe there may be small red spots at the vestibule and inside the vagina that are the result of extremely fragile capillaries that have leaked blood into the tissues.

The vaginal microbiome undergoes a dramatic shift away from a lactobacillus dominant environment to a variety of other bacteria. For some women this can result in subtle changes in their normal vaginal scent. The pH rises, often it's 5.5 or higher (the pH before menopause is typically 3.8–4.5), and there is a decrease in lubrication. The vagina also shrinks a little in length and width, likely due to changes in blood flow and collagen, but there may be other reasons. All of these changes, in addition to the loss of tissue elasticity and increased fragility, can lead to pain with sex. Interestingly, the penis also shrinks with age due to declining testosterone levels, decreased blood flow, and collagen production. We just don't hear about that as much.

There's a myth that with age the vagina risks a "use it or lose it" scenario—meaning without the potency of a penis the vagina may shrink permanently. It's simply shocking (imagine my voice dripping in sarcasm) that there's no similar myth that the penis can avoid shrinkage with regular vaginal contact. The "use it or lose it" theory was based on lower quality data that wouldn't be accepted today. Loss of estrogen and age-related changes are what affect a vagina; it's not a lament for the touch of a man. Rarely, when a woman has significant inflammation from low estrogen and the tissues have become so fragile that they bleed with touch, the walls of the vagina can fuse together. In thirty years of running a vaginal and vulvar clinic, I have seen this once or twice. Even if the vagina closing up from lack of sex with age were a thing, a penis couldn't mechanically prevent this from happening, because for these women vaginal sex would be too painful, and a penis can't reduce inflammation to the tissues or repair blood vessels. It's a penis, not a magic wand.

With age the clitoris reduces in size and the amount of erectile tissue also decreases, but whether this is age-specific or estrogen-related isn't known. The labia minora can reduce in size and the labia majora may flatten a little and even appear a little larger due to looseness in the skin and the shifts in location of adipose tissue. Pubic hair graying typically starts after the age of forty-five and is an age-related phenomenon.

During the menopause transition and shortly after menopause, women are at increased risk of developing autoimmune skin conditions that involve the vulva and/or vagina—the most common are lichen sclerosus and lichen planus. These conditions don't just cause troubling symptoms, such as itching, burning, and pain with sex, they are also associated with physical changes. For example, the skin can turn white and become extremely fragile, the labia minora can shrink and even disappear, the tissue over the clitoral glans can fuse so the glans is no longer visible, scar tissue can narrow the vagina—and when advanced and untreated may progress to the point where the vagina fuses shut.

These skin conditions affect 1 percent to 3 percent of women, and while they can occur at any age, the risk seems especially high during the menopause transition, possibly due to the impact of hormones on the immune system. Lichen sclerosus and lichen planus can cause simi-

THE VAGINA AND VULVA — 165

lar symptoms to GUSM—itching, dryness, pain with sex, a feeling of tightness or loss of elasticity in the tissues—so they may be erroneously diagnosed as GUSM. Lichen sclerosus and lichen planus are associated with a higher risk of cancer of the vulva and require specific treatment, so it's important for women with these conditions to see a knowledgeable practitioner.

Symptoms of GUSM

The most common symptom of GUSM is vaginal dryness, but other symptoms include vaginal burning or a sandpaper-like feeling, pain with vaginal penetration, vaginal and vulvar itching, irritation with wiping after using the toilet, decreased lubrication with sex, a change in odor and a change in discharge. The loss of elasticity may make vaginal penetration painful or more difficult and this pain with sex can affect libido. GUSM also increases the risk of urinary tract or bladder infections (see chapter 14).

Over time women can also develop perianal dermatitis, which is chronic redness and inflammation and sometimes even skin breakdown around the anus, and it's very irritating and even uncomfortable. Perianal dermatitis is the combination of increasing skin fragility with age combined with the repetitive trauma of wiping and exposure of the skin to stool, which is chemically very irritating. This is likely less related to GUSM and more a phenomenon of aging skin.

Some women report a decrease in orgasm strength or a longer time to achieve orgasm. There could be many reasons, including reduced blood flow to the tissues, changes in size and erectile tissue of the clitoris, age or estrogen-related changes in how nerves communicate with the brain, or even weakness or decreased responsiveness in the pelvic floor muscles (these are the muscles that physically contract during an orgasm), which—like all muscles—will lose mass with age. These muscles also respond to estrogen, so it's possible there may be combined effects of aging and loss of estrogen. It's not uncommon for women to need a vibrator to achieve orgasm after menopause where they didn't before, and this is *not* a failing. Some women may also find that working on their pelvic floor strength with Kegel exercises (see chapter 14) can benefit their orgasm.

Attention to Vulvar Care

The foundation of managing GUSM is vulvar and perianal skin care. With increased fragility the skin is more apt to become dry, further increasing the risk of microscopic trauma, starting a cycle of irritation and inflammation that can progress to the point that gentle attempts at masturbation, oral sex, or even wiping can be enough to cause discomfort. Key recommendations for good vulvar care include the following:

- **USE A CLEANSER:** Soap can damage the acid mantle, the protective layer of fat and other microscopic substances that coats the skin. It can also react with the vulvar skin raising the pH from a typical 4.0–5.2 to 10. Soap can also be drying. An unscented facial cleanser—inexpensive drug store brands are just fine—is the best option.
- **AVOID WIPES:** These may be valuable for women with incontinence to help clean up when they are out of their own home, but most contain irritants and they are hygienically unnecessary. They are a common source of vulvar irritation and perianal dermatitis. I could write a ten-thousand-word essay on how wipes are a combination of infantilizing women (they're meant to remove stool from a baby's bottom; women are not babies and are capable of wiping with toilet paper or using a bidet), a remnant of purity culture (the cleanliness, or faux cleanliness of wipes, means a woman is "good"), and the obsession of a patriarchal society with degrading women based on their normal bodies (if women need their skin prepped for men and the reverse isn't true, then the conclusion is women are inherently dirty). If wipes were about genital hygiene and not oppressing women, then there would be shelves of these products for men with scents such as Dick's Delight, Sunset Escape, and Puppy Paws.
- **USE INCONTINENCE PADS FOR INCONTINENCE, NOT MENSTRUAL PADS:** Menstrual pads can't handle the volume of urine, and consequently the pad stays wet leading to skin irritation and, if this happens enough, skin breakdown.
- **MOISTURIZE:** Dryness is the enemy of the skin. Coconut oil, olive oil, and petroleum jelly are all good low-cost alternatives. There

are more expensive alternatives that claim to be made for vulvar skin, although none have published any meaningful results. While proving their claims isn't possible, based on the ingredients it's unlikely they offer a true advantage. A moisturizing product is more about what you like—the feel of a product is a very personal thing. Some women like beautiful jars, and buying these products may feel like self-care. As long as the product is unscented and doesn't irritate, most are likely fine. However, some of the companies promote these products not just for dryness, but as tools to prevent against the perils of feminine odor, which is not a medical thing and is harmful messaging. That may factor into the decision to use certain products for some women. (When I'm in a mood I call out these manufacturers on my Instagram. At some point they will tire of me and remove the destructive messaging about "feminine odor.")

- **TRIM PUBIC HAIR, DON'T REMOVE:** Pubic hair increases humidity and hence traps moisture against the vulva. Removing hair—whether it's waxing, shaving, or any other method—damages the top layer of the skin, increases the risk of cuts, and as skin ages the consequences may increase.
- **IF YOU SMOKE, DO YOUR BEST TO QUIT:** Smoking has anti-estrogenic effects and impairs blood flow to all skin.

Lubricant

These products are used during sex, either self-love or with a partner. Many women and their partners like these products regardless of age or menopausal status, but for some women they may become necessary if they have GUSM. For many women with mild symptoms, lubricants may be all that is needed.

There are three types of lubricants: water based, silicone based, and oil based. The desired feel or what I like to call the slip of a lubricant is very personal. Some women will love how one product feels against the skin and another might find that same product sticky. Overall, women with GUSM tend to do best with a silicone lubricant, so if a woman hasn't used lubricant before or the last time was several decades ago, then silicone is a good place to start. They all contain a combination of one or more silicones, such as dimethicone, cyclomethicone, and dimethiconol, meaning there isn't an organic, bespoke silicone business. Some silicone lubes may also have small amounts of coconut oil or vitamin E, which is also an oil. Following are some common products that seem well tolerated:

- Astroglide X—silicone only
- Astroglide X Silicone gel—silicone and coconut oil
- Über Lube—silicone and vitamin E

While Astroglide and Über Lube both claim the small amount of oil doesn't change their compatibility with latex condoms, I can't locate any publicly available studies supporting that statement. Astroglide did respond to my request for more information; they indicated they had done testing to determine compatibility, but could not share the documents. Über Lube did not respond to my email.

I have a large stash of single-use Über Lube packets in the office for pelvic exams, and I don't think any patient has told me she found it uncomfortable on her vulva or vagina; in fact many are surprised when it doesn't irritate. While I appreciate that observation reeks of bias, I do make notes of products I use and recommend as well as any feedback I receive. Some people find silicone lubricants harder to clean out of sheets, and these lubricants may not be compatible with all silicone sex toys.

Water-based lubricants require more knowledge about ingredients, and the wrong choice here is more likely to be irritating. Here are some considerations:

- **pH:** This is the acidity of the product. It's best to aim for one that is close to vaginal pH, meaning 3.5–4.5, even though the pH of the vagina rises with menopause. Most products unfortunately don't list their pH.
- **OSMOLALITY:** Best thought of as concentration. When the osmolality is higher than that of vaginal secretions the product will draw water out of the vaginal tissues, potentially causing irritation and even increasing a woman's risk of acquiring a sexually transmitted infection (STI) if exposed. The osmolality of vaginal secretions is 260–280 mOs/kg, and it's best to use a product with

an osmolality <380 mOsm/kg. The World Health Organization (WHO) recommends against lubricants with an osmolality >1,200 mOsm/kg.

- **CERTAIN PRESERVATIVES:** Products with clorhexidene gluconate, polyquaternium, and more than 8.3 percent glycerin should be avoided as they can irritate tissues and/or damage the vaginal ecosystem.
- **FRAGRANCE, FLAVORING, AND WARMING:** Avoid. The ingredients can be irritating and these products often have a very high osmolality.

Given all the ins and outs of the lubes listed above and knowing that product labeling isn't always complete, here are a few water-based lubes in the recommended ranges:

- Good Clean Love, pH 4.73 and 240 mOsm/kg
- Yes Baby Vaginal-Friendly Lubricant, pH 4.22 and 249 mOsm/kg
- Yes Water-Based Intimate Lubricant, pH 4.08 and 154 mOsm/kg

Oil-based lubricants are another option; just remember they're not compatible with latex condoms. Some women find coconut oil or olive oil—just the kind from the grocery store—work well. Olive oil has specifically been evaluated in one small study and no adverse effects were noted. Anecdotally, I have a lot of patients who use coconut oil and have yet to hear that it has been irritating.

Vaginal Moisturizers

These products rehydrate vaginal tissues and are formulated to be bioadhesive, so the product stays on the vaginal tissues and lasts for several days. They are generally well tolerated. In addition, often these products are the placebo arm in studies that evaluate vaginal hormones, and at times they perform as well as lower-dose estrogen! They are most effective when the issue is dryness, but they can also help many women who have pain with sex.

Moisturizers can be water-based (glycerin is a common ingredient, so when present it needs to be in a concentration of 8.3 percent or less), silicone, oil, or hyaluronic acid-based or a combination. Hyaluronic acid is a large molecule that is found in and around skin cells that lubricates and hydrates cells. The impact of moisturizers isn't cumulative, so if you try one of these products and don't see a benefit after four weeks of regular use as directed, then consider switching to a different active ingredient, for example from silicone to hyaluronic acid. (See supplemental table 2, p. 338, for a list of products, pH, and osmolality.)

Hormones

Vaginal estrogen is considered the gold standard for GUSM, meaning that of all the pharmaceutical and over-the-counter options, it's by far the most well-studied and effective. Another hormone called dehydro-epiandrosterone or DHEA is a recent addition to prescription vaginal therapies for GUSM. DHEA is one of the hormones in the process that converts cholesterol to estradiol (see chapter 3). DHEA doesn't have any direct effect on tissues itself; it's useful because it's converted inside the cells into testosterone and estrogen. Vaginal estrogens and DHEA increase blood flow, reverse tissue fragility, restore lubrication, and repopulate the vaginal microbiome with beneficial bacteria. They're effective at treating vaginal dryness, vaginal itching, pain with sex, and may help with changes in odor.

Traditional menopausal hormone therapy or MHT is only effective about 50 percent of the time for GUSM as the resulting levels of estrogen are often not high enough in the vaginal and vulvar tissues. (MHT is taking hormones by mouth or transdermally; see chapter 17.) As there are greater risks with MHT (albeit those risks are small) compared with vaginal therapy and MHT is only helpful approximately half the time, MHT is not recommended for the sole purpose of treating GUSM. However, a woman starting MHT for other reasons, for example hot flushes, may wish to wait two to three months to see how that therapy helps her vagina and vulva before deciding on adding other approaches.

Vaginal estrogen products in the United States and Canada are either estradiol or conjugated equine estrogens or CEE. The brand name is Premarin (see chapters 17 and 18 for more on these estrogens). Vaginal estrogen comes in a wide range of doses as well as methods of application, including creams, a vaginal ring, vaginal tablets, and vaginal suppositories, so customization to an individual woman's needs is possible. Vaginal DHEA is a vaginal suppository and is available in one dose. (See supplemental table 3, p. 338, for a list of the products and doses.)

Estrogen and DHEA will take at least six weeks to work, but may take two to three months to get the full effect, so it's worth completing a three-month course and then re-evaluating. All of the products, with the exception of the estrogen ring and DHEA, are typically dosed initially every day for fourteen days and then twice weekly thereafter. If women prefer to just use a twice-a-week dose, they will get where they need to be; it just may take longer. There may be a transient increase in blood levels of estrogen in the first few weeks with estradiol cream, CEE cream, and DHEA, and possibly intermittently thereafter. This isn't high enough to lead to health concerns—the estradiol cream and CEE especially have decades of data, but this may be why some women initially report breast tenderness. Once the estrogen treats the vaginal inflammation the levels drop. If higher doses of the cream than listed in supplemental table 3 are given, then estrogen levels may be more likely to rise.

There's no increased risk of breast cancer, heart attack, stroke, or dementia with vaginal estrogen or DHEA despite the Black Box Warning required by the Food and Drug Administration (FDA). The warning is based on studies of oral and transdermal therapy and isn't appropriate for vaginal therapy. Several good studies have shown these concerns are not an issue when vaginal estrogen is used appropriately. Unlike estrogen given by mouth or transdermally, no progestogen (progesterone or hormone with similar properties to progesterone) is needed.

Vaginal hormones haven't been studied head to head (or perhaps vagina to vagina?), so it isn't possible to say product A is superior to product B. Pharmaceutical companies rarely put their product on the line with a direct comparison to a competitor—what if their product comes out the same or inferior? Consequently, we typically only see studies from drug companies that compare their results with placebo, and almost always these results show benefit. When independent researchers with funding from non-Pharma sources look at pharmaceuticals, their results are not always as impressive. For example, when the 10 mcg estradiol tablet was studied by independent researchers, it didn't perform any better than the placebo moisturizer. It's unknown if this is formulation-specific (some women report the tablets don't always dissolve well) or if there is another reason.

Another issue with Pharma studies is how the data is presented. Often the outcome has statistical significance, meaning the effect that was found didn't happen by chance, but whether that effect was meaningful to those women isn't always revealed. For example, the estradiol vaginal inserts sold under the name Imvexxy come in doses of 4 mcg and 10 mcg. These very low doses of estradiol performed better than placebo when looking at the changes at a cellular level in a study called the REJOICE trial. This study also tells us that women who used Imvexxy had more improvement in their pain with sex than the women who used a placebo insert. Pain with sex was recorded with a 4-point scale, with 4 being the highest. At week twelve the average pain with sex score was 1.1 for the 4 mcg dose and 1.0 for the 10 mcg dose respectively and it was 1.4 for women assigned to the placebo.

What the study doesn't tell us is if a pain with sex score of 1 or 1.1 out of 4 is meaningfully different from a score of 1.4 out of 4. This doesn't mean that women shouldn't try the lowest dose of estrogen; it just means that studies don't always provide the answers that help us most when we are speaking with women about their medical concerns. For many women this lowest dose of estradiol may work well, but if it doesn't after three months, then a higher dose may be needed.

How to choose a product? For many women price will be a consideration and for others it's the application process. For example, the idea of a ring that's left in for three months at a time greatly appeals to some women, and it elicits a "No way!" from others (you can leave the ring in during sex or take it out). The mess of creams may bother some yet feel soothing to others. The idea of a product that hasn't been shown to budge estradiol levels above the menopausal range—the 4 mcg and 10 mcg vaginal inserts and the ring—may feel comforting for some women, while others may be happiest with the creams as they have the longest track record of safety (as long as they are dosed correctly). Women with a lot of irritation on their labia minora and at the vestibule may need a cream as the vaginal inserts or ring might not provide enough estrogen to cover those tissues. Choices are good and remember it's not a tattoo—if you choose one and it just doesn't seem right, you can easily switch.

What about compounded products? The concept and the myriad of concerns and disadvantages are addressed in detail in chapter 20. The only time I suggest compounded vaginal estrogen is when the pharmaceutical grade is too expensive. In the United States the pricing is currently outrageous—one tube of generic estradiol cream can be over $300 US dollars. While one tube should last at least 3 months, but often up to 6 months depending on the dose, it is a a lot of money up front if not covered or poorly covered by insurance. Many compounding pharmacies can make the same amount of vaginal estradiol for $100 or possibly less. The issue here is compounded creams can contain more estradiol than advertised, which could be a safety concern for some women. If the alternative is to go without, then a compounded cream may be an option as long as it is part of shared decision making.

Women who continue to have pain with sex, itching, or more generalized pain after an adequate trial of vaginal hormone therapy need to be evaluated for other causes of these symptoms. A review of these is beyond the scope of this book, but it is the exact scope of *The Vagina Bible*.

Nonhormonal Medications

Ospemifene (*Osphena*) is an oral medication in the class of drugs called selective estrogen receptor modulator (SERM), meaning it acts like an estrogen on some tissues and like an anti-estrogen on others. On vaginal tissues it acts like an estrogen. It is FDA approved to treat vaginal symptoms of GUSM.

Ospemifene is a good option for women who dislike vaginal products, who find vaginal application painful, or who are looking for something that isn't technically a hormone. The dose is 60 mg per day. Ospemifene acts like estrogen on the uterus, and although the product labeling indicates a progestogen may be needed to protect the lining of the uterus as with MHT (see chapter 17), there is some data that suggests it may not be necessary and that the decision should be individualized. Side effects include hot flushes and a slightly increased risk of blood clots.

Minimally Invasive Energy-Based Therapies

These are lasers or radio frequency devices that heat the vaginal tissues, increasing blood flow and promote remodeling of tissues. Some small studies indicate they can restore glycogen in the tissues and improve the vaginal microbiome as well as lower the vaginal pH to the premenopausal range. Despite their growing popularity there is very little quality data about the safety of these devices and how well they perform when compared with estrogen, DHEA, ospemifene, or even against a placebo gel. If these products were medications, they would not yet be approved by the FDA as the data would be considered insufficient.

One of the most popular devices is called a fractional carbon dioxide laser, but to date there are only two small studies comparing it with estrogen. These studies did not enroll enough patients to answer the question about the effectiveness of the laser for GUSM or the safety. The larger of the two studies enrolled sixty-five women, thirty-two of whom received the laser, so not a lot of data to go on. The study also wasn't blinded, so the women knew which treatment they were receiving, and there was no placebo arm. To truly know if this laser is effective one group of women should receive the laser and a placebo cream, another a sham laser treatment and vaginal estrogen cream, and a third group a sham procedure and a placebo cream. This is especially important given how well the placebo creams and moisturizers work in many studies. In addition, the follow-up from these two small studies has not been long enough to determine risks. The FDA has received reports of women being injured with these lasers—and I've seen it as well. Based on the low quality of the studies and the lack of good safety data, these energy-based therapies are currently not recommended by the American College of Obstetricians and Gynecologists (ACOG) and the North American Menopause Society (NAMS).

The hypothesis behind the energy devices isn't unsound and it deserves testing, but it's infuriating that they have been in use for five years or so and yet here we are with essentially no quality data and unanswered questions about safety remain. Women deserve better. It's shameful when you consider that women have borne a huge burden from undertested medical devices—from the Dalkon Shield (an intrauterine device), the Rely tampon, the Essure device for sterilization, and some types of mesh used for vaginal surgery—and we are still having conversations about untested procedures creeping into women's health care. Years of being used on women and less than one hundred women in inadequately designed prospective studies is simply awful.

How do these devices get approved? Well, they're not approved for treating GUSM in the United States and Canada. These machines are approved for other uses and along the way they were used off label, meaning not for their intended purpose. Though I'm not privy to the internal documents at any company, a typical pathway for devices like these is low-quality studies (which don't offer the kinds of conclusions we want to have before exposing women to this therapy) are generated from the off-label use. These studies should really just be hypothesis generating and lead to more studies so that the device can be evaluated appropriately. Instead, somehow a buzz is created among physicians, in social media, and in the press. The equipment may even be displayed at conferences or promoted to doctors via email campaigns, word of mouth, and other strategies—although everyone is careful about not making claims that the therapy actually works as it's not approved for this reason. Once the device is purchased or leased by providers it gets offered more and more as a therapy. And voilà! There is a new treatment that exists without quality studies and no expensive submission process to the FDA.

These new energy-based therapies could be exciting game changers with a low risk of complications when used by a well-trained provider; they could be moderately helpful, but require re-treatment on a fairly regular basis to maintain effect; they could be relatively harmless and no more effective than placebo; and they could be less effective and more harmful than we know. At this point it's only possible to say that these devices are almost mainstream, they have been inadequately studied, we don't know how well they work compared with the products that are available, and there are unanswered safety concerns.

What's frustrating and awful is in the several years these devices have been used off label, the study to answer these questions could have been performed and we'd have the answer.

What if a woman wants to try an energy-based therapy? People look at risk differently, and the potential that it may not be as effective as claimed or may have more risks than we know may not bother some women. Some individuals are really interested in novel therapies, and there are women who just don't want to use vaginal products at home. As long as a woman is fully informed of the unknowns, it is her body and her choice.

Women with Cancer

Some cancers are estrogen sensitive and so for these women there are concerns that the estrogen in vaginal therapies, including that from DHEA, could hasten a recurrence and worsen their prognosis. The most common cancers that fall in this group are breast cancer, endometrial cancer (the lining of the uterus), uterine sarcoma (the muscle of the uterus) and several types of ovarian cancer.

Women with these cancers should first try the nonhormonal options discussed. For some of these women applying a topical anesthetic (a numbing medication, most commonly lidocaine) at the vestibule (vaginal opening) several minutes before sex can be helpful for pain with sex. Sex therapy and physical therapy may also be helpful for some women. Other women may wish to explore anal sex. I've spoken with several women in the office who had considered this option, but it wasn't part of their sexual repertoire so they appreciated the safe space to discuss.

When those options fail to provide relief or aren't acceptable, then for some women estrogen therapies that don't result in a bump in estrogen levels may be an option, but this requires a consideration of all factors involved, such as type and stage of cancer and time from diagnosis, so this can't be generalized. The products that may be an option in this situation are the low-dose estrogens: the 4 and 10 mcg capsules, the 10 mcg tablets, and the vaginal ring. The creams can occasionally result in detectable estrogen levels, so they should be avoided. Estradiol levels may also rise with DHEA, although they typically remain in the postmenopausal range, so DHEA is less optimal than the low-dose estradiol.

Many women with breast cancer have an additional concern—they may be taking medications to prevent a recurrence. These drugs are tamoxifen and a class of medications called aromatase inhibitors, discussed previously in chapter 5. Tamoxifen blocks the action of estrogen on tissues, and aromatase inhibitors prevent the production of estrogen in every tissue. Tamoxifen is an interesting drug, because on some tissues it may act like an estrogen. Consequently, not all women get symptoms of GUSM with tamoxifen or if they do they may not be as bad.

For women with breast cancer, those with a hormone-receptor-negative cancer are likely at the lowest risk, and most guidelines suggest that in consultation with their providers and as part of a shared decision a low-dose vaginal estrogen is acceptable. Women with hormone-receptor-positive breast cancer who are taking tamoxifen may be a candidate for a low-dose vaginal estrogen; theoretically if any estradiol is absorbed it should be blocked by the tamoxifen from affecting breast tissue. Again, this requires discussion with a woman's gynecologist and oncologist (cancer specialist).

Women with breast cancer who are taking aromatase inhibitors face unique challenges—the point of the aromatase inhibitor is to prevent the production of *all* estrogen. This is why the effects on GUSM are so profound. As aromatase inhibitors block the enzyme that produces estrogen, if any estrogen were absorbed from vaginal therapy it won't be blocked and is free to act on tissues. One option, if all the nonhormonal options fail, is to consider a switch from an aromatase inhibitor to tamoxifen, although this switch may not always be in a woman's best interest medically, so this approach needs to be individualized.

Another option for women for whom low-dose estrogen is not advised is the energy-based therapies just discussed. A woman who is unable to have sex because of an aromatase inhibitor who may be looking at five or even ten years of this therapy, may consider the unknowns with this energy-based therapy worth the risk.

Every woman views risk differently, so how one woman might feel about a device that hasn't been adequately tested versus a low dose of estrogen that to the best of our knowledge isn't absorbed may vary. Women also have to balance any risks against their quality of life. For too long women who survived a cancer were made to feel that their survival was enough, that they should just be happy, that they are alive and need to just suck up their vaginal symptoms. But quality of life is very important, and so women with a history of cancers that could be affected by hormones deserve to hear the options and in collaboration with their medical providers make the choices that work for them.

BOTTOM LINE

- GUSM affects up to 80 percent of women, and for some women the symptoms can start during the menopause transition.
- Common symptoms of GUSM are vaginal dryness, pain with sex, burning, and itching.
- Nonhormonal options include appropriate vulvar care, lubricants, and a moisturizer.
- Topical estrogen and DEAS are effective therapy for GUSM and they result in little to no absorption of estrogen.
- Energy devices are understudied and not yet recommended by major medical societies given the paucity of data.

Chapter 14

Bladder Health:
Breaking the Culture of Silence

IT'S TYPICAL FOR WOMEN TO develop bladder conditions with both menopause and age, but it's not normal, and there is an ocean of difference between those two words. *Typical* means it's no surprise that a medical condition happens, but it doesn't mean that condition is safe or unproblematic or needs to be tolerated. In contrast, normal sounds as if the experience is something to be tolerated. Many women suffer from bladder health concerns, and yet they are often told this is "normal" and "just part of being a woman." This is unacceptable. Imagine if we told men with erectile dysfunction that it's "not bad enough to need treatment" or "that it's just part of being a man"? And with erectile dysfunction, no one is leaking in public. Women are constantly expected to tolerate the consequences of their biology, and it's unacceptable.

One common theme in bladder-related concerns is their near-absence from public discourse. I think of all the magazines with their headlines that prophesize vaginal doom should the wrong pair of lace underwear touch the skin or the seemingly constant discourse about vaginal discharge, and yet with the bladder it's mostly silence. This can't be because people are squeamish; after all both vaginal discharge and urine are bodily fluids from "down there." Female currency in a patriarchal society is a prepped and cleaned virginal vulva and vagina—the literal incarnation of purity myths. So society can have a discourse about the vulva and vagina because the shaming is useful, but bladder concerns are linked with senescence, which means irrelevance for women.

Recurrent Urinary Tract Infections

A urinary tract infection or UTI is the overgrowth of bacteria in the urine that leads to inflammation. The main symptoms are pain with emptying the bladder (dysuria), having to go more often (frequency), and when you gotta go you gotta go (urgency). Some women may also have blood in their urine (hematuria). Recurrent UTIs are diagnosed when a woman has two infections in six months or three in a twelve-month period of time.

UTIs are fairly common. Between the ages of twenty and fifty-nine approximately 2 percent to 4 percent of women will have at least one a year, and the risk of infection starts to increase around age sixty. Recurrent UTIs also increase with age—before menopause up to one-third of women will have a second infection within twelve months, but for women after menopause that number jumps to 55 percent. Despite the increased risk of recurrent UTIs for women after menopause, this area remains poorly studied.

The increased risk of UTIs after menopause is largely related to low estrogen, which results in a variety of changes that facilitate these infections such as a reduction in blood flow to the tissue, the tissues themselves become more fragile, and the protective bacteria in the vagina is replaced with bacteria more likely to cause infection—so this becomes a source of infection for the bladder. The loss of estrogen may also negatively impact the immune system. In addition, there are age-related changes to collagen and the immune system that likely also play a role.

Strategies to prevent recurrent infections are important, not only to reduce pain and suffering, but to reduce exposure to antibiotics as these medications can cause collateral damage to the body (for example, antibiotic-related diarrhea and an increased risk of developing antibiotic-resistant bacteria).

When a woman thinks she may have recurrent infections, the most important first step is to get a urine culture. The culture can confirm a correct diagnosis as well as inform the provider which organism is causing the infection and if it has become resistant to any antibiotics. Without the right antibiotic, treatment is destined to fail. Strategies that have been shown to be effective in preventing recurrent UTIs include:

- **VAGINAL ESTROGEN:** Some data suggests the cream may be better, but it's not definitive. Women should try whatever vaginal estrogen product or DHEA that appeals to them (see chapter 13 for options). If an option other than estrogen cream option is selected and there isn't a reduction in UTIs over the next six to twelve months, it may be worth considering the cream to see if that is more effective.
- **ANTIBIOTICS:** These can be taken daily (or every few days depending on the antibiotic) to prevent infection. For women whose infections are triggered by sex, use can be limited to after sex to reduce the cumulative antibiotic exposure. Typically antibiotics are given for three to six months and then the need is reassessed. The antibiotics commonly used are trimethoprim, trimethoprim combined with sulfamethoxazole, nitrofurantoin, cephalexin, and fosfomycin.
- **METHENAMINE HIPPURATE:** An oral medication that is converted in urine to formaldehyde, which prevents bacteria from growing. It appears to be safe with few side effects.
- **D-MANNOSE:** A sugar that may inhibit how bacteria binds with bladder tissue. There is one well-done study that indicated 2 g of D-mannose a day was as effective as a daily antibiotic.

There are other interventions for recurrent UTIS that are often recommended but have little or no evidence to back their use:

- **CRANBERRY:** Most of the work here has been funded by—surprise—the cranberry industry. There is really no quality data supporting its effectiveness, which is somewhat surprising given how often it's recommended. A large review of the data available where cranberry products were compared with placebo found no benefit.

- **VITAMIN C:** The hypothesis is it acidifies the urine to the point that bacteria are unable to grow, but there isn't really any supporting data.
- **PROBIOTICS:** The idea with probiotics, which are beneficial bacteria, is to recolonize the vagina, either restoring defense mechanisms and/or replacing the bacteria that can cause UTIs. The data is very low quality and you may not always be getting what the label claims—in one study of probiotics in general 44 percent of products tested were incorrectly labeled, meaning they contained species not on the label or had missing ingredients. Probiotics are also typically very expensive, so it appears the money people are paying isn't always going into quality control.
- **WIPING:** Many women are told to be careful to wipe from front to back after going to the bathroom, but there is no evidence this practice is beneficial.
- **EMPTYING THE BLADDER RIGHT AFTER SEX:** Not supported by data. This one always surprises people!

Women who have recurrent UTIs may wish to have a consultation with an expert to ensure they are getting all the right preventative therapies and that other less common causes of recurrent infections have been considered.

Incontinence

Urinary incontinence is the involuntary leakage of urine, and although it affects women of all ages, the risk increases with age. Approximately 25 percent of young women, 50 percent of middle-aged women, and 75 percent of older women have urinary incontinence. Unfortunately, less than 50 percent of women who leak urine at least once a week seek care.

Stress Urinary Incontinence or SUI

This is the leakage of urine with activities that put more stress on the bladder. Normally when we cough, sneeze, or lift something heavy—any activity that increases the pressure in the abdomen—those forces are also transmitted equally to the bladder and the urethra. So while the additional stress or pressure on the bladder is trying to push more urine out, the urethra is also squeezing even tighter to keep it in, and the net result is no leakage. With SUI the forces that are transmitted to the bladder overwhelm the forces that help the urethra close, and leakage occurs.

The best way to think about SUI is to consider a garden hose pouring out water (our proxy for the urethra) laying on the ground (the supporting tissues). The normal mechanism for continence is a foot stomping on the urethra—the flow of urine is stopped. With SUI the supporting tissues are changed, so instead of a cement backstop think of a muddy, slippery ground. Now when the foot stomps on the hose, the hose may slip and slide, and the seal from the pressure of the foot is poor, so leakage occurs.

The reasons for SUI are varied. Genetics clearly plays a role in tissue strength and support. The loss of estrogen also affects the integrity of the tissues; however, taking systemic menopausal hormone therapy or MHT (meaning by mouth or transdermally, see chapter 17) is actually associated with an increased risk of SUI, so clearly the role of estrogen is complicated. Age negatively impacts collagen as well as muscle mass, including the muscles of the pelvic floor that surround and support the bladder and urethra. Tissue damage from birth is a factor and obesity also plays a role. Smoking is a risk factor for SUI as is constipation, as straining repetitively can injure the tissues.

Some women leak only while jumping on a trampoline or during weight lifting. This is because these activities put so much force on the bladder that the urethra doesn't really have a chance. Women who only leak in these situations may be helped by any of the therapies for SUI.

Women who think they have SUI should be evaluated for a bladder infection as that can cause incontinence. Once they get the all-clear, incorporating some basic strategies, such as being mindful of water intake (eight glasses of water a day is a myth) and working on exercises to strengthen the pelvic floor—often called Kegel exercises—are good places to start. Many women can learn to do these exercises on their own, but some may need help from a pelvic floor physical therapist.

Kegel exercises are sustained contractions (holding the squeeze or contraction in the pelvic floor muscles, working up to ten seconds) as well as quick flicks, a simple contraction and release that takes one to two seconds. With greater strength and control of their pelvic muscles women can also learn what is called the Knack maneuver, which is contracting their pelvic floor before and during a cough. A more detailed review of how to start a Kegel exercise practice can be found in *The Vagina Bible* and at the American Urogynecological Association at augs.org (click the Patient Services tab).

Timed voiding, which means urinating on a schedule, can also be helpful. The reasons this works are likely more complex than simply never getting to the point where the bladder is full. Voiding is a complex reflex that involves many behavioral factors, and cues and timed voiding may help strengthen other brain-bladder pathways. When pelvic floor exercises are combined with timed voiding, incontinence can improve significantly.

Even a small amount of weight loss can have a big impact on SUI—losing about 8 percent of body weight can reduce the number of incontinence episodes by 50 percent, and quitting smoking can also be helpful.

Interventions for SUI involve supporting the backstop that we discussed with our garden hose analogy. This can be accomplished with pessaries or vaginal incontinence devices, which are objects placed lengthwise in the vagina and provide support for the urethra. Some women find a tampon can be helpful, and there is also an over-the-counter tampon-like device called an Impressa. A medical provider can do a fitting for an incontinence ring, which has the advantage of being reusable and can be worn for longer periods of time than the tampon or Impressa. There is also an over-the-counter vaginal incontinence device called the Uresta and no physician visit is needed. Vaginal incontinence devices can be very helpful for SUI, and women are generally very satisfied with these options.

What about estrogen? We've already addressed how MHT can make stress incontinence worse—so women who choose to start MHT should be aware of this—but vaginal estrogen (see chapter 13) may help some women and the reasons aren't known. It's possible estrogen in low amounts in the urethra and vagina (as would be typical with MHT) could have one effect and the higher doses to the vaginal tissues and bladder achieved with vaginal hormones may have another effect.

Surgery can also be helpful for SUI. The most common procedure is called a midurethral sling and involves a strip of mesh placed beneath the urethra that provides the same kind of backstop as a pessary. There are other surgical options for SUI and a discussion is beyond the scope here.

Many women have heard concerning stories and reports about vaginal mesh, and so may be surprised to read an endorsement for a mesh procedure for SUI. Not all mesh is the same, an important factor that is consistently neglected when I read stories about mesh in the press. Lumping all mesh together is like lumping every motor vehicle together, from cars that have passed safety inspections and get high ratings from *Consumer Reports* to dune buggies with no air bags or seat belts. Yes they are both motor vehicles, but they are not the same thing.

A lot of issues with mesh are related to products that were inadequately tested and should never have come to market, and I am fortunate that the bladder specialists I have worked with for many years never considered using those products because the data was so poor. Because these mesh products were heavily advertised by pharmaceutical companies as being "easy"—traditional surgery for incontinence and prolapse (discussed later) requires additional training beyond residency—they were often used by surgeons who should never have been doing the surgery in the first place. I am not excusing these doctors, rather, trying to explain the difference between bad mesh and mesh that has been studied and found to be safe when used by trained surgeons.

Midurethral slings, the most common mesh surgery for SUI, is perhaps one of the most studied procedures in gynecology. The wealth of data here is impressive and is a testimony to those doctors who are committed to women's health. It has a high satisfaction and low complication rate. Like all surgery there are risks, and a good surgeon should run through them all so each woman can decide her personal risk-benefit ratio. Unfortunately many women with SUI don't learn enough about the surgery, so as soon as they hear "mesh" they just don't want to hear anymore.

Overactive Bladder

Overactive bladder is exactly how it sounds—the bladder is being triggered to empty at lower volumes than typical. With OAB the bladder is twitchy and contracts without receiving a signal that it is getting full and needs to empty. OAB isn't a menopause-specific condition; it's just a common condition.

Normally the volume for emptying is 180–240 ml (6–8 ounces), but with OAB the urge to go happens with lower volumes. For some women the urge may have triggers—such as heading to the bathroom or pulling down their clothes, but other times it can just happen. With OAB it may simply be the urge that is bothersome, meaning a woman is able to get to the bathroom in time, she just has to go a lot and it's uncomfortable and annoying. But the urge can also be so great that the bladder empties and she is incontinent of urine, and this may be a little or a lot. If women lose mobility, what was once OAB that didn't leak may end up becoming incontinence because they can't get to the bathroom in time.

Women who suspect they have OAB should complete a bladder diary, meaning recording everything they drink and urinate for at least twenty-four hours to monitor how often they go to the bathroom, the volume of urine when they do, and whether they leak and if it's a little or they are very wet. This is helpful for tracking progress as well as making sure a woman truly has OAB, as opposed to drinking so much fluid throughout the day that her multiple trips to the bathroom are her bladder working normally. It's also important to rule out a bladder infection.

The therapies for OAB supported by medical evidence include:

- **BLADDER TRAINING:** This is a mind over bladder technique as it is the brain that tells the bladder to relax so it can fill and tells the bladder to contract or empty. Bladder training means increasing the time between trips to the bathroom to train the brain-bladder connection to accept more urine before sounding the "I gotta go" alarm. It also incorporates techniques to control the urge, such as relaxation or distraction. Strengthening the connection between the brain and bladder is effective because most signals from the brain to the bladder are those that promote bladder relaxation. Bladder training outperforms medications for OAB in studies.
- **DIET:** Some foods can irritate the bladder contributing to spasm. Foods to limit or avoid include coffee, tea, sodas, artificial sweeteners, fruit juices, and alcohol.
- **REVIEWING MEDICATIONS:** Some women take diuretics or water pills, which increase the volume of urine. Sometimes it may be possible to switch this medication to one that doesn't increase the volume of urine.

- **PELVIC FLOOR PHYSICAL THERAPY:** Squeezing the pelvic floor sends a signal to the bladder to relax. This can help reduce OAB overall, and with training women can also learn a maneuver to help reduce the urge on command. Doing a set of five quick flicks—quickly contracting and releasing the pelvic muscles—as soon as the urge to empty strikes can relax the bladder and give time to get to the toilet without leaking.
- **MEDICATIONS:** These help reduce bladder contractions. There are a variety on the market. If one is ineffective or had intolerable side effects, another medication may be more effective or better tolerated. Common medications for OAB include oxybutynin, solifenacin, tolterodine, darifenacin, fesoterodine, and tropsium. In general, if a woman has tried and failed one medication for OAB, then she should see a specialist.
- **INJECTIONS:** Botulinum toxin A (Botox) injected into the bladder muscle is very effective.
- **SURGERY:** This involves implanting a device that stimulates a nerve that supplies the bladder. This is typically reserved for women who have failed several other options.

There are a variety of other therapies for OAB that are less well studied, such as energy devices and an acupuncture-like procedure known as peripheral-tibial nerve stimulation.

Caruncles

This is a condition where the loss of tissue support causes cells of the urethra to protrude and become irritated. A caruncle is a red lesion about 1 cm in size at the opening of the urethra, but given how hard it is to look at your own vulva, for some women who are using their phone as a virtual selfie stick a caruncle may look like a mass protruding from the vagina. They can look scary—angry is actually a good description—so much so that it can even resemble a cancer, but they are not cancerous.

A caruncle is related to loss of estrogen on the supporting tissue at the opening of the urethra and responds well to topical estrogen cream, either estradiol or CEE (combined equine estrogens).

Pelvic Organ Prolapse

Pelvic organ prolapse or POP is the descent or dropping of the vagina, uterus, bladder, or bowel or a combination of these. Visualizing POP can often be hard, so think of a sock on a hand—if part of the inside of the sock is grasped and pulled downward toward the opening that's a representation of POP.

Some POP is normal with age as sagging tissues are synonymous with aging collagen. The vagina is literally designed to stretch (a good thing when trying to deliver a baby), but that leaves it more vulnerable to the unique effects of aging on stretchy tissues. Mild POP is so common that 40 percent to 50 percent of women who have no symptoms will have it on exam, so it isn't whether a woman has POP that matters, rather it's whether she has bothersome symptoms that are due to her POP.

The most common symptom of POP is a bulge at the vaginal opening that may be felt with wiping or even sitting. Increased pressure or the feeling that something is falling out are also symptoms, and when POP is severe the part that has prolapsed may have descended so much it is outside of the vagina (think of a sock pulled halfway inside out). Other symptoms of POP are difficulties having a bowel movement, and occasionally POP can obstruct the flow of urine. POP doesn't cause pain with sex or pelvic pain.

POP isn't a menopause-specific condition. It's related to changes in collagen with age, genetic susceptibility, and any activity that can damage collagen in the tissues, such as smoking, chronic constipation, and childbirth.

Some women are distressed by their POP and others aren't at all. This is a very important point, because unless POP is obstructing the flow of urine or the prolapse is so severe that the tissues are hanging through the vagina and are getting ulcerated from exposure (they aren't meant to be external), no treatment is needed medically. POP typically is only treated if it bothers a woman. That is an important quality of life concern, but it's an important distinction—treating POP is a valid option, but not usually a medical necessity.

Many women can get significant improvement in their symptoms with pelvic floor muscle exercises (Kegel's as discussed) and a pessary—device that sits in the vagina to support the tissues and is like an incontinence ring on steroids. They do require a little more expertise to fit than an incontinence ring—a provider has to be knowledgeable about the range of pessaries as well as understand how each pessary may work given a woman's anatomy and the type and severity of her prolapse. Pessaries are highly effective for POP and have very high satisfaction rates. Even with advanced POP, a correctly fitted pessary will be successful for approximately two-thirds of women.

Surgery for POP is beyond the scope of this book. Women should be encouraged to try all the nonsurgical options first, and if those options fail or their prolapse is still bothersome, then surgery might be a viable remedy. Prolapse surgery is big surgery and recurrence rates are high— the core issue is weakness of the tissue, and surgery can't repair that problem. Prolapse surgery can sometimes cause pelvic pain or pain with sex; often this can be treated, but not always. Any woman considering surgery for POP should have an evaluation with a surgeon—either an OB/GYN or a urologist—who is board certified in urogynecology so they can weigh the risks for them versus the benefits.

BOTTOM LINE

- The risk of recurrent UTIs increases with both menopause and age and vaginal estrogen is an effective preventative strategy.
- Incontinence is common and it increases as women age, mostly due to age-related issues rather than the hormonal changes of menopause.
- Many women have their incontinence concerns dismissed and unfortunately go without treatment.
- SUI occurs when the urethra is unable to close and prevent leakage; there are many effective nonsurgical therapies, but there is also highly effective surgery.
- Overactive bladder is a twitchy brain-bladder connection and there are many effective treatments.

Chapter 15

Let's Talk About Sex:

The Complicated Story of Desire

DISCUSSING SEX IS COMPLICATED; WE are constantly bombarded with images that tell us our lives should be all about sex. Sex! And more sex! Anything less is abnormal. But studies show there is a big disconnect between what people say they want sex-wise (A Lot! More!) and the amount of sex most people are actually having (once a week, a little more for married people).

Why people who could be having more sex but don't (meaning those with partners) is complicated. Some people aren't good sexual communicators—a person shouldn't assume what their partner wants sex-wise just as they shouldn't assume what their partner might want for dinner. Others may feel societal pressure to say sex is what matters above all else, even on surveys. Being untruthful on surveys about intimate things happens, because admitting something to yourself can be hard. Also, many of us want more of the things we like, so when asked on a survey we may rank something higher than what is practically achievable in real life.

And finally there are mistaken ideas about sex. Many people erroneously think that having sex in a coupleship is one of those spontaneous things that happens without planning. And while passion, lust, and the thrill of someone new may be a more spontaneous driver of sex at the beginning of a relationship, the truth is a successful long-term sex life requires cultivation. Many people put more effort into organizing their after-school activities for their kids, cleaning their house, posting on social media, or grocery shopping than they do into their sex lives. No judgment. These are just all important facts to acknowledge. Sex has to be a higher priority for it to *be* a higher priority.

In addition, there is a pharmaceutical industry as well as many doctors who want women to think that their lack of being horny (a high spontaneous desire or sex drive) is a medical condition. What I mean by this is the normal sexual response of many women has been medicalized and turned into a disease and the only way to treat it is with medications. This skews the messaging that women receive because it is drugs for sex that make headlines, not the normal sexual response.

Several years ago a drug called flibanserin was introduced for hypoactive sexual desire disorder (HSDD, a condition that no longer exists and is probably best described as lack of spontaneous horniness), and it was heavily promoted by a group of Pharma funded sexual medicine physicians who called their campaign *Even the Score*. Men get all kinds of drugs for sex, this group claimed, but women are left out in the cold. And this was a crisis as 43 percent of women were suffering from lack of desire. A literal epidemic of desire disorders!

I remember first reading these numbers and being aghast. I know a lot of women, and I speak with women daily about sex and almost half of them weren't upset with their sexual relationship. In reality, the number of women with desire disorders was in the 7 percent to 10 percent range. Still significant, but a lot less headline grabbing. The other issue was Even the Score's facts. Women do have medications for sex that are equivalent to phosphodiesterase inhibitors (drugs like Viagra)—vaginal estrogen and DHEAS, transdermal and oral estrogens, and oral osphemine. Like phosphodiesterase inhibitors they increase blood to the genitals. Phosphodiesterase inhibitors improve the mechanical ability to have sex—like estrogen, DHEAS, and osphemine—not desire.

EVEN THE SCORE's mission to get flibanserin approved for women was covered fairly heavily by the media and they were involved with petitioning the Food and Drug Administration. Who was funding Even the Score? Yes, the company who made the drug.

This backstory is important, because sexual difficulties are common, but a difficulty doesn't make something dysfunctional or a disease. The reality of women's sexuality has been fictionalized to serve a patriarchal script and medicalized to support pharmaceutical industries. A medical model doesn't work well for desire because the reasons people engage in sex are complicated, numerous, individual, and influenced by multiple factors. Low sexual desire can't use a medical model, like appendicitis. After all, whether your partner is attentive to your appendix, whether you can talk with your partner about your appendix, and how your partner speaks with you, and whether your partner does their fair share around the house don't influence whether or not you get appendicitis.

Deconstructing Desire

Before we can discuss desire and how that might affect women in their menopause transition and beyond, we should have a clear idea of what we are discussing—like the Cheshire Cat says, *If you don't know where you are going, how will you know when you get there?*

Desire can mean actively wanting to engage in sexual activity or being receptive to engaging in physical activity. Meaning the lack of spontaneous desire is not a medical condition. The traditional model of sexual response starts with spontaneous desire, which leads to arousal and then orgasm. Like many things in life and in medicine, it was based primarily on the sexual responses of men. What we know now is this model doesn't apply to many women and it also doesn't work for all men. This is a good place to add that the patriarchy hurts men as well as women, because men who don't follow the *always thinking about sex and always ready* model are viewed as being lesser, when they are just following the sexual script that works for them.

Dr. Rosemary Basson introduced a new model in 2000 that suggests desire is far more complicated than a straight line from wanting to orgasm. Desire, it turns out, isn't always spontaneous and it isn't the only reason people engage in sex. Sex is multidimensional just like the people who have it. Spontaneous desire or libido may be a reason some people have sex, but people may also decide to engage in physical intimacy for reasons other than desire—for example, comfort, or satisfying their partner—and then once things get started desire kicks in. Desire often comes after arousal and it's important to normalize this arousal-then-desire experience.

Think of sex like a party and lack of spontaneous desire is sitting on the couch not thinking about a party at all. In fact, it's movie night in pajamas and a retainer. Your person says, "Hey, want to go to a party?" And you reply, "Meh."

But then your person reminds you how much fun you had at the last party. And it was true, you did. And they remind you how pretty you always look, not just at parties. And how much you say you won't dance, but always do. So you think, okay, I'll try the party for five minutes, but I'm not changing my clothes! You are willing.

Your person says, "Wonderful, you always look beautiful, so pajamas it is!" And off you head to the party. And yes, you hit the dance floor soon after you got there and had a great time. Afterward, you spent time cuddling and talking about the party and yes, you were glad that you went.

That's a model for responsive desire. Rather one model, because relationships are complex. But needing someone to stoke your fire isn't abnormal; that's the way it works for some women all the time and episodically for others.

Before this model was widely accepted, the standard desire disorder was called hypoactive sexual desire disorder or HSDD. It was discarded as it focused on spontaneous desire, medicalizing what is a normal experience for many women—responsive desire. It probably doesn't surprise you to learn that even though the diagnosis of HSDD has been abandoned as it over medicalized a normal experience, it is still used today in articles that promote medications for yes — HSDD.

The new term for a desire disorder is sexual interest/arousal disorder (SIAD) and a woman must experience three of the following for at least six months to meet the criteria:

- Reduced or absent desire for sex
- Reduced or absent sexual thoughts/fantasies
- Reduced or absent initiation *and r*eceptivity of sexual activity
- Reduced or absent sexual pleasure
- Reduced desire triggered by sexual triggers or stimulation
- Reduced or absent genital or nongenital sensations

In addition, a woman must be distressed by these symptoms—if only her partner is distressed it is not a diagnosis. And there must be no other cause for the symptoms, such as relationship distress, inadequate sexual technique, medication side effect, or pain with sex.

It's also important to note that desire is almost always higher at the beginning of a relationship and drops in about 50 percent of relationships that last three years or more. Yes, 50 percent and in just three years. With these kind of stats a drop in desire is often a natural consequence of long-term relationships. An important consideration is that the beginning of a relationship is typically when more people are putting in an effort to cultivate desire.

Menopause and Desire

The menopause transition is associated with a decline in desire. In one study 12 percent of women ages forty-five to sixty-four had desire disorders, and for women over the age of sixty-five that number was 7.4 percent greater. Interestingly, this is unrelated to hormone levels, meaning there are many women with lower levels of estrogen and testosterone with high levels of desire, and the reverse is also true. As such, hormone levels are not indicated in an evaluation of desire concerns.

Desire issues in menopause can be confused with sexual difficulties. What I mean by this is if sex is painful a reduction in desire is expected. This holds true for any cause of pain with sex, and there are many. Genitourinary syndrome of menopause (GUSM), a common cause of pain with sex is addressed in Chapter 13 and those wanting to learn more about other causes of pain with sex may wish to read *The Vagina Bible*, which has several chapters that address the subject. Women with incontinence may also have a reduced desire for sex if they fear leaking urine or stool during sex.

It's also important to consider medical conditions and medications that can affect desire. For example, if a woman is sleeping poorly or has depression, her desire to have sex may be affected. In addition, some medications can directly affect desire or they can lead to difficulties achieving orgasm, which is a problem in itself and may also in turn reduce desire. These medications include (but are not limited to) many antidepressants, spironolactone, beta blockers, trazodone (a sleep aid), and opioids. Oral MHT can theoretically affect desire as it produces more sex hormone binding globulin (remember, Seats Handy on the Bus, Girl?), so there is less active testosterone available. Even though testosterone levels don't predict libido, sometimes switching from oral to transdermal estrogen can be helpful. Admittedly the role of testosterone and desire is complicated because women with polycystic ovarian syndrome (PCOS) have higher levels of testosterone and yet they don't report an increase in desire, in fact they often report the opposite. When an antidepressant is believed to be the cause of low desire, switching to bupropion (Wellbutrin), an antidepressant that is less likely to have that side effect, or adding that medication to the other antidepressant (if safe depression-wise), are possibilities. Another option is a trial of the phosphodiesterase inhibitor, such as Viagra.

So when desire feels dead, the first step is to look at medications, medical conditions, life in general, and communication with your partner. Relationship problems, financial stress, or stress from work or other sources may also affect desire.

As women age it isn't uncommon to need more physical stimulation to become aroused and achieve orgasm. Remember, all of the wiring and parts age. Some women need glasses, some may need hearing aids, so a boost to get enough stimulation for arousal and orgasm can be normal for many women. The reason is unknown, but some possibilities include a reduced blood flow, decrease in clitoral size, loss of muscle mass in the levator ani (the muscles that physically contract during an orgasm), or general aging of the nervous system.

Consequently, some women find that whereas they were once able to achieve orgasm with masturbation, oral sex, or vaginal penetration now they can't. If sex is less physically satisfying that could impact desire. The first step is to pump up the sensory volume with a vibrator if one isn't being used (as long as there is no pain with sex, that should be investigated first). If women are already using a vibrator, investing in one that can deliver more stimulation or one that can stimulate other areas (for example vaginally or anally) may be helpful. For example, I regularly recommend that my patients visit a local sex shop, Good Vibrations. Their staff are incredibly helpful and know everything about all the vibrators on the shelf and are happy to help! They are docents of sexual pleasure. Many cities have similar shops and for those uncomfortable making an in-person visit, a conversation over the phone may be helpful to make the right choice with online shopping.

Another consideration is to work on strengthening the pelvic floor muscles; these are the muscles that physically contract during orgasm. For more on a pelvic floor practice, head back to chapter 14 or check out my book *The Vagina Bible.* In addition, a visit to a pelvic floor physical therapist for a formal assessment and treatment plan may also be helpful. Consider contracting the levator ani during foreplay to increase blood flow and stimulation.

Developing Desire

So how do people maintain desire? In one study researchers surveyed people who still had desire in a long-term relationship and compared them with those who did not. Sexual satisfaction and passion were higher among people who had sex more often, had more orgasms, received more oral sex, tried a variety of positions, worked on setting the mood, and who communicated about their sexual needs and desires. It's unlikely that different positions lead to magical sex endorphins; rather, many of these factors associated with maintaining desire seem to be related to having sexually curious conversations and being willing to try different things to pleasure your partner. Think of sex in a relationship as you would movie night. If you chose from a small repertoire of movies every movie night and never asked what kind of movie your partner liked, or if they said what they wanted to watch and you didn't listen, the idea of movie night might become stale over time.

Other work has shown that women who believe that sexual enjoyment will decrease with age are twice as likely to have a decrease in sexual desire than women who don't share that belief.

With that in mind, it may be an idea for women heading into their menopause transition to challenge any beliefs they may have about age being synonymous with the death of sex and, to think how they can be proactive in cultivating desire, and to work on communication about their relationship and sex before a problem develops.

Nonmedication Options for a Decrease in Desire

As communication is the cornerstone of a satisfying long-term sexual relationship, it's important for a woman to consider how she and her partner communicate as a couple as well as if her sexual needs—meaning what she wants—are being met. Because talking about sex seems harder than having it, a sex therapist, a psychologist, or a marriage and family therapist may be helpful. They can introduce both communication and sexual techniques, and also help people learn skills to tolerate distress in a relationship. There will be times when desire and sexual frequency ebb and flow in a relationship, and tolerating the lows is as important as celebrating the highs.

Consider cognitive behavioral therapy or CBT—the goal-oriented therapy we've discussed for hot flushes and insomnia, but it's also very effective for cultivating desire and is more effective than medications. Think of CBT as strengthening desire pathways in the brain. One of the world experts on the subject and a friend of mine, Dr. Lori Brotto, has written a fantastic book on desire and CBT, *Better Sex Through Mindfulness.* I strongly recommend this book for any woman who is struggling with a lack of desire or heading into her menopause transition so she has a robust skill set to prevent against the possibility of a menopause-related drop in desire. There are apps that claim to improve or enhance sex-life, but it's important to note that they haven't been studied and so we don't know if they truly have a meaningful effect. One of these apps is called Rosy, which includes information about many mindfulness techniques, facts about sex, and even access to sex therapists and other professionals.

Strategies that can help cultivate desire include:

- **FANTASIES:** For some people this may be watching erotica or porn, but for others it may be reading erotica. Another option is to get a good sexual fantasy book (e.g. *Garden of Desires*) and take turns reading it to each other. I personally like to create historical fan fiction with my partner and imagine us meeting at different points in our lives and what the sex might have been like. It's like revisiting the start of our relationship over and over again.
- **FOREPLAY:** Is important for good sex, especially for arousal. But foreplay starts when you wake up—it's not just the physical acts, but also how you are made to feel and are treated. Take time to

use more foreplay before sex starts, for example, sexts or notes left around the house. Once I was traveling and came back to my car in the airport parking garage to find my partner had tracked down my car and left a love note tucked under the windshield wiper. Knowing someone is thinking about you when you least expect it creates intimacy. Foreplay may mean different things for different people, hence why good communication matters. However, most studies tell us people would like more physical foreplay as part of sex.

- **AFTER PLAY:** Cuddling, kissing and pillow talk. If this is something you enjoy it may improve sexual satisfaction, which may in turn help with desire. If your partner doesn't do this, ask. You may be surprised.
- **SETTING TIME FOR INTIMACY:** Many people think they "shouldn't" have to do this, but that is simply the wrong attitude. This can be a date night or a romantic getaway. Even in the time of pandemic lockdown people can find ways. For example, my partner formally invited me to watch a classical piano concert via zoom. We got dressed as if we were going to the symphony and enjoyed cocktails and hors d'oeuvres.
- **MIX IT UP:** Try different positions and try more oral sex. I once had a partner tell me he had been reading *Cosmopolitan* at the gym and realized he was neglecting my mons, and the idea that he had read something and specifically considered how that might increase my sexual pleasure was a huge turn-on, as was the additional attention to my mons.

Who has the time for cognitive behavioral therapy (CBT) or to cultivate desire? Think about the time people spend grocery shopping, preparing a meal, getting their kids ready for school, or preparing for a presentation at work. We spend a lot of effort doing a lot of things. The more effort we put into it, the better that outcome. Many people don't realize that good sex is like any other task. The more effort you put in, the more likely you will see rewards. Talking about sex, what you like and don't like, and trying new things is the oxygen that keeps a sex life going. Some of these strategies we've discussed to increase desire—reading erotica or more foreplay or adding new positions—aren't taking hours out of the day.

Medications

Before embarking on medications for desire, women in the late menopause transition and those who are past menopause should consider a trial of medication for GUSM (chapter 13) as this will increase blood flow to the vagina, vulva, and clitoris and this may improve sexual pleasure, and people are more likely to desire sex when it feels good.

Women should also consider maximizing the non-medication options, what they can do regarding medications that may be affecting desire, explore CBT as well as fantasies and intimacy building, speak with a sex therapist or other relationship professional, and consider using a vibrator to improve blood flow and orgasms as well as strengthening the pelvic floor muscles. The studies with these medications tend to be lower quality and there may be some unresolved risks.

For women who find these options are ineffective and who do not have pain with sex, medications can be considered. It is important to remember, however, that in most studies for medications for desire, women are already having two or three sexually satisfying episodes of sex each month, and so the women in these studies reflect a very narrow group of women with desire disorders. In addition, these medications are typically tested for HSDD, meaning a lack of spontaneous desire, and not how we now think about desire disorders. How these medications work for women who are having sex a few times a year or for women who have an issue with receptive desire—if they even work for these women at all— isn't known.

Bupropion

The antidepressant known as Wellbutrin is not approved for desire disorders, but it does share many properties with a drug that is approved (flibanserin, see below), has extensive safety data with a known risk profile, and a generic is available. Bupropion can be effective in helping women who have low desire caused by other antidepressants. In addition, one study indicated that 300 mg a day increased sexual pleasure and arousal.

As bupropion is a well-known medication with no unresolved cancer issues, it may be a good first start medication for women with desire concerns even though this is an off label indication. It may not be an option for some women with depression or for those taking other medications for mood.

Testosterone

Testosterone levels slowly decline with age. Testosterone is not approved for low sex drive, but there are enough studies to give some advice about its use. There is not enough data to recommend testosterone for desire disorders before the final menstrual period, but it may help some women who are postmenopausal.

All of the data on testosterone is short term, and there are unresolved issues with heart disease, uterine cancer, and breast cancer—in one study over twenty-four weeks there were three new cases of breast cancer in the women who took testosterone versus none in the placebo group. Safety concerns with testosterone could be from the testosterone itself or because testosterone is metabolized to estradiol, or the studies we have may not accurately reflect concern—either overestimate or underestimate. This is very important for women to understand, because when we want a medication to work it is human nature to think those risks won't happen to us, but that should not be the assumption. Unknown means we don't really know how often these concerns could happen, we just know concerns have been raised and the medications are insufficiently studied to answer the safety questions.

The other issue with testosterone is that there are no commercial products specifically formulated with the low doses needed for women. Consequently, women must use compounded products or low doses of products made for men, and so there is a risk of receiving too much testosterone—leading to side effects such as a deepening of the voice (permanent), unwanted hair growth on the face and elsewhere, acne, enlargement of the clitoris, and a negative impact on lipids.

At most it seems testosterone in a dose of 300 mcg/day may increase the number of sexually satisfying events by one or two per four weeks versus placebo (these studies used a patch). Another study, however, looked at a testosterone gel and found no change versus placebo.

Testosterone pellets should not be used; the dosing is too high and they cannot be removed, and there are reports of harm with these products (see chapter 20).

For women who very much want to explore testosterone when other treatments have been ineffective, options include the following:

- **COMPOUNDED 1 PERCENT TESTOSTERONE CREAM, OINTMENT, OR GEL:** This includes all the inherent dosing issues with compounded products, see chapter 20. The dose is 0.5 g per day applied to the arms, legs, or abdomen.
- **A TOPICAL PRODUCT DESIGNED FOR MEN AT 10 PERCENT OF THE DOSE:** This can be challenging as the metered dosing and packets are not designed for dividing the dose this way.

Women who decide that testosterone is right for them should have normal lipids and blood pressure before starting, and this should be monitored during therapy. They should know that there is no good data to guide risks and benefits after twelve months of use, so whether risks accumulate with duration isn't known. Women on testosterone should have their free testosterone level and or free androgen index monitored after starting and while on therapy with the goal of keeping the levels in the normal range for women. If there is no improvement after 12–24 weeks the testosterone should be stopped.

Flibanserin

This is sold under the name Addyi; it acts on the brain in a way similar to many antidepressants—on the neurotransmitters dopamine, serotonin, and norepinephrine. It is only approved for use for women before menopause (how well it may help women after their final menstrual period—if it does at all—isn't known).

Compared with placebo, flibanserin has a small effect on desire. In studies 100 mg a day of flibanserin appears to lead to 0.4–1 additional episode of satisfying sex per four weeks and it takes at least four weeks to start to work (but more likely after 8 weeks of daily use). Dizziness, fatigue, and nausea are common side effects—about 18 percent of women stop flibanserin due to side effects. Flibanserin can also lower blood pressure and women should not have alcohol for 2 hours before taking a dose and should not have alcohol again until the next day.

Bremelanotide

The trade name is Vylessi. It likely works in the brain, but the true mechanism of action is unknown. Bremelanotide is given by injection at least forty-five minutes prior to anticipated sex and alcohol must be avoided for two hours before and two hours after using the medication. Side effects are common: 40 percent of women have nausea—in one study 13 percent of women taking the drug requested a medication for nausea (not especially sexy). Other side effects were fairly common, and 18 percent of women elected to stop the drug during one study versus 2 percent of women taking the placebo. Women with cardiovascular disease should not use bremelanotide.

Okay, so how well does it work? At best it's only mildly more effective than a placebo. In the two studies used to get approval by the Food and Drug Administration, the drug company used a standard scoring system for desire that involves two questions:

> Over the past four weeks, how often did you feel sexual desire or interest?
> Over the past four weeks, how would you rate your level (degree) of sexual desire or interest?

It's important to note this is only measuring spontaneous desire, so not the ideal questions to ask. The answers to both questions are scores from almost never or never (1 point) to almost always or always (5 points). So the lowest score possible is 2 and the highest is 10.

Bremelanotide increased desire on that scale by an average of 1.2 points for 25 percent of women who received the drug versus 17 percent who took a placebo. To me that is underwhelming. These two studies also surveyed how distressed women were with their low spontaneous desire. At baseline they had equal distress scores; bremelanotide reduced distress by 1 point or more on a 10 point scale for 35 percent of women and the same decrease was seen by 31 percent of women using placebo. So it seems that doing something that feels constructive for low sex drive—taking a medication—makes some women feel less distressed. This study was just for premenopausal women, so we have no idea how this medication would perform for women who are in postmenopause.

Whether bremelanotide has a meaningful impact on one's life can't be answered with the data available, but it seems minimally effective for a decrease in spontaneous desire, which is no longer considered a medical condition. The cost is currently approximately $250 a dose for people paying cash.

Imagine the impact of spending $250 on erotica or a fancy dinner or a new vibrator. Or all three?

Scream Cream

This is a topical preparation made by compounding pharmacists. It is completely untested (honestly, women deserve so much better than these untested products). It also is a hodgepodge of ingredients depending on who writes the prescription or what pharmacy is used. This *cough* product has been around for years in one formulation or another and includes a variety of ingredients that are supposed to improve blood flow. None of which has been evaluated for this method of delivery—rubbing into the clitoris. This is a very important point. The instructions for *Scream Cream* state to rub it into the clitoris for fifteen minutes.

I mean come on (or rather, cum on). Rubbing the clitoris for fifteen minutes is masturbation and that has shown to be very effective in improving desire and arousal. Rubbing coconut oil or a silicone lube on the clitoris will almost certainly produce the same results.

The ingredients that are supposed to increase blood flow to the clitoris or perform some other kind of sex magic include some or all of the following:

- **AMINOPHYLLINE:** A medication for asthma that dilates the airways
- **L-ARGININE:** An amino acid that is found in many protein-rich foods
- **SILDENAFIL-CITRATE:** Viagra
- **PENTOXIFYLLINE:** A medication used to increased blood flow for people who have peripheral artery disease
- **TESTOSTERONE:** Topical testosterone can be absorbed as we have previously discussed, but the impact is not immediate. One

does not apply testosterone and then magically fifteen minutes later it is rutting season.

Sometimes I wonder if this drug gets prescribed because providers are uncomfortable or don't know how to discuss masturbation?

What I want to say about Scream Cream is this isn't how it works. Any of it. Medications, sex, and science. Giving women unstudied topical medications with false promises is abysmal and the name "scream cream" sounds like locker room talk. "I'm gonna make her scream and moan."

Definitely do rub your clitoral glans and lots of other parts, but until Scream Cream is tested against placebo I'd personally give it a pass. We also have no idea if these medications can irritate the vulva when used topically.

A final note about medications: they all involve planning and more attention to sex, so they are incorporating a mindfulness component.

BOTTOM LINE

- Desire is complicated and is related to many factors, including social, relationship, and health.
- Desire decreases with age and also decreases for some women due to the menopause transition.
- Levels of estrogen and testosterone do not correlate with desire and testing is not indicated.
- Cognitive behavioral therapy, as well as mindfulness, and learning to cultivate desire—with communication skills, apps, books, erotica, foreplay, and after play—are important strategies for low desire.
- Medications for desire are at best moderately effective and many have side effects, but they may be an option for women who have found other choices ineffective and who understand the potential risk-to-benefit ratio with these therapies.

Chapter 16

Will I Ever Feel Rested Again?

Sleep Disturbances and How to Tackle Them

As many as 40 percent to 60 percent of women report difficulties with sleep during their menopause continuum, and the most common disturbance is waking up during the night, meaning women have trouble staying asleep. Though some women may report trouble falling asleep and others wake up earlier than desired, these sleep disturbances are less common. Many women also report they feel unrested with the sleep they are getting. Sleep disturbances increase during the menopause transition and peak during the last few years before the final menstrual period (FMP) and the first year or so after.

Insomnia is a description of difficulty sleeping, but it's also a disorder that involves difficulties falling asleep and staying asleep despite the opportunity to have a full night's sleep three or more times a week. Insomnia, the disorder, affects approximately 25 percent of women in their late menopause transition/early postmenopause. This isn't just important because such disordered sleep causes distress; insomnia is also associated with poor health outcomes, such as increased risk of heart disease and lung depression. Interestingly hot flushes, insomnia, and cardiac disease are all linked. It's unknown if there is cause and effect here or an underlying shared biological vulnerability.

It's not surprising that there is a link between menopause and poor sleep. Areas of the brain that are influenced by estrogen and progesterone are also important in sleep regulation, and fluctuations in hormones during the menstrual cycle are known to affect sleep patterns. Estrogen and progesterone and possibly other reproductive hormones appear to influence circadian rhythms—our natural sleep-wake cycles—by influencing part of the brain called the suprachiasmatic nuclei, which is thought of as the sleep pacemaker. The hormone progesterone also has a mildly sedative effect.

In addition to these hormonal effects, there are vasomotor symptoms (hot flushes and night sweats) and depression—both of which are menopause-related and can affect sleep. And at the same time as a woman is going through her menopause transition she is also aging, and age negatively affects sleep. Finally, as women age they are more likely to develop sleep apnea and other medical conditions that impact sleep.

There is clearly a hormonal component as the women who report the most sleep disturbances are those who have their ovaries removed before menopause (surgical menopause), but how much is hormones and how much is everything else can sometimes be difficult to determine.

Hot Flushes, Hormones, and Sleep

During the late menopause transition and early postmenopause are when women report the greatest impact on sleep. Medically what is happening is best described as an excessive arousal, meaning the sleep is just not as deep as it should be, and much of this may be due to hot flushes. In other words, for some women hot flushes are enough to disturb how deep they sleep but not enough to wake them up. My partner and I have definitely experienced this phenomenon. There have been nights where I have given off so much heat from my hot flushes that it woke my partner from sleep yet did not wake me.

Sleep disturbance can also happen when hot flushes/night sweats wake women from their sleep—in one study, up to 69 percent of the hot flushes at night resulted in the woman waking up. It isn't surprising that this is more likely to occur for women who have more vasomotor symptoms during the day. Interestingly, women with higher levels of follicle stimulating hormone are more likely to wake at night, and women with lower levels of estradiol are more likely to have difficulties falling asleep.

While insomnia affects many women in their late menopause transition/early postmenopause, that doesn't mean that all insomnia is caused by menopause. Insomnia can be its own independent condition, related to age, or linked to such medical conditions as depression. But untangling cause and effect is challenging because depression can affect sleep and lack of sleep can affect depression and the menopause transition can affect both. What we do know is that women who report sleep disturbances during menopause should always be screened for depression.

Sleep Hygiene and Cognitive Behavioral Therapy

These are the modifications to set you up for optimal sleep and to condition your brain and body to sleep at the appropriate time. We've addressed cognitive behavioral therapy or CBT before, and when it's specifically designed to treat insomnia it is known as CBT-I. It involves challenging cognitive distortions—meaning the fear that you might never get back to sleep or that insomnia will never go away, scheduling sleep to train the body, and specific responses to waking.

CBT-I is one of the most effective therapies for sleep disturbances and has been evaluated for women in the menopausal transition, and an eight-week program was not only effective, but the benefits were still maintained at six months.

A psychologist or other therapist with training in this area can be very helpful. If these things were easy to do on their own everyone would be doing them. CBT-I is more effective than sleeping pills (hypnotic medications), which typically only give about thirty minutes of additional sleep a night, meaning they are less effective than most people think. Some basic, introductory components of CBT-I include:

- **MAKE A SLEEP SCHEDULE:** Wake at the same time each day regardless of plans and have a set bedtime.
- **ELIMINATE DAYTIME NAPS:** It's hard, but it helps.
- **LIMIT ANXIETY-PROVOKING OR STIMULATING ACTIVITIES BEFORE BED:** This typically means no screen time; it can be the light from the

screen itself that has an impact, but also a bad email before bed may live rent-free in your head all night.

- **ESTABLISH THAT BED IS FOR SLEEP AND SEX:** No TV or snacking in bed; you want your brain to only think of your bed for two reasons.
- **WHEN YOU WAKE AND CAN'T GET BACK TO SLEEP:** Don't check the clock; lay in bed until it seems as though fifteen minutes have passed. If you get to what feels like fifteen minutes, get up and go to a dimly lit room and read a boring book. Once you feel sleepy head back to bed. This helps to limit the anxiety from tossing and turning in bed worrying that you will never get back to sleep, and also helps with not associating your bed with poor sleep.

Does Menopausal Hormone Therapy (MHT) Help Sleep?

Overall, women who take MHT are no less likely to report sleep issues than women who aren't, but that may not be the best way to look at the issue. Some studies that have followed women with sleep disturbances have concluded that MHT may bring a modest improvement in sleep when vasomotor symptoms are a problem. So for a woman who is experiencing vasomotor symptoms, it may be worth giving MHT a try to see if it helps sleep, especially given how low risk three months of MHT is medically speaking (see chapters 17 and 18). Women who decide they want to try MHT to see if that improves their sleep may wish to keep a sleep diary before starting. Doing so will give them an objective measurement of what is happening and then they can re-evaluate their sleep with the diary after two or three months. Women who are not bothered by hot flushes can also consider a trial of MHT, although there is less data on effectiveness.

Another option for hot flush–related sleep disturbances is the medication gabapentin (see chapter 9). This is a nonhormonal medication that can significantly help hot flushes and has also been shown to reduce insomnia. There is also the hormone progesterone. When taken in a dose of 300 mg at night it can help with sleep (see chapter 18). While progesterone is a hormone in MHT, this is a sleep specific dose and higher dose than typically used for MHT.

If a woman is struggling with sleep it's also important that she knows there are specialty sleep clinics that can do more formal testing and make precision recommendations after considering all the factors—medical and environmental—that could be impacting sleep.

Other Sleep Disorders and Menopause

Sleep apnea, known medically as sleep disordered breathing or SDB, is airway obstruction at night that results in daytime sleepiness. Before menopause, sleep apnea is more common among men, but after menopause the risk for women increases significantly. The main reasons are believed to be the drop in the production of progesterone and the increase in visceral fat seen in the menopause transition. Risk factors for sleep apnea include high blood pressure and and an increased waist circumference >88 cm (55 inches).

As many people erroneously think of men with sleep apnea, women often go undiagnosed and undertreated. Women with sleep apnea are more likely to experience other medical complications, for example, heart disease, lung problems, and depression, so diagnosis and treatment are essential.

Sleep apnea should be considered for women with daytime sleepiness who are snoring at night or whose partners tell them that they sometimes wake up and appear to be choking. Another symptom of sleep apnea is having to wake up a lot to go to the bathroom at night to empty your bladder. This is because the changes in oxygen and carbon dioxide levels with sleep apnea trigger signals that tell your body that you are overloaded on fluid when you are not. The kidneys are then stimulated to get rid of fluid and that means a greater need to get up and go to the bathroom at night.

When there is any suggestion of sleep apnea there are some simple screening questionnaires to complete, and if they are positive more formal testing can be arranged. The initial tests for sleep apnea no longer require a visit to a lab and are done with devices that are worn at home. Restless leg syndrome (RLS) and periodic limb movement disorder (PLMD) are two other conditions that disturb sleep, but they do not appear to be menopause-specific but rather are age-related. Treatment for sleep apnea, RLA, and PLMD are beyond the scope of this book.

BOTTOM LINE

- Approximately 50 percent of women report sleep disturbances during menopause; the most common is waking during the night, and this seems to be related to vasomotor symptoms.
- MHT may help women with sleep who are experiencing moderate or severe hot flushes.
- Gabapentin and the hormone progesterone can also help with sleep disturbances.
- Cognitive behavioral therapy is very effective for insomnia and is generally more effective than sleeping pills.
- Sleep apnea is a cause of sleep disturbance that is often under-diagnosed in women and increases in prevalence after menopause.

Part 3

Therapy for the Change:

Hormones, Diets, and Supplements

Chapter 17

Menopausal Hormone Therapy:

The Messy History and Where We Are Today

MENOPAUSAL HORMONE THERAPY OR MHT is the use of hormones to manage symptoms and/or prevent certain health complications related to the menopause transition and/or postmenopause.

MHT was called hormone replacement therapy or HRT for years, but that name falsely implies that estrogen or other hormones are missing because of a medical problem, and the low levels of estrogen after menopause are biologically abnormal. Some may argue that the increased risk of cardiovascular disease after menopause suggests it's a disease, but they're going to lose that argument. As discussed previously if you follow that logic to its conclusion, then being a man is a disease.

The messaging matters. "We're just replacing what your body should be making," is very different from the more accurate, "You have symptoms and may be at risk for several health conditions. The hormone estrogen may be one option. Let's review your concerns, what you should know about your health, and then discuss the risks and the benefits as they apply to you."

It's fair to use the term "replacement" for women with primary ovarian insufficiency (see chapter 6) or for those women who have their ovaries surgically removed before natural menopause (see chapter 5) as estrogen production has stopped prematurely, but otherwise MHT should be discussed for what it is—a medical intervention, not a replacement.

The Origins of MHT

The first documented use of MHT was in 1887 when Dr. Hubert Fosbery used an ovarian extract to treat Mrs. C, a fifty-two-year-old woman with hot flushes. Mrs. C had been subjected to all manner of awful nineteenth-century remedies for heavy periods, such as arsenic, ergot, ground thyroid gland, potassium bromide, and twice daily plugging of her vagina alternating with iced douches. When her periods finally stopped, she had "frequent and violent flushing." When standard therapies failed, an ovarian extract was administered and by the third day she was feeling better. Three weeks later she was cured, requiring only occasional doses thereafter to keep her symptoms at bay.

The hypothesis of an ovarian extract for hot flushes was based on sound evidence. Removing the ovaries was known to cause symptoms of menopause, and animal studies had shown the effects of castration could be reversed by transplanting ovaries from another animal. However, interpreting Mrs. C's results as anything more than placebo isn't possible. Resolving hot flushes in three weeks is impressive, although not impossible. Considering she was treated orally, the amount absorbed would likely have been negligible as pharmaceutical modifications are typically needed to improve absorption and achieve therapeutic levels in the blood. Oral estrogens also needs to be given daily to maintain levels; so Mrs. C dosing herself every few weeks seems unlikely to be successful even if any estrogen were absorbed. It's also worth noting that her violent flushing could have been a side effect of the therapies used to try to stop her bleeding, either the ergotamine, the thyroid hormone in the gland, or arsenic poisoning or possibly a combination of all three.

Regardless, the idea of treating menopausal symptoms with ovarian extract was introduced to the medical world, and by 1899 formulations for powdered cow ovary, called Ovarin, were commonly available. Most often the powder was placed into capsules or flavored with vanilla; apparently the taste of cow ovaries was unpleasant.

The first hormone was identified in the early 1900s, and then the search was on to identify reproductive hormones. Researchers began injecting extracts of ovary, placenta, and amniotic fluid into castrated rats and mice to look for an effect on tissues, thereby proving that these extracts had hormones. Although reproductive hormones had yet to be identified, that they likely existed let to a variety of different therapies and by the 1920s various extracts were used for symptoms of menopause: an extract from the corpus luteum in the ovary (what we know today produces progesterone—it proved to be ineffective); amniotin, made from the amniotic fluid from fetal cattle; and theelin, an extract from the follicular fluid from hog ovaries. Amniotin and theelin were apparently moderately successful.

Estrogen Therapy: The First Wave of MHT

In 1929 a significant leap forward occurred when estrone was identified simultaneously by Dr. Edward Doisy in the United States and Dr. Alfred Butenandt in Germany. Dr. Doisy believed this hormone so potent that "one gram could restore the sex cycle in more than 9 million rats." I'll just let that statement speak for itself. Dr. Doisy and his team also discovered what we now know as estriol in 1931, and estradiol in 1940. Dr. Butenandt isolated progesterone in 1934 and later identified testosterone. Given the equipment of the day, the work identifying and purifying these hormones was an amazing achievement.

Preparations of estrone and estradiol soon appeared in the 1930s to treat symptoms of menopause, such as hot flushes, headaches, sweats, joint pain, insomnia, and "nervousness." These medications didn't have the uniformity or stability of modern pharmaceuticals. The estrogens were suspended in oil and administered as injections and likely would have produced large swings in hormones.

It's fascinating to read the medical research using these early formulations. I'm struck by the moments of distress and suffering captured in the many articles on menopause in medical journals from the 1920s and 1930s—before the estrogen industry took off. Instead of the deidentified tables and charts of the articles of today there were snippets of lives. Such as: "H.L., aged 31, married, artificial menopause November, 1925 (intrauterine and vaginal radium for endometriosis) who has hot flushes every 5 minutes" as well as "headaches, and backaches who was admitted to hospital in 1929 and studied and finally discharged, with no diagnosis being made," who finally found her way to a menopause clinic for treatment in 1932. Or A.S. who was fifty, and married and having twenty to thirty hot flushes a day.

Another issue with this first wave of therapeutic hormones was availability of the raw product and the effort it took to isolate the estrogens. There was still no way to synthesize hormones, meaning making them in a lab, so they were extracted from the urine of pregnant women (high levels of estrogens spill into the urine during pregnancy) or from animals. These estrogens were natural chemicals, meaning they were obtained by extraction from a natural source, remaining unchanged by the process. Think boiling salt water for the salt. The salt was always there; boiling removed the water and didn't alter the salt.

Extracting natural estradiol and estrone from urine, amniotic fluid, and hog ovaries was, as one might expect, time consuming, expensive (about $300 a gram at the time), and large volumes of raw product were required for a small amount of usable material. So much urine was needed that one of Dr. Doisy's assistants was transporting jugs of urine from a prenatal clinic to their lab when he was stopped by the police. This was during prohibition and the volume and color of the liquid in the containers made the police suspect he was a bootlegger. I imagine the officer was quite surprised when he smelled the contents of the containers.

In the late 1930s and early 1940s several discoveries were made that greatly advanced the ability to mass-produce hormones. Estrogens were isolated from horse urine, known chemically as conjugated equine estrogens or CEE, becoming the drug Premarin, *pregnant mares urine*. Urine from pregnant mares is easier to source than urine from pregnant women. CEE contains at least ten different estrogens. Premarin was approved for use for menopausal symptoms in 1941 in Canada and in 1942 in the United States. CEE are the only natural estrogen—meaning extracted from nature—available today.

At the same time, new methods for synthesizing hormones in the lab were also discovered. There's often confusion about the word "synthetic"—not only is it often used incorrectly but it's become a derogatory term regarding hormones. As the misuse of this term features heavily in the marketing of certain forms of MHT, it's worth investing some time to get the language right.

Synthetic chemicals are made by humans using methods different from nature. When the starting compound for a hormone is found in plants or animals and then altered through chemical steps, the process is known as semi-synthesis; when the starting compound is smaller molecules not typically found in nature, the resulting compound is made by synthesis. Synthetic has nothing to do with the end product being identical to a human hormone or not. Admittedly the language is confusing as synthetic means made by either semi-synthesis or synthesis.

The chemical structure is what matters because that is how a hormone works, so whether estradiol is extracted from urine, made by semi-synthesis or synthesis, the chemical structure is the same. Going back to our key and lock analogy for hormones, natural, semi-synthetic, and synthetic estradiol are all the same key. The method of production also has nothing to do with safety. After all, estradiol made by the ovaries—the most natural of all—is a cause of breast and endometrial cancer. When there is a need to distinguish between an estradiol made by the body and that made by semi-synthetic methods, it's best to use human estradiol and therapeutic (or prescription) estradiol, respectively.

In 1938 two novel synthetic estrogens were identified—ethinyl estradiol (still used today in MHT and the most common estrogen in oral contraceptive pills) and diethylstilbestrol or DES. Both of these estrogens were more potent than estradiol and easily absorbed from the intestine. In 1941 DES became the first medication approved by the FDA to treat symptoms of menopause, although its use was often hampered by the side effects—nausea and vomiting. Ethinyl estradiol was approved for this use in 1943. The production costs with DES were especially low compared with extracting natural estrogens, about $2 versus $300 a gram. The research was funded by the UK government, so any company was free to produce it. At one point DES was available under two hundred different brand names.

DES was also widely prescribed to prevent miscarriages, despite the fact that Dr. Dobbs, the lead researcher on the team, advised against it. Not only would DES prove ineffective for preventing miscarriages, it caused cancers of the reproductive tract and birth defects for the women whose mothers took it during pregnancy. Even though research proved that DES was ineffective for miscarriage in the 1950s, the FDA didn't caution against its use until 1971 and it was still prescribed in the United States until the early 1980s. The tragedy of DES isn't an indictment of synthetic hormones or novel compounds; rather, it highlights the problems of rushing a product to market without testing and oversight as well as issues regarding off label use with no supporting data.

Today, all medications approved by the FDA are required to have appropriate studies for approval as well as postmarketing surveillance—meaning studies that follow people who are taking the medication to observe for side effects or complications missed in the original studies. With each new product that comes to market we must always ask ourselves: Is this the next DES?

A different method of making hormones was also invented in 1938 (a big year in hormone discoveries) by a chemist named Dr. Russell E. Marker, who devised a way to make progesterone from a plant steroid called sarasapogenin (found in sarsaparilla), with a process that now bears his name—the Marker Degradation. This is considered semi-synthesis because the starting compound is found in nature. Sarasapogenin didn't prove to be an economical option, so Dr. Marker began a quest for a different steroid, eventually finding it in a yam from Veracruz, Mexico, called *Dioscorea mexicana* that contained diosgenin. Eventually, another yam called *barbasco*, which contained even more diosgenin, became the source and by the mid to late 1940s there was large-scale production of progesterone. In 1950 the ability to make estradiol and estrone from diosgenin was discovered. Today, yams and soybeans are used as the source or the raw material that will be converted into most hormones.

The 1950s and 1960s:
The Glamorous Age of MHT

By 1947 there were fifty-three different formulations of estrogen on the market in the United States, and, as expected, the use of MHT increased. Many women suffer from symptoms, so the emergence of treatment that worked and didn't require injections of fluid from hog ovaries likely had appeal. However, there was also a shift in medical attitudes toward MHT, likely driven in large part by pharmaceutical advertising that switched from ads that targeted doctors to those aimed at women and their husbands. Through these advertisements MHT was linked with glamour, sophistication, and youth. And for men, well "Husbands, too, like Premarin." Premarin was significantly more expensive that its counterparts, so the move was advertising brilliance.

Pre-1950s menopause was something to be managed, but once there were reliable pills instead of painful and dodgy injections, menopause was something to be cured. This shift in attitude was achieved with significant help from Dr. Robert Wilson, a medical doctor who wrote a series of academic articles extolling the benefits of MHT in the early 1960s. His thesis revolved around the false belief that menopause was a disease that only existed because women were finally able to live long enough to have it (a hypothesis we dispatched in chapter 4) and that menopause was particularly horrific as not only was it bad for women medically speaking, it was also a desexed state, so it made women undesirable to men. A double horror. The cure was estrogen, which Dr. Wilson claimed was 100 percent safe. Estrogen, from puberty to grave!

Wilson's work was picked up by a variety of publications, including *Newsweek, Time, Vogue, Ladies' Home Journal,* and *Cosmopolitan.* Public discussions about menopause were likely nonexistent before Wilson, so whatever he called it—and he chose menopause—was going to stick. Wilson quickly translated his menopause moment into a book, *Feminine Forever,* that was published in 1966. It was serialized in *Vogue* and sold one hundred thousand copies in the first seven months. According to Wilson, with menopause women were "condemned to witness the death of their own womanhood," but with estrogen they could have an "age defying youthfulness" and at fifty "still look attractive in tennis shorts or sleeveless dresses, and of course regain 'supple breasts.'" So yes, estrogen was a ticket to the hot enough World Championships. Step right up!

Despite the fact that in Dr. Wilson's hands the experience of being a woman was distilled into sexual currency, *Feminine Forever* advanced some forward-thinking ideas for the time on sex, such as women shouldn't be ashamed to be sexual and the desire to take medication to continue having sex was valid. It's likely Dr. Wilson did create a space for more women to have conversations about sex.

In a 2002 interview, Wilson's son, Ronald Wilson, told the *New York Times* that Wyeth-Ayerst financed Dr. Wilson's research as well as the promotion of *Feminine Forever.* I'll always wonder if Wilson's jump from medical journals to *Newsweek* and *Vogue* was courtesy of an assist by Big Pharma. It wouldn't have taken much on their part to get the first journalist interested and create buzz. After all, that's why publicity departments exist. Whether the pharmaceutical industry adopted Wilson's ideas or he was translating pharmaceutical talking points isn't known. Ever heard the phrase, "By the time you're thirsty you're already dehydrated" or "Drink to stay ahead of your thirst"? These untruths are derivatives of marketing created by the Gatorade Sports Science Institute (GSSI). The ultimate goal in marketing is for the message to become so-called common knowledge. Catchy science-ish phrases require constant vigilance, because they are most often hype that originated in a marketing department, not health.

Wilson's incorrect theories of menopause being a disease and estrogen the cure clearly struck a cord with the medical community and the public, and it was quickly accepted as canon.

The Forgotten Uterus

The role of progesterone in protecting the lining of the uterus from cancer wasn't well understood before the 1970s. Even if doctors had known about the importance of progesterone, they were limited to injections pre-1957 because the technology to allow for absorption of progesterone from the intestine (oral) or across the skin (transdermal) was still unknown. Injections also didn't fit well with the modern glamorous, portable lifestyle branding of estrogen pills.

Emerging technology allowed manipulation of chemical structures, producing a new class of hormones called progestins that worked like progesterone on tissues, but chemically looked more like testosterone. Progestins are in a class of drugs call progestogens. Yes, the language is a bit of a mouthful. Progestogen and progesterone and progestin, oh my! Think of progestogen as an all-girl rock band featuring progesterone (the hormone made by the body) and the progestins.

Progestins were added to MHT in the 1960s to control the bleeding produced by MHT, thereby making it more palatable to women. (Estrogen causes the endometrium to build up and without a progestogen to offer support, this uterine lining will eventually become unstable and break off irregularly producing unpredictable bleeding.) A regular period induced by a progestin also fit with the "natural" marketing of MHT—the idea the hormones were replacing what a woman was *supposed to* have. This is a great example of how the word "natural" can be absurd because the least natural thing is for a woman in menopause to have a menstrual period. In *Feminine Forever,* Dr. Wilson wrote that a period was a "token of femininity."

Yes, a menstrual period was a curse until menopause—when it becomes a blessing and a sign of being desirable to men. This constant moving of the goal posts is enraging. A woman's body can simply never be just right.

In the 1970s a jump in the rate of endometrial cancers was identified and eventually the failure to include a progestogen or a sufficient amount of progestogen was identified as the cause. Remember back to chapter 3, estrogen stimulates the lining of the uterus (endometrium) and progesterone curtails that process. Over time without a progestogen that unchecked estrogen-fueled growth results in cancer. Progestogens in the right doses were added to MHT regimens in the 1970s, removing the risk of endometrial cancer, and the product labeling for estrogens was changed to reflect the risk of endometrial cancer. It wasn't until the 1980s that progesterone could be manipulated in such a way that it could be absorbed orally. This involved decreasing the size of progesterone particles to <10 µm, hence oral progesterone is called oral micronized progesterone.

Estrogen as Wonder Drug

During the 1980s multiple observational studies suggested MHT could prevent cardiovascular disease. The idea that estrogen might be protective for the heart had been around for a while. In the 1970s, Premarin was even studied for men with heart disease—doses up to 5 mg a day (a high dose, as in birth-control-equivalent dose) were used. However, the study was stopped due to an increase in blood clots.

There was also growing observational evidence that estrogen could protect the bones as well as the brain. The hype was huge, as heart disease, osteoporosis, and cognitive impairment were and still are three of the biggest health conditions that impair and/or shorten women's lives. If estrogen could do all this, it would be a wonder drug indeed. Promises of looking younger were generally abandoned or downgraded in pharmaceutical messaging, and living longer and healthier, the literal fountain of youth, took center stage.

An observational study means researchers look at women taking hormones and compare their outcomes with those not taking the medication. As these women aren't randomized in a study, many factors could have been involved in whether they chose to take hormones, so proving that a good outcome was due to the hormones or these other factors wasn't possible. Almost all of these observational studies involved White, educated, upper-middle-class, thin women. Considering the impact of social determinants of health on outcomes, this was a group of women who, on average, would have a lower risk of many medical conditions. Studies that don't account for diversity harm the groups of women excluded from the study as opportunities are lost to advance their health, and the studies harm the women who are enrolled because the results are contaminated with confounding variables and are potentially less reliable.

The observational data poured in and everyone was on the estrogen express. In 1992 the American College of Physicians recommended all postmenopausal women take estrogen therapy as did almost every other medical professional society. I remember this time well, as my OB/GYN training was 1990 to 1995. In clinic it was typical to start three or four women a day on MHT. We were trained to discuss MHT in much the same way we talk about other preventative therapy, such as mammograms. It was also common for women to make appointments specifically to discuss their menopause concerns. Women heard about medications for menopause from their doctors, but also a friend, a sister, or even their own mother.

Whether we like it or not, the Golden Era of MHT made menopause a milestone and created a space to talk not just about MHT, but menopause itself. While it's true that most of those conversations ended in MHT—and so the prescribing was likely excessive because after all we even started seventy- and eighty-year-olds on MHT—we were at least having conversations about menopause. What I hear now from women is no one is listening, that there are no stories and limited opportunities to learn.

In 1992 Premarin was the number one selling prescription drug in the United States. Sales were >$1 billion in 1997 and by 2001 42 percent of menopausal women in the United States—15 million women—were taking MHT. A single drug Prempo, a convenient pill with both an estrogen and a progestin, was taken by almost 50 percent of women on MHT.

The WHI—A WTF for MHT

Given that the data on MHT was largely observational, the Office of Technology Assessment (OTA) correctly highlighted the need for a clinical trial as well as the need to research alternatives for menopausal symptoms. Hence the Women's Health Initiative or WHI was born.

Funded by the National Institutes of Health, the WHI enrolled over 64,000 women who were randomized to taking a drug or a placebo as well as an observational study of approximately 100,000 more women across forty centers in the United States. This was a massive undertaking—clinical trials of this size are rarely possible. The goal of the WHI was to evaluate MHT as prevention for cardiovascular disease and fractures due to osteoporosis, while monitoring for an increased risk of breast cancer, endometrial cancer, blood clots, and dementia. Other arms of the WHI evaluated the value of calcium and vitamin D supplementation in preventing fractures and colorectal cancer, and the role of a low fat eating pattern on prevention of breast cancer and colorectal cancer.

The trial enrolled postmenopausal women ages–fifty to seventy-nine years, with an average age of sixty-three (this will become important shortly, so hang on to the age). Women with a uterus took 0.625 mg of combined equine estrogens or CEE (Premarin) and 2.5 mg of medroxyprogesterone acetate (a progestin, trade name Provera) a day. Women without a uterus took CEE alone. Over 27,000 women were randomized to the hormone/placebo arm of the WHI.

The NIH halted the hormone arm in 2002, five years into the study and three years earlier than planned, due to an increased risk of breast cancer and what seemed clear evidence that the study would not prove MHT reduced cardiovascular disease; in fact the opposite seemed the case. The initial findings indicated an increased risk of invasive breast cancer, coronary heart disease, stroke, and pulmonary embolism, but fewer cases of hip fractures and colon cancer.

There was a press conference to discuss the findings, which isn't typical. The journalist Tara Parker-Pope in her 2007 book *The Hormone Decision* quotes Dr. Rossouw, the director of the WHI as saying the NIH was going for "high impact from its press conference" and the goal was "to shake up the medical establishment and change the thinking about hormones."

I dunno—I think the goal should be to report accurately on data so women and their providers can make the best health care decisions. Study results by press conference don't sit right with me. Medicine doesn't need drama, it needs quality, unbiased data, and the ability to put that data into perspective. Hormones relieve symptoms. Heart disease matters. Preventing osteoporosis is important. We don't want to cause cancer. This needed to be done right and explained well.

But shake things up they did. And what followed was a clusterfuck.

It's hard to explain what it was like to be a physician prescribing MHT at the time of the WHI press conference and the resulting media frenzy. It would be like a study today telling us that the human papilloma virus (HPV) isn't the cause of cervical cancer. The headlines were frightening and there were lots of them—in 2002 over 130 major new stories were devoted to MHT, most with an emphasis on risks. What were the WHI findings? A 41 percent increased risk of heart attacks and a 26 percent increased risk of breast cancer. Of course people were alarmed. That sounds alarming!

Things were not quite what they seemed in WHI-land. Some issues included the following:

- **CONFUSING COMMUNICATION ABOUT RISKS:** The WHI identified a 26 percent increased risk of invasive breast cancer, which sounds scary. In practical what-does-this-mean-for-me terms this means 6 additional women with breast cancer a year for every 10,000 who took MHT, which is a slightly less than 0.1 percent of women on MHT a year. What are some other factors that similarly increase the risk of breast cancer? Two to three glasses of alcohol a day increase the risk by 20 percent, obesity 20–40 percent, and giving birth after the age of thirty-five is a 40 percent increased risk versus giving birth before the age of twenty. Imagine if we cajoled women into a pregnancy before the age of twenty to lower their risk of breast cancer?!
- **THE WHI DATA SHOULDN'T BE EXTRAPOLATED TO ALL FORMS OF MHT:** The hormones CEE and MPA are one type of estrogen and proges-

togen, respectively. The risks and benefits from these hormones may not be the same as with other hormones or delivery systems.

- **THE WHI DATA SHOULDN'T HAVE BEEN EXTRAPOLATED TO ALL WOMEN:** The average age of women starting the WHI was 63. The breakdown: 33 percent of women were 50–59 years, 45 percent were 60–69 years, and 21 percent were 70–79 years. Cardiovascular disease increases significantly with age, so two-thirds of the women in the WHI who were 60 years or older were at higher risk for estrogen-related heart complications. The risk of estrogen on the heart may not be the same for women who start MHT at a younger age.
- **THE BAR FOR DETECTING BREAST CANCER WAS SET LOW:** This means the WHI could detect a minute change in breast cancer to stop the trial. This is a good thing, however, telling the public the study was stopped because the plan had always been to detect a very small increase in breast cancer sounds very different from the study was stopped due to an increased risk of breast cancer.
- **THE SMALL RISK OF BREAST CANCER WITH MHT WASN'T A NEW FINDING:** This was rarely mentioned. For example, one of the largest reviews of the data published a few years before the WHI indicated the increased risk of breast cancer with five years or more of MHT was 35 percent—exactly in line with the WHI findings.
- **THE LACK OF DIFFERENCE IN MORTALITY WASN'T EMPHASIZED:** While rates of breast cancer were higher, overall women taking MHT weren't more likely to die than those who were not taking MHT.

The consequences were profound. For the medical community the biggest shock was the complete dismantling of the canon that estrogen protected the heart. For over ten years I'd told my patients that the small increased risk of breast cancer was outweighed by the large protective effect on the heart, and that mattered because heart disease was the number one cause of death for women. Now estrogen didn't just protect the heart it might actually hurt it?

It felt like a nanosecond before the medical malpractice lawyers started in with the "WERE YOU HARMED BY HORMONES?" advertising (the ads are always very shouty, hence the capitals). Patients were calling in a panic. Some doctors insisted that women who refused to stop their hormones sign liability wavers—how enforceable, who knows—but it gives you an idea of the level of alarm. As OB/GYNs are among the most sued physicians and they prescribed the bulk of the MHT, fear of litigation likely played a significant role in stopping MHT.

At first I, like many of my colleagues, had no idea what to tell women suffering with symptoms—largely women in their mid to late forties and early fifties and therefore not represented by the WHI. At the time only one nonhormonal medication for hot flushes—clonidine—was used. The data on the many nonhormonal medications for hot flushes we have today was in its infancy in 2002.

MHT use plummeted, by some reports up to 80 percent. Women with symptoms suffered because many doctors were afraid to prescribe MHT. Reasons doctors stopped prescribing MHT were fear they were harming their patients, fear of malpractice lawsuits, or both. Professional societies scrambled to make sense of the data and provide some perspective on the WHI, but often when MHT was offered many women were too afraid to take it. As there were very few nonhormonal alternatives to offer, conversations about menopause seemed to disappear. I remember a lot of "I'm sorry" and shoulder shrugging on my part. I felt helpless and enraged, because women were suffering and it was hard to apply the WHI data to most women who were in need of help with symptoms.

When 42 percent of the population are taking a drug for menopause, it legitimizes conversations and stories about menopause—it invited women to talk about what was happening to their bodies, and that needs to be acknowledged. When a medication exists for hot flushes—even if you don't want to take that medication—it vindicates the ones that you're experiencing. Many of my own patients told me they suffered at home because they believed hormones weren't safe, so I never even had the chance to have a conversation with them about their bodies, to try to put the risks of estrogen in perspective, or to consider other nonhormonal options which were becoming more available.

It's not possible to overstate the impact of the WHI on how we view MHT today, and I suspect its reverberations will likely be felt for decades more. Not just because of the results, but how they were communicated by the investigators and the press, and how they have been interpreted and reinterpreted ad nauseam—and will likely continue to be reinterpreted. Since the first paper from the WHI was published in 2002 the findings have been the subject of more than a hundred papers, and at times it feels as if the data generated has been broken down to the molecular level and reassembled multiple times. Making sense of it all is hard.

There are other implications as well. I wasn't brought up, medically speaking, to fear MHT, so as more safety data became available it was easy for me to quickly readjust. I felt comfortable prescribing sooner than many younger colleagues who were in training when the WHI was published. It took a good ten years for new data and policy statements to permeate, so two generations of doctors went through their residency exposed to largely negative attitudes to MHT, and some of them still have reservations about MHT today. In addition, multiple important studies were also stopped due to fear about cardiovascular disease and breast cancer.

A New Window on MHT

In 2007 the data from the WHI on cardiovascular disease was reviewed looking at women by age groups. Women who started MHT within ten years of their final menstrual period actually had a lower than expected risk of coronary heart disease, and those who started ten or more years after their final menstrual period displayed a slightly increased risk. Women using MHT between the ages of fifty and fifty-nine also had a 30 percent lower risk of dying versus those women given placebo.

This idea that there was a window of safety for starting MHT—meaning starting hormones closer to the final menstrual period is different risk-wise from starting later—was born and is now supported by an increasing amount of data.

Today approximately 5 percent of women take MHT, a big drop from the hormone heyday of the late 1990s. The recommendations regarding MHT have been consistent for the past eight years, which is reassuring. The North American Menopause Society (NAMS) guidelines, which have been endorsed by almost every major American and international medical society dedicated to women's health, state that for women under the age of sixty or who are within ten years of menopause and have no contraindications, MHT is an appropriate choice for treating vasomotor symptoms (hot flushes and night sweats), preventing osteoporosis, and treatment of genitourinary syndrome of menopause (GUSM, although as discussed in chapter 13 starting with GUSM-specific therapies is recommended). There are other potential benefits of MHT that aren't in official guidelines, but may end up being factors that help women and their providers make decisions. As we have discussed MHT can help some women sleep better, can improve mood for those with mild to moderate depression, and reduces the risk of colon cancer and type 2 diabetes (see chapter 18 for more). Over the age of sixty the risk of a negative outcome for MHT rises, and so starting MHT for women over age sixty or when they are ten years from menopause is generally not recommended. This is due to increased risks of coronary artery disease, stroke, blood clots (venous thromboembolism), and dementia.

What happens on the sixtieth birthday for women who started MHT during that critical window of safety after their final menstrual period? Do those women now assume the risks of starting later or are they protected by starting earlier? There are very few clear answers here, so how to forge a path going forward will be based on a hard look at what MHT is really doing for a given woman, her risks of osteoporosis, and her risk of other medical conditions that could be helped or hurt by MHT.

MHT—The Risks

Most risks from MHT are in the 1–10/10,000 women/year range and in medicine this rate is considered rare (very rare is 1–10/100,000). However, if a complication happens to you, then that risk to you is now 100 percent. Remember rare or even very rare doesn't mean never, so there will always be small numbers of women with complications. Knowing these risks is part of informed consent, so women can weigh them against the potential benefits and decide what serves them best.

Discussing risk is difficult, because what risk means to a woman contemplating MHT is very different from looking at that same risk for a population. If 10 million women take MHT and the risk of a negative event—we'll pick breast cancer—is 6 per 10,000 women/year, that means 6,000 women will develop breast cancer each year. It would be wrong for those invested in the health of the public to not mention those 6,000 women with breast cancer. But statistics are tricky. Population level data is also what typically generates headlines as large numbers amplify perception of risk, making a treatment sound scarier than it is because fear sells. *I mean, 6,000 women, a year? My god. Are you trying to kill me?* But 6 women per 10,000 women a year is also 0.06 percent of women a year, and that sounds like a much safer medication, even though it's simply the same risk explained in different ways. *I mean, 0.06 percent of women a year, that's it? Why won't you just give me the hormones already?*

For me the answer is simple. Explain this issue to women. It took me less than 200 words in the preceding paragraph. Women are very capable of understanding risk. After all, most are familiar with weighing whether they should walk down a specific street at night or whether it's better to take the bus.

It feels as if we overemphasize risks related to MHT, and to me it seems as if it even goes beyond the concept of infantilizing women and their decision-making skills. Medications for erectile dysfunction cause blindness for 3 out of every 100,000 men who take them, and yet society trusts men to decide if those risks are worth it. Treating erectile dysfunction may be helpful for a man's well-being, but it will not prevent him from getting osteoporosis, help with his sleep, or treat mild depression. Estrogen, on the other hand—which offers more than quality-of-life improvements—is viewed as risky. I'm not sure I have the answer for the warped differences in perspective beyond misogyny. Perhaps men view risk differently, so fear-driven headlines have less of an impact. Maybe fear of breast cancer is such a driver that articles on the subject are more likely to be published. I do not wish to downplay the significance of breast cancer at all, but if one only read the popular press one wouldn't be faulted for thinking that heart disease and osteoporosis are minor concerns for women.

The risk of venous thromboembolism (a potentially dangerous blood clot, also known as VTE) with oral MHT is approximately 9 per 10,000 women per year (it's not increased with transdermal estrogen). The risk of VTE in pregnancy is 5–20 for every 10,000 pregnancies, and during the postpartum it's 40–65/10,000 pregnancies, yet there are no guidelines telling women not to get pregnant because of the risk of blood clots. When we say it's acceptable for a woman to assume the risk of a VTE with pregnancy and not assume a lower risk than that with MHT, what are we saying about the worth of women? That as long as she's in servitude to her uterus the risk is acceptable and once her natural resources have been consumed by society her health concerns are barely worth a mention? Because that is exactly what it sounds like to me.

If a woman can decide whether she should get pregnant or drink milk (head to chapter 19 to learn more about the observational data that links milk with cancer) or drive a car for that matter, then we can in truth let them decide whether MHT is right for them. Here are the risks of MHT based on the available data for women of average risk derived from the ashes of the WHI and from many other studies. Many of the potential benefits have been explored in previous chapters and will be discussed in chapter 18. Women at higher risk of these conditions will need different conversations.

The main risks of MHT are as follows:

- **BLOOD CLOTS:** Overall risk with oral MHT risk is 8–9 per 10,000 women per year. The risk of blood clots with MHT is related to age. For women ages 40–55 the risk is 5/10,000 women per year, and for women ages 56–64 the risk is 15/10,000 women per year. With transdermal therapy the risk isn't increased.
- **BREAST CANCER:** For women ages 50–59, combined MHT (an estrogen and a progestogen) is associated with an additional 6–15 breast cancers per 10,000 women per year. Use for more than 5 years is associated with the greatest risk. The breast cancer risk is lower without a progestogen. The risk may be higher for older women.
- **CHOLESTEROL:** Oral estrogen can worsen triglycerides, but improve HDL-C, LDL-C, and total cholesterol. Transdermal estrogen has no beneficial effect on cholesterol and no negative impact on triglycerides.
- **GALLBLADDER:** With oral estrogen the risk of gallbladder disease ranges from 47–58 additional cases per 10,000 women per year. This is the highest risk of all complications with MHT. Transdermal therapy is associated with no increased risk.
- **HEART HEALTH:** As we gather more information on the cardiovascular effects, a more complicated picture emerges. The risk of coronary heart disease or CHD—plaque buildup in the arteries of the heart that can cause angina and heart attacks—isn't increased for women who start MHT before the age of sixty or

within ten years of menopause, in fact the risk is lower. Over the age of sixty the risk definitely increases.

- **STROKE:** The risk is approximately 8 per 10,000 women per year with oral MHT.

Other potential risks that are less well described, meaning they seem to be associated with MHT but the actual risk is unknown—include the following: potential for worsening incontinence (see chapter 14); contributing to hearing loss; increased risk of dry eye syndrome, or keratoconjunctivitis sicca (this can affect the ability to wear contacts); a change in vision prescription as estrogen can increase elasticity in the cornea; and a potential role in affecting sense of smell, although this isn't well described.

BOTTOM LINE

- Prior to the discovery of estrogens, women were treated with a variety of extracts made from animal ovaries or amniotic fluid.
- The only natural estrogen is conjugated equine estrogens (CEE or Premarin).
- Most estrogens and progestogens (think of progesterone and the progestins as an all-girl band) are made by converting a steroid in yams or soybeans via a multistep process to hormones.
- MHT is FDA approved for prevention of osteoporosis and for treatment of hot flushes, and GUSM and is associated with a small but definite increased risk of stroke, blood clots, breast cancer, and gallbladder disease.
- There is a window before the age of sixty or before ten years have elapsed from the last menstrual period where MHT offers the most benefits and the lowest risks.

Chapter 18

The Cinematic Universe of Hormones:

What MHT Is Right for You?

BEFORE WE GET TO THE hormone talk, it's important to remember the three healthiest things a woman can do for her menopause have nothing to do with menopausal hormone therapy (MHT)—they are quitting smoking, getting the recommended amount of exercise, and eating a diet that meets nutritional needs. While MHT can help many women with quality of life and sometimes longevity, greater gains can be made with these other changes. This doesn't mean women shouldn't use MHT; rather, it's important to put the benefits of MHT into perspective as it's only one piece of the menopause puzzle. Many women start MHT with overly high expectations, but that can lead to disappointment and stopping prematurely or unnecessary changes in therapy, sometimes even leading them to less safe compounded options. Another consideration is MHT isn't permanent; if you don't like how it makes you feel, you can switch to another product or stop altogether.

Can MHT Help Me?

The approved indications are treatment of hot flushes and night sweats, prevention of osteoporosis, treatment of genitourinary syndrome of menopause (GUSM), and treatment of primary ovarian insufficiency. This means MHT is effective for these conditions and for most women the benefits outweigh the risks. Women don't have to be postmenopausal to start; remember, symptoms of menopause can start years before the final menstrual period (FMP) during the menopause transition.

Women with primary ovarian insufficiency (see chapter 6) don't need symptoms to start MHT. Unless contraindicated, these women should take MHT until the average age of menopause, fifty to fifty-two years, and then make a decision about continuing the therapy or not. MHT is also recommended for women whose final menstrual period is between the ages of forty and forty-five because it helps to mitigate their increased risk of heart disease, and for these women MHT has been shown to reduce mortality.

What about other symptoms or conditions? MHT can also be used for reasons other than the four approved indications. This is called an off label indication, meaning data hasn't been submitted to the Food and Drug Administration (FDA) to prove MHT works well enough for these reasons and/or to prove the benefits outweigh the risks. It's possible the data may exist—meaning studies have been published —and the pharmaceutical company just hasn't submitted it to the FDA or it could mean there is no quality data. Fortunately, there are expert guidelines that have looked at the body of literature to make recommendations for many of these in between situations. The classic example of off label use endorsed by multiple guidelines is using MHT to control irregular bleeding during the menopause transition.

Other potential health benefits seen with MHT that aren't covered by the FDA approved guidelines, but may be a consideration for some and something for women to consider in their personal risk-to-benefit ratio, include the following:

- **COLON CANCER:** Studies have shown a reduced risk for this type of cancer with MHT.
- **DEPRESSION:** MHT may improve mild or moderate depression that begins during the menopause transition.
- **EYES:** MHT reduces risk of cataracts and open angle glaucoma.
- **METABOLIC SYNDROME AND WEIGHT:** MHT shows a favorable effect on metabolic syndrome and may slow accumulation of visceral

fat (the active or harmful fat, see chapter 7). MHT is not associated with weight gain.

- **MOOD AND DEPRESSION:** MHT may help some women; see chapter 12 for more.
- **MUSCLES:** Estrogen combined with exercise *may* help slow the loss of muscle mass with age and menopause (not definitive). May also help balance.
- **SKIN:** May slow the appearance of wrinkles and be beneficial for skin moisture due to a positive effect of estrogen on collagen. Estrogen does not impact hair loss related to menopause or aging.
- **SLEEP:** MHT reduces waking due to hot flushes.
- **TYPE 2 DIABETES:** There is a 19 percent to a 40 percent reduction— this translates to approximately 16 fewer women per 10,000 per year on MHT.
- **VAGINAL SYMPTOMS DUE TO GUSM:** MHT can help 50 percent of women with GUSM. Consider GUSM-specific therapies over MHT as they're 100 percent effective, and the vaginal options are as risk free as a medication can be when prescribed and used correctly (see chapter 13).

MHT is not currently recommended for prevention of dementia or Alzheimer's disease for women at average risk (see chapter 12 for more).

There are many symptoms that are menopause-adjacent, and it can be hard to know if they're menopause, age-related, or perhaps something else (remember back to the M diagram in chapter 1). If a woman decides that MHT may be an option for other symptoms or conditions—for example, a persistent flare of another medical condition, such as an autoimmune condition, or worsening of migraines—during the menopause transition it's important she be clear about her definition of an acceptable benefit and a stopping point if MHT doesn't appear to be helping. While the risks of MHT are very low—especially for the first four to five years of use—no one should be taking a medication that isn't helping. It's also important to look for other causes of symptoms as there is a tendency to blame hormones for everything that happens to a woman between the ages of forty and sixty.

All the symptoms and conditions listed above combine to make what we could call "quality of life," and that's difficult to study as it can mean different things for different women. When a woman is suffering, a trial of MHT may be reasonable. It can be helpful for every woman to write down the health concerns she hopes MHT will help before embarking on therapy and to be as specific as possible and then revisit that list periodically to ensure she is truly getting the benefit that she had hoped. Build time into the expectations of improvement. It may take a minimum of six weeks or more to see a true benefit, so waiting at least ten to twelve weeks to assess for the desired effect is a good idea. Download the MenPro app from the North American Menopause Society (NAMS) to check what your provider recommends in the office against the society's guidelines.

Getting Started on MHT

To consider MHT a woman should be younger than sixty years or less than ten years from her final menstrual period and not have a personal history of breast cancer, stroke, or heart attack. Some women who have had an early-stage endometrial cancer (cancer of the uterus) that has been treated and are considered cured may be able to consider some forms of MHT after a discussion with their oncologist (cancer specialist).

As the major health risks associated with MHT are related to blood clots, cardiovascular disease (heart attack and stroke), and breast cancer, it's important to thoroughly review a woman's risk factors for those conditions. Some women with milder conditions that increase the risk of blood clotting may be able to take some forms of MHT, but this requires an in-depth consultation with their provider. Women can assess their risk for heart disease (atherosclerotic and cardiovascular disease or ASCVD) and breast cancer using free online calculators: ASCVD at tools.acc.org/ASCVD-Risk-Estimator-Plus/#!/calculate/estimate/at (cholesterol levels are needed) and breast disease risk calculator, bcrisktool.cancer.gov. If a woman's risk of ASCVD in the next ten years is >10 percent or her risk of breast cancer is >5 percent, then MHT is generally not recommended. Women at moderate risk for these conditions should have more detailed discussions with their providers so they can assess their own risks and how to weigh them against potential benefits.

Screening for health conditions that could influence the decision to start or affect hormone choice is recommended before starting. This is also a good opportunity to review non-menopause-related health care screenings. Women should consider the following in their pre-MHT evaluation:

- **BLOOD PRESSURE CHECK:** High blood pressure increases the risk of stroke and heart attacks.
- **A BLOOD TEST FOR DIABETES:** This blood work is recommended every year starting at the age of forty-five and younger for those with risk factors. Diabetes is a risk factor for stroke and heart attack. Women with diabetes should only use transdermal therapy.
- **A BLOOD TEST FOR CHOLESTEROL, LIPIDS, AND TRIGLYCERIDES:** Elevated cholesterol and triglycerides are risk factors for stroke and heart attack. Oral estrogen can worsen triglycerides, so women with high triglycerides should choose transdermal therapy.
- **BREAST CANCER SCREENING:** Estrogen in MHT could make some breast cancers grow. Make note of the breast density on your mammogram as MHT can increase breast density for some women, which in turn can impact screening for breast cancer on future mammograms.
- **EVALUATION OF ABNORMAL UTERINE BLEEDING:** An evaluation by a medical professional can ensure any irregular or unanticipated bleeding isn't due to endometrial cancer (see chapter 10 for more on testing). Pregnancy should also be ruled out as a cause.
- **BONE HEALTH:** Women should evaluate their risk of an osteoporosis-related fracture (see chapter 11). If their risk is elevated, that may impact their choice of hormones and how long they wish to stay on MHT.
- **CERVICAL CANCER SCREENING:** Cervical cancer isn't affected by menopause, but it's always a good idea to make sure your screening is up to date.
- **SCREENING FOR DEPRESSION AND ANXIETY:** Women ages forty to fifty-nine have the highest rate of depression (12.3 percent). Although MHT may help some women with mild to moderate depression, severe depression may require other therapies and follow-up. Objectively measuring depression and anxiety before starting can also help women determine a pre-existing condition, and not wonder whether they are developing depression while on MHT.

- **SCREEN FOR INTIMATE PARTNER VIOLENCE (IPV):** Every visit is an opportunity to screen for IPV.

Choosing MHT

There are so many choices it can feel like the Cheesecake Factory—how does one navigate such a massive menu? The number of pharmaceutical-grade MHT products is overwhelming, but this also means among this wealth of options is a regimen that can be tailored to fit almost every woman's individual medical needs. The goal here is to provide a solid background of facts to prep for informed discussions with your own health care provider. This chapter is a practical internship in hormones.

And remember if you start on one therapy and find there may be side effects or using it is a nuisance (after all, quality of life is part of the goal), this isn't Tinder and you haven't swiped left.

The Estrogen

It's the estrogen that provides the therapy. The biggest difference between the estrogens isn't between the types; rather, it's the route of delivery: oral versus transdermal (which includes topical applications to the skin as well as vaginal). Transdermal estrogens have the lowest risk of blood clots and stroke; in fact they don't increase the risk of these major complications over the baseline risk associated with age.

There are some other smaller differences between the estrogens that will be discussed later, but one of the most important is not all estrogens are approved for osteoporosis, an important consideration for many women.

The reason for the relative safety of transdermal versus oral estrogens is a phenomenon known as the first pass (see figure 14). Most of the medications absorbed through the intestine enter a specific group of blood vessels that head directly to the liver for processing and from there head to the bloodstream. So the liver gets the first pass at the medication. With transdermal delivery the estrogens enter directly into the bloodstream through the skin or from the vagina, so when the hormone reaches the

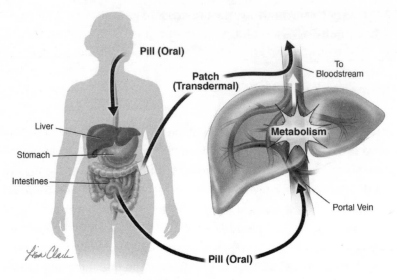

Figure 14: Oral vs. Transdermal Therapy

liver it has been diluted by the greater volume of blood in the body. The first pass effect means the liver sees a much larger dose of the hormone with oral therapy as compared with transdermal therapy.

When estradiol is taken by mouth the liver converts most of it to estrone. While estrone is a weaker estrogen, it triggers the liver to make more proteins that cause the blood to clot, hence the increased risk of clots with oral estrogens. Oral estrogen also causes the liver to increase production of SHBG (remember the Seats Handy on the Bus, Girl? mnemonic), binding more testosterone so it can't be active. This may be one reason why some women find oral estrogen has a negative effect on libido. It's also possible that estrone may have other negative effects on the liver. The first pass effect is also the reason that oral estrogen lowers cholesterol but raises triglycerides. Transdermal estrogen doesn't have these effects.

Other advantages of transdermal therapy are steady levels of hormones, especially with the patch and the vaginal ring. Oral therapy produces more ups and downs in the levels as a large amount of estrogen is absorbed all at once as opposed to a constant low level of delivery to the blood with transdermal therapy. This effect may not be noticeable for most women, but it could have an impact on mood for some who are sensitive to hormone fluctuations. Transdermal estrogen is also less likely to cause high blood pressure. Women who may have difficulties absorbing medications, for example, after weight loss surgery or those with inflammatory bowel disease, will not have that concern with transdermal therapy.

In 1978 the labeling of estrogen was changed to reflect the increased risk of blood clots, which was seen in the high doses of ethinyl estradiol used in the oral contraceptive pill. When one form of medication is associated with a risk, all forms of the drug are required in the United States to carry the same warning label, so even though transdermal estrogen in MHT is not associated with an increased risk of blood clots the labeling has that listed as a risk because of the issues seen with oral estrogens.

All transdermal therapy is estradiol. The options are as follows:

- **PATCHES:** Typically applied to the lower abdomen or back and changed once or twice a week depending on the product. They produce the most stable levels of estradiol, so may be a better option for women whose mood is more sensitive to hormone fluctuations. Doses range from 0.014 mg a day to 0.1 mg a day, so there are a wide range of options. Side effects are reactions to the adhesive and the annoyance of removing the leftover adhesive. Patches may not stick as well for people who spend a lot of time swimming or in a hot tub. If there is an issue with the adhesive of one patch, another brand may be less irritating.
- **GELS, SPRAYS, AND EMULSION:** Applied daily to the arms. Like patches there is also a very wide dosing range, although with some products at the mid to upper dosing range there is a fairly large surface area needed for application. These products tend to cause less skin irritation than the patch and have none of that gross leftover patch adhesive that seems so tarlike it could be used for road repairs. The downside is the application site shouldn't be washed (lowers the estrogen absorbed) or have moisturizer applied (raises the estrogen level) for at least an hour after application.
- **VAGINAL RING:** Replaced every ninety days, so very user-friendly. There are two dosing options, 0.05 mg a day and 0.1 mg a day, which is a disadvantage as some women can control their symptoms and protect their bones with lower doses of estradiol.

If a transdermal option isn't possible due to cost or has been tried, but there are ongoing issues with skin irritation the ring isn't acceptable, then oral estrogen therapy is an option. Oral estrogens have a risk of 8–9 blood clots per 10,000 women per year, so they are still very safe, but the risk is higher than the patch. Oral estrogen options include the following:

- **ESTRADIOL:** The main estrogen produced by the follicles, made by semi-synthesis.
- **CONJUGATED EQUINE ESTROGENS OR CEE:** Contains more than ten different estrogens, the most plentiful being sodium estrone sulfate and sodium equilin sulfate. It's only available as an oral therapy. It is the only natural therapy and is extracted from horse urine.
- **CONJUGATED ESTROGENS OR CE:** A synthetic (lab-created) version of CEE. Some of the many estrogens in CEE are replicated, but not all. In the United States conjugated estrogens aren't considered an equivalent to CEE, but in Canada they are. Only available as oral therapy. They're an option for women who prefer CEE, but don't want a product made from horse urine. CEs aren't approved for prevention of osteoporosis in the United States.
- **ETHINYL ESTRADIOL:** More potent than other estrogens, so doses are typically lower. It's metabolized slower, producing less variability in hormone levels.
- **ESTROPIPATE:** Estrone that has been modified by combining it with piperazine. Approved for osteoporosis.
- **ESTERIFIED ESTROGENS:** A mixture of estrone sulfate and equilin sulfate, but higher levels of estrone and lower levels of equilin than CEE or CE. Only available as oral and not approved for osteoporosis.

Estetrol is an estrogen currently under investigation, but not on the market. It's only produced by the fetal liver during pregnancy. Some interesting preliminary research suggests estetrol may has some unique properties including less of a negative effect on breast tissue. As of September 2020 there isn't enough human data to support or refute this hypothesis, but it's an avenue of research. Estriol, the estrogen made primarily by the placenta, is used in MHT in Europe, but no data supporting estriol has been submitted to the FDA in the United States. It is a much weaker estrogen than estradiol and CEE.

The goal with estrogen is to give the lowest amount that manages symptoms and/or prevents osteoporosis. When symptoms are severe some providers may start with a moderate dose to aim for the fastest improvement, while others may recommend starting lower and increasing if ineffective. It's worth mentioning that lower doses can often be effective. The goal is not to mimic hormone levels before the FMP—remember this isn't replacement therapy—rather to give what is needed. For perspective, during ovulation the amount of estradiol in the blood typically ranges from 70 to 300 mcg of estradiol (sometimes even higher) and after menopause estradiol levels are <25 mcg/l. A 0.05 mg estradiol patch results in blood levels of approximately 50 mcg/l and a 0.0375 mcg patch is 37.5 mcg/l, and so on.

Estrogens haven't been studied in a way that direct comparisons are possible, but supplemental tables 4 and 5, pp. 339–40, provide a best guess on comparing estrogens based on hormone, route of administration, and source.

The Progestogen

Progestogens include progesterone and progestins (remember our all-girl band?). Progestogens protect the lining of the uterus from the effects of estrogen by reducing the number of estrogen receptors in the uterine lining and by increasing the activity of the enzyme that converts estradiol to the much weaker estrone. The risk of precancerous changes and cancer with estrogen are very real, and the longer a woman takes estrogen without protecting her uterus the greater her risk, so the correct dose of a progestogen is important. There are claims online that "estrogen stimulates and progesterone calms," meaning all women need both hormones, but that's not true. The reason for a progestogen is the uterus, although there are some exceptions (always the exceptions with menopause).

Some of the breast cancer risk with MHT is due to the progestogen, although how much is still a source of controversy. With CEE and medroxyprogesterone acetate (MPA, the progestin used in the WHI study) the risk of breast cancer increased after three or four years with an estrogen-progestin compared with estrogen by itself. Other studies have shown that progesterone and dydrogesterone (a progestin with a very similar chemical structure to progesterone) doesn't raise the risk of breast cancer for the first five years of use, but after five years the risk starts to rise, eventually becoming similar to other progestins—around 1 case per 1,000 women per year. When estrogen is used alone the risk of breast cancer may not rise for seven years on the therapy. There are also some small studies looking directly at breast tissue suggesting progesterone may have less of a negative effect than the progestins. Based on this data, the North American Menopause Society (NAMS) favors progesterone (dydrogesterone isn't available in the United States) to start, but also stresses there may be reasons that progestins may be preferable for an individual woman. Breast cancer risk with the levonorgestrel IUD in MHT isn't known. What is definitely unsafe is transdermal progesterone, as it isn't absorbed well and so cannot protect the uterus.

In the United States and Canada there are six different progestogens and four different routes of administration—transdermal, oral, vaginal, and intrauterine. So lots of choices. Prescription progesterone is medically known as oral micronized progesterone, but we'll refer to it as progesterone for the sake of simplicity.

Most progestogens are made by semi-synthesis (see chapter 17 for a review). Some are derived from progesterone and others from testosterone or from another steroid hormone called spironolactone, but ultimately they come from diosgenin or a similar plant compound that has been modified in a lab. Progestins were initially the only option for oral therapy as the chemical changes required to alter progesterone so it could be absorbed when taken orally hadn't been invented. Other modifications made some of the progestins more effective at suppressing the effect of estrogen on the uterine lining to reduce irregular bleeding patterns with oral contraceptives.

Progestins derived from testosterone may retain some testosterone-related properties, but it isn't known if these are clinically meaningful for most women. It's always possible for some women one type of progestin could cause more bloating or acne than another. Drospirenone, derived from spironolactone, has properties that reduce the effect of testosterone, and this hormone may be especially useful for women who have issues with bloating on MHT.

To protect the uterus a progestogen must be given for a minimum of twelve days per "cycle," where a cycle is twenty-eight days of therapy. This mimics the exposure during an ovulatory cycle as progesterone is only released with ovulation.

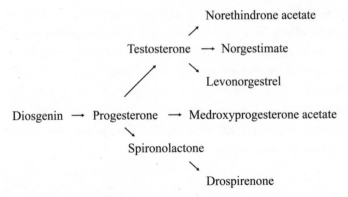

Figure 15: Origin of progestogens.

Progestogens are available in combination products, and individual progestogens can be mixed and matched with the estrogen of choice. There are too many individual products to list, but here are some general considerations and nuances to consider:

- **PROGESTERONE:** Hormone of choice for starting, but the progesterone advantage over other options is small.
- **IN THE MENOPAUSE TRANSITION:** A levonorgestrel IUD or low-dose birth control pill (combination estrogen and progestogen) can control irregular cycles and provide contraception if needed.
- **PREVIOUS OR CURRENT HISTORY OF DEPRESSION:** Progesterone is likely the best option to start MHT.
- **EASE OF USE:** The levonorgestrel IUD is the most user independent; a combination patch is also convenient (changed weekly).
- **THE ROUTE:** Some women prefer the idea of a combination product, some love the idea of a patch with both hormones, others the idea of an IUD, and some think a vaginal product is better for their needs.
- **SLEEP:** Progesterone can make some women sleepy, which may or may not be helpful depending on the individual circumstances. See chapter 16 for more.
- **PEANUT ALLERGY:** The oral formulation of progesterone in the United States still has peanut oil listed on the product monograph; however, in Canada it's now available in sunflower oil.
- **IRREGULAR BLEEDING:** Progestins typically provide better control.

- **HOT FLUSHES:** Progestins can be helpful; this may be of value for women who wish to stay on a very low dose of estrogen or for whom estrogen isn't working sufficiently. Progestins may be an option for some women who are unable to take estrogen because of risk of stroke or heart attack as they don't affect blood clotting.
- **OSTEOPOROSIS:** Progestins help maintain bone health; progesterone has no impact. This may be valuable for women using a very low dose of estrogen.

A Nonprogestogen Option

Protecting against the negative effect of estrogen on the lining of the uterus can also be achieved with a medication called bazedoxifene, which is a selective estrogen receptor modulator or SERM. This means it acts like an estrogen on some tissues and on other tissues it opposes the effect of estrogen. We've discussed SERMs before—tamoxifen in chapter 5 for breast cancer. Bazedoxifene is useful because it acts like an estrogen on bone and opposes the effect of estrogen on the lining of the uterus and on breast issue. It has no risk of breast cancer and doesn't increase breast density, which is an issue for some women with MHT. The downside is that bazedoxifene slightly increases the risk of blood clots and hot flushes.

Combining a SERM with an estrogen creates a new class of drug called a tissue-selective estrogen complex or TSEC. The idea is to get benefit from both drugs and have the drugs cancel out any negative side effects of the other. The only TSEC currently available as of September 2020 is 0.45 mg of CEE (combine equine estrogens) with 20 mg of bazedoxifene known as CEE/BZA (Duavee in the United States and Duavive in Canada). It's approved for treatment of hot flushes and for prevention of osteoporosis—the CEE cancels out the effect of bazedoxifene on hot flushes and the bazedoxifene cancels the effect of the CEE on the lining of the uterus and the breasts, so there is no risk of endometrial cancer and no increase in breast density (something that affects the quality of a mammogram). While it's not FDA approved for GUSM, it may help vaginal dryness although it's less clear if it helps pain with intercourse as the dose of estrogen may be too low. The data on CEE/BZA doesn't show an increased risk of blood clots over estrogen alone, but there is not enough long-term data to be 100 percent sure.

CEE/BZA is a good option for women who desire MHT for hot flushes or prevention of osteoporosis and who don't tolerate a progestogen, either due to effects on mood or bleeding. It shouldn't be considered a safer form of MHT, meaning the risks of breast cancer and blood clots and dementia are the same as other MHT. A woman with very dense breasts who has already had a biopsy or two but who doesn't have breast cancer may wish to consider this product so not to make breast screening even more challenging. If the primary goal is treatment of pain with sex, then CEE/BZA is probably not the best option.

There is ongoing research looking at CEE/BZA for women with ductal carcinoma in situ or DCIS, a noninvasive form of breast cancer that can become breast cancer. It's theoretically possible that bazedoxifene could cancel out the negative effect of CEE in breast tissue, so it's possible a TSEC could be an option for these women one day.

Troubleshooting MHT

More common side effects include bloating, irregular bleeding, breast tenderness, mood changes, nausea, and migraines. Migraines and nausea are typically due to the estrogen and mood changes and bloating more likely the progestogen. Bleeding and breast tenderness can be caused by either. The options to mitigate these issues is to either change the medication or dose. A medication switch could be to a different class of hormone, for example, from a progestin to a progesterone or from estradiol to CEE. Another option is to change the route or delivery—for example, from a patch to vaginal, or to raise or lower the dose. This is a process of trial and error and requires a knowledgeable provider. It may take three months to see the desired change depending on the side effect. More on mood-related complications in chapter 12.

When Do I Stop?

Previous guidelines suggested women stop MHT at sixty-five, but as long as blood pressure, cholesterol, and triglycerides are stable there is no medical need to stop, and continuing may be a fine option. There is ongoing research into the long-term effects of estrogen on dementia and so we may know more about potential safety issues in time.

Whether a woman should consider stopping MHT also depends on why she started. If it was for symptoms such as hot flushes, sleep disturbances, or mood changes those symptoms may not be as severe once the hormonal chaos of the menopause transition years have passed. Stopping estrogen at age fifty-five (or any time after the final menstrual period) doesn't reset the menopause transition; MHT allows women to bypass those extreme hormone fluctuations and step back in, as it were, after they have passed. Hot flushes can sometimes persist for years after the final menstrual period and the risk of osteoporosis doesn't go away, so each woman will need to decide with her provider when and if she should stop MHT.

BOTTOM LINE

- While oral estrogens are low risk, transdermal estradiol offers the lowest risk and is the preferred method to start.
- Transdermal estradiol is available in pharmaceutical patches, creams, lotions, sprays, and a vaginal ring—all have minor advantages and inconveniences associated with use, but there are a wide variety of doses and so therapy can be customized to suit almost every woman's need.
- Progesterone or oral micronized progesterone may have the lowest risk of breast cancer and the lowest risk of negatively affecting mood, so it's the preferred progestogen for oral therapy.
- The Mirena IUD is an excellent choice for progestogen for women who don't want to take progesterone orally, but vaginal progesterone and a progestin patch are other options.
- A tissue-selective estrogen complex or TSEC is a good option for women who wish to avoid a progestogen.

Chapter 19

Phytoestrogens, Food, and Hormones:

Facts and Fads

THE INTERACTION BETWEEN HORMONES AND food is complex and at times the language and the medicine can be very confusing, so it's no wonder there's a lot of misinformation here.

There are many people who claim various foods or diets can provide hormone fixes, cures, and resets for women in the menopause continuum. But food doesn't change hormone levels in an eat-this-change-that-hormone kind of way. If plants contained hormones that could be digested and used by humans, then we'd know by now because these foods wouldn't just improve symptoms of menopause they'd also cause premature puberty, irregular menstrual cycles, infertility, as well as breast development for men. And those who ate the most plants—vegetarians and vegans—would have more of these health concerns. But that isn't the case.

Humans don't get hormones from plants and we're not able to convert plant compounds into hormones. We make all our estrogens, testosterone, and progesterone from cholesterol. This is a complex, multistep process (see chapter 3) and not a conveyor belt where adding more raw ingredients results in more end product. Also, the gut can't tag a specific molecule in a meal as soon as it hits the stomach with a "Don't touch, for ovary use only!" sign.

Misperceptions about plants and hormones likely stems in part from many people not understanding how hormones are made and the knowledge that plants have compounds known as phytoestrogens. The word "phytoestrogen" is very similar to estrogen, so it's easy to understand any confusion between the two, but phytoestrogens aren't estrogens and they're not converted into estrogens. Another source of confusion is the fact that most hormones in menopausal hormone therapy (MHT) are synthesized in a lab from a substance found in a specific type of yam or soybeans. That transformation involves a multistep process and is hardly natural, and our bodies are not able to convert these substances from yams or soybeans into hormones. See chapters 17 and 18 for more.

Hormone levels can be affected by malnutrition and/or changes in eating patterns that lead to rapid or extreme weight loss due to the impact on the complex, coordinated hormone signaling required for regular ovulation. Some women are more sensitive to dietary changes than others. Dietary patterns that increase visceral fat can affect sex hormone binding globulin (SHBG, the protein that carries hormones that we've discussed throughout the book with the Seats Handy on the Bus, Girl? analogy). Fiber can also affect how estrogen is reabsorbed (see chapter 6), but if this produces an effect it's over the long-term.

Phytoestrogens

Phytoestrogens are compounds found in plants that can mimic estrogen or interfere with estrogen. Hormones interact with receptors on cells—remember the lock (receptor) and key (hormone) model we've discussed previously (chapter 3). An estrogen molecule is a perfect fit with estrogen receptors. With phytoestrogens, part of the key is similar. As they're not identical, phytoestrogens aren't as strong or as *estrogenic* as estrogens. Think of estrogens and phytoestrogens like cow's milk and soy milk. There are similarities—soy milk can sometimes replace cow's milk in recipes—but they're decidedly different products. And cow's milk most definitely can't be made from soy milk.

Phytoestrogens can also be antiestrogens by occupying a receptor, in the way the wrong key stuck in a lock prevents other keys from accessing the lock. This may explain why some studies have suggested phytoestrogens may protect against some hormonally sensitive cancers, such as breast cancer and endometrial cancer (cancer of the lining of the uterus), as they may reduce the effect of circulating estrogens on tissues.

Phytoestrogens are often called "plant-based hormones," but this is inaccurate and confusing terminology. Not only are phytoestrogens not hormones for people, they're not even hormones for plants. Some plants do contain minute amounts of progesterone, but the levels are too low to have an effect on humans—why plants have tiny amounts of these hormones isn't fully understood.

So why do plants have substances that can sometimes act like an estrogen and sometimes block estrogens? The main theory is phytoestrogens evolved as defense mechanisms for plants—basically contraception for herbivores. Grazing herds can strip fields, so contraception reducing the number of herbivores is a nifty evolutionary adaptation. Sheep grazing in clover-rich fields have been documented to have higher rates of infertility, spontaneous abortion, and offspring with birth defects due to high levels of phytoestrogens in the clover. This theory would also explain why phytoestrogens can be absorbed from the gastrointestinal tract.

Evolution, hey?

Phytoestrogens may also provide defense for plants against certain mycotoxins, which are harmful toxins produced by fungi that can harm plants. One mycotoxin, zearalenone, is such a potent endocrine disruptor that it is even stronger than manmade ones such as per- and polyfluoroalkyl substances (PFAS, see chapter 5). There are many harmful mycotoxins. Ergot is perhaps the most infamous example, produced by a fungus that grows on grain. It can cause hallucinations, burning skin, gangrene, miscarriages, and even death. In the Middle Ages it was called St. Anthony's fire. Interestingly, ergot is also used in medicine (see chapter 22 for more). Given these health concerns there are strict guidelines for limiting mycotoxins in food.

There are five major classes of phytoestrogens: isoflavones (the most well-known are genistein and daidzein), coumestans, prenylflavonoids, lignans, and stilbenes (see table 3, p. 250). Before you get carried away, drinking red wine and beer isn't the cure for hot flushes!

Some phytoestrogens must interact with bacteria in the bowel to be absorbed, and some people may be more efficient at this process. For ex-

Table 3: Phytoestrogens

PHYTOESTROGEN CLASS	PHYTOESTROGENS	COMMON SOURCES
ISOFLAVONES	Genistein Daidzein Glycerin Formononetin Biochanin A	Soy Soy-based foods Legumes
COUMESTANS	Coumestrol 4' methoxycoumestrol Repensol Trifoliol	Split peas Pinto beans Lima beans Alfalfa sprouts Clover sprouts
PRENYLFLAVONOIDS	8-prenylnaringen	Beers, hops
LIGNANS	Enterodiol Enterolactone	Flaxseeds Whole grains Fruits Vegetables Sesame seeds Legumes
STILBENES	Resveratrol	Red grapes Red wine

ample, only 30 percent to 40 percent of people have bacteria capable of converting daidzein into equol, an even more potent phytoestrogen. Individuals of Asian origin are more likely to have this bacteria. Age reduces the ability to convert phytoestrogens into active forms as do antibiotics, which can negatively affect intestinal bacteria and prevent the conversion of phytoestrogens to bioactive forms in the gut.

Are Dietary Phytoestrogens Beneficial for People?

Technically phytoestrogens are endocrine disrupting chemicals (EDS), although that term is usually reserved for synthetic endocrine disrupting chemicals such as PFAS that have negative effects (for example, increasing the risk of an earlier menopause). However, as natural endocrine disrupting chemicals in plants can have negative effects on the animals that eat them and mycotoxins that are phytoestrogens can have serious health consequences, it's important not to give phytoestrogens a pass on safety. Turning estrogen receptors on or off, especially chronically for foods that may be dietary staples, could theoretically have consequences.

The good news is extensive studies haven't linked diets high in phytoestrogens to hormonally responsive cancers or other negative health outcomes. In fact, many studies show that traditional diets with high phytoestrogen intake may have a protective effect. Although it's important to remember these studies looked at diet as a whole, so the phytoestrogens came with plenty of vegetables and fish—meaning foods that are beneficial for health.

The Osteoporosis Prevention Using Soy or OPUS study randomized postmenopausal women to a high dose of phytoestrogens from soy, up to four times higher than typically found in a traditional Asian diet, and followed these women for two years. There was no increased risk of any negative health outcomes related to estrogen, such as increased thickness of the lining of the uterus (a potential sign of precancer), breast cancer, or uterine fibroids (benign tumors of the uterus). Whether this amount of phytoestrogens might cause an issue with longer term consumption isn't known.

Some studies suggest that a diet high in isoflavones from childhood may protect against breast cancer, but increasing isoflavone intake later in life doesn't appear to confer that same benefit. The European Prospective Investigation into Cancer and Nutrition (EPIC) study followed women with moderate and low intakes of isoflavones (10.8 mg/day vs. 0.23 mg/day) for an average of seven years and found no difference in rates of breast cancer for women who ate more phytoestrogens.

Early data suggests no negative interaction between aromatase inhibitors (drugs used for hormonally responsive breast cancer, see chapter 5) and phytoestrogens may possibly reduce the risk of breast cancer recurrence among breast cancer survivors, but before adding large amounts of dietary phytoestrogens, women with breast cancer, especially those who are taking aromatase inhibitors, should first talk with their oncologist.

Consumption of foods rich in phytoestrogens varies dramatically around the world, with the highest levels in Japan and China (varies sig-

Table 4: Phytoestrogen Consumption

COUNTRY/REGION	AVERAGE ISOFLAVONE/DAY
Japan	26–64 mg
China	18–41 mg
South Korea	24 mg
UK Healthy Diet	22.4 mg
UK Regular*	4 mg
Europe–Mediterranean	1.5 mg
Europe–Non-Mediterranean	2.1 mg
Canada	1.2 mg
United States	1.1–2 mg

* The average UK diet likely has more isoflavones than Europe, the United States, and Canada as flour often has added soy flour

nificantly by province, but overall still higher than the West) and the lowest in Mediterranean countries (see table 4). This is typically recorded by isoflavone consumption, the most common dietary phytoestrogen.

Here we have two traditional diets both associated with health and longevity—one in Japan that's very high in isoflavones and another diet in the Mediterranean (see chapter 21) that's very low in isoflavones. It's not the dietary conundrum that it first appears to be as there are some core similarities between these traditional diets—no processed foods, low in added sugar, lots of vegetables, and fish. Humans are pretty efficient omnivores, and perhaps as long as the diet is balanced and has the core important elements, we can otherwise adapt to what is made locally.

This is a very important point that's often lost when people focus on so-called super foods. Clearly phytoestrogens can be part of a healthy diet, but they're not essential nutrients. It makes sense, evolutionarily speaking, that in different regions the foods most associated with health and longevity became staples, considering the people who ate these foods—or were most able to extract benefit from them due to genetic differences—were the healthiest and hence more likely to reproduce and pass along those genetics. The diets that were most likely to lead to longevity allowed grandmothers to live long enough to help ensure the reproductive success of the next generation. Food can provide an evolutionary pressure by favoring people with more efficient enzymes or different intestinal bacteria, and this is often forgotten when looking at traditional diets. Women in Asia coevolved with their locally available foods as did women in the Mediterranean, so it's possible the ability to benefit from a given diet may also be tied to genetics.

Many people who make dietary changes that increase their phytoestrogen intake are also eating more vegetables and whole grains, so sorting out what benefits come from phytoestrogens and what comes from the dietary overhaul or the weight loss that may have resulted from the change in diet is challenging.

Overall, a diet with <100 mg of isoflavones a day (to get to that level would take a dedicated effort) offers no health risks and for many people is part of a very healthy, balanced diet. Diets with levels of isoflavones >100 mg a day have not been well studied.

Can Dietary Phytoestrogens Improve Symptoms of Menopause?

While some people point to a lower rate of hot flushes among women in Japan who eat a traditional Asian diet, it's very hard to sort out what benefit is from phytoestrogens in food versus the genetic ability to convert phytoestrogens into a more bioactive form versus overall quality of diet versus cultural attitudes toward menopause and aging or other unknown factors.

Most studies with phytoestrogen supplements, meaning more than can typically be consumed in a diet, don't seem to have a significant (or they have any) impact on hot flushes, sleep quality, or vaginal dryness, so it seems unlikely that phytoestrogens in diet could have an impact. One study suggested supplementing with soy flour may have a minor beneficial effect on vaginal cells under the microscope, but this study didn't ask women if they had a reduction in vaginal dryness or pain with sex so it's not possible to know if the intervention was helpful. Another study of postmenopausal women given 100 mg of isoflavones in diet via soy found no effect on hormones (as expected) and no improvement in menopausal symptoms.

Even knowing the data doesn't support increasing dietary phyto-estrogens as a treatment for symptoms of menopause, some women still want to make a switch to see for themselves if there is a change in their well-being or a reduction in bothersome symptoms. There appears to be no harm in increasing dietary phytoestrogens, but it's important to keep in mind that switching to a diet with more phytoestrogens usually in-volves more vegetables, whole grains, and fish and fewer ultra-processed foods—and as these are all good changes determining any effect from phytoestrogen-rich food isn't possible.

Hormones in Food: Milk

Estrogens are naturally found in milk and hence all dairy products, but how much and is it significant? And what about the hormones given to animals to improve milk production?

These are important questions as a recent study that followed over 52,000 women for eight years linked three glasses of milk a day with an 80 percent increased risk of breast cancer. Even one glass a day was asso-ciated with a 50 percent increased risk. This is a scary sounding statistic, but it doesn't mean 80 percent of women who drink three glasses of milk a day will get breast cancer. For example, at the age of fifty if a woman has approximately a 1 in 42 or 2.4 percent risk of breast cancer in the next ten years, with an 80 percent increased risk means her risk is now 4.3 percent. That's still a big jump and needs further attention, but it's critical to have the right perspective. This association with breast cancer wasn't seen with cheese or yogurt in this study.

It's important to point out that the association between milk and breast cancer has been controversial with some data showing no in-creased risk. This new study is observational, so it's not definitive, but it does present some very compelling data given the number of women en-rolled and the length of time.

Some have postulated that the estrogen in cow's milk could be the culprit for raising the risk of breast cancer. Cow's milk naturally has some estrogen and with modern dairy methods most cows are pregnant, but their milk has very little estrogen—three glasses of whole milk a day has 0.01 percent to 0.1 percent of the average estrogen produced during ovulation. Given estrogens are poorly absorbed from the gastrointesti-nal tract, it seems unlikely any could make it into the bloodstream to have an effect.

The potential impact of estrogen in cow's milk has been studied on mice fed milk supplemented with very high levels of estrogens. There was no negative effect when mice were fed milk with 100 times more es-trogen than commercially available; only milk with 1,000 times more estrogen led to changes and it's not possible to have milk with this much estrogen. The researchers postulated that the estradiol and estrone in cow's milk didn't have an effect until truly massive doses, because these hormones aren't well absorbed, so if milk has a negative effect it's un-likely to be the estrogen.

Most dairy cows have been bred to produce more insulin-like growth factor (IGF-1), which increases milk production and has been hypothe-sized to encourage the growth of cancers. As milk has also been linked with nonhormonally dependent cancers, IGF-1 seems a more plausible cause. Another possibility is lactose, the protein in milk. It's digested into D-glucose and D-galactose—D-galactose is inflammatory and may pro-mote oxidative stress and aging in tissues, increasing the risk of both cardiovascular disease and cancer. It may even paradoxically increase age-related bone loss. As yogurt would be expected to contain similar hormone levels as milk but it doesn't have the same levels of D-galactose due to fermentation, this could explain why milk may pose a risk and fer-mented milk and cheese don't. Yogurt also has the advantage of being beneficial for intestinal bacteria.

Milk is a very complex subject nutrition-wise (see chapter 11 for more on the effect of dairy on bones). A lot of research has been funded by, sur-prise, the dairy industry, so sorting best evidence from bias is challenging. Also, like all foods, milk isn't consumed in a vacuum. It's a good source of protein, calcium, phosphorus, and vitamin D, so for someone strug-gling to get enough of those in their diet milk may be an inexpensive, readily available, and palatable option. Milk and milk products have been a staple in many thriving cultures for thousands of years, and so it's im-portant not to extrapolate.

I've long been a big milk drinker. As I love my high-fiber cereal for breakfast, I've switched to having that with yogurt instead of milk and am currently investigating—somewhat unsuccessfully—the most palatable non-milk options for my latte addiction. I'm trying to keep my milk consumption to one cup a day.

Hormones in Food: Animal Meat

Because cattle are often fed hormones for growth, questions arise regarding beef and reproductive hormones. To address this concern a group of researchers looked at several foods with an assay designed to test the estrogenic activity of a substance on tissue, so they could compare foods with estrogens as well as foods with phytoestrogens. The foods evaluated included beef from cattle with hormone implants and those without, commercial eggs, rice from a boil-in bag (the rice was tested as prepared in the bag and then the rice and bag separately), and a soy burger.

Unsurprisingly, beef from cattle fed hormones had twice the amount of estrogen activity than cattle not fed hormones, 5 ng per 250 g serving versus 2.5 ng per 250 g serving. A medium egg had 6.5 ng. As hens make estradiol in their oocytes just like humans and the oocyte is incorporated into the egg, this isn't unexpected.

Interestingly, the different rice samples had a large range in estrogenic activity, from 0 to 66 ng per 250 g, yet rice has no known phytoestrogens. After further evaluation the investigators discovered the rice with estrogenic activity was contaminated with tiny amounts of the estrogenic mycotoxin called zearalenone (discussed earlier). The soy burger had the highest amount of estrogenic activity, 300,000 ng/g. The researchers then created a model to try to determine how much of these estrogenic compounds would be absorbed and impact tissues. The most estrogenic? The soy burger.

None of this means soy burgers or meat from cattle fed hormones are good or bad; rather, the idea of food being estrogenic can be looked at in a variety of ways and it's important to compare not just levels, but absorption and impact on tissues. It's also important to know that some foods that don't have any natural estrogen or activity could be contaminated with estrogenic mycotoxins. And when there are scary headlines about food, it's important to step back from the panic and make sure there's perspective.

BOTTOM LINE

- The best foods for hormone health are simply the best foods for health.
- Phytoestrogens are compounds found in plants that mimic or block the activity of estrogens.
- Phytoestrogens may have evolved as a defense mechanism against herbivores by affecting fertility.
- Increasing dietary phytoestrogens is unlikely to help symptoms of menopause or reduce risk of breast cancer; however, it's not associated with harm and many diets rich in phytoestrogens have other health benefits.
- Milk is associated with an increased risk of breast cancer, but it seems unlikely that estrogen is the cause as it's absorbed poorly from the gastrointestinal tract and yogurt and cheese aren't linked with breast cancer.

Chapter 20

Bioidenticals, Naturals, and Compounding:

Separating the Medicine from the Marketing

How so-called bioidentical, plant-based, and custom-compounded hormones took root and became the financial behemoths they are today is an even messier story than the one behind menopausal hormone therapy (MHT). What women are really getting with a compounded product is the same hormone as can be prescribed in a pharmaceutical product, with none of the precision or safety monitoring.

The term "bioidentical" is used by some to describe hormones that are supposedly identical to those made by the body, typically estradiol, progesterone, estrone, and testosterone. The word is a portmanteau of biologic or biology and identical. It's not a medical term, but has been used so often it has forced its way into the lexicon.

Bioidentical is problematic on several fronts. First of all, it's medically unnecessary—estradiol made by the ovaries is the same as estradiol made in a lab. The term "therapeutic" or "pharmaceutical" can be used if necessary to emphasize when estradiol is made in a lab. I trust women can learn that difference when it's necessary. Those who use the term "bioidentical" either don't trust women or they don't want them to know this truth.

The term bioidentical also evokes nature, and so we tend to assign a positive meaning to words and phrases that use it. It's important to remember that natural doesn't mean safe. Oleander, the plant, is highly toxic, every part of it. It's so dangerous that a case of oleander poisoning related to eating snails that had eaten oleander has been reported! The estradiol made by our bodies is natural, but it's also responsible for blood clots and breast cancer—even in the amount that is *naturally* produced by the ovary. This doesn't mean that estradiol is unsafe in MHT, but it's an example of how natural means nothing safety-wise, what matters is the science and rigorous evaluation.

And speaking of the science...the term bioidentical isn't even accurate as hormones made in the lab aren't identical on a bimolecular level to those made by the ovary. I know, right? This is possibly the most complicated medical concept in this book, but it's important because women need medicine, not marketing. All chemical elements have isotopes, which are variations with a different number of neutrons (a neutron is one of the subatomic particles in the nucleus of an atom). Carbon, the atom that forms the backbone of steroid hormones, has two naturally occurring isotopes, 12C and 13C. Steroid hormones made by semi-synthesis from steroids in plants have a different ratio of 13C/12C ratio compared with steroid hormones made by the body, so they are not biologically identical. Very close, but not identical. This is because plant steroids like diosgenin, the substance that will be chemically converted into a hormone, have a fixed 13C/12C ratio. Cholesterol, the raw product humans use to make hormones, such as estradiol and progesterone, has a range of different 13C/12C isotopes because humans don't get cholesterol from one source; it comes from a variety of different animal and plant sources. So estradiol made from a single source from yam or soy is like a bag of Halloween candy with one type of candy and estradiol made by the body is the bag with five varieties of candy. As far as the body is concerned, it doesn't matter as the surface of the bag is what counts. So no, hormones made in the lab cannot be biologically identical to what is made by the body; they can be essentially the same as far as your body is concerned, but that doesn't make good marketing.

Estradiol and progesterone made from diosgenin or other plant steroids are also often inaccurately advertised as plant based. This term evokes drying and grinding leaves or plants with a mortar and pestle, whereas the truth is these hormones are manufactured in a multi-step process in a lab from diosgenin or similar compounds (see chapter 17). At one point a part of a plant was involved, but by this same logic gasoline is natural. The other issue with this term is people confuse plant-based estrogen with phytoestrogens, which are plant-based compounds that act like estrogen (see chapter 19). I've spoken with many women who believed their compounded plant-based hormones were an extract of wild yam root, not a hormone, and so didn't have any safety concerns. It's not uncommon for women to hear that so-called plant-based hormones are 100 percent safe, which is no different from what Dr. Wilson was claiming in the 1960s.

Bioidentical and plant-based also imply a lifestyle connection that's no different from marketing Premarin with glamour. Speed boats and cocktails parties are simply replaced with a cornucopia of fruits and vegetables and a stunning woman with ash blond hair striking a yoga pose on a beach at sunset under #naturallife.

Twisting words and presenting half-truths can dramatically alter the information presented about hormones. Consider this statement about progesterone, the first entry in a Google search on the subject:

> Natural Micronized Progesterone is a form of the hormone progesterone derived from plants, that matches the human progesterone, unlike synthetic forms you would find in birth control pills and many forms of synthetic HRT used for menopause [like Provera].

This implies that progesterone is extracted from plants and is good, while other hormones are synthetic Frankenchemicals made in a lab and are a one-way ticket to unmentionable harm. Here is the paragraph rewritten with correct information and terminology:

> Therapeutic progesterone is a semi-synthetic form of the hormone progesterone, meaning it's made in a lab from diosgenin, a compound found in some plants. Therapeutic progesterone has the same chemical structure as human progesterone. Other semi-synthetic hormones with different but related chemical structures to progesterone can be found in birth control pills and many forms of MHT [one is Provera, which is medroxyprogesterone acetate and like therapeutic progesterone is also made in a lab from diosgenin].

Sounds a bit different, hey? Accuracy matters; it's medicine not alchemy.

Compounding

Compounded hormones are made by a pharmacy instead of a pharmaceutical company. The end product can be a pill, cream, or implanted pellet. Compounding pharmacies fill important gaps; for example, when there is an allergy to an ingredient in the pharmaceutical option, when no commercial pharmaceutical option exists, or the commercial product is exorbitantly expensive.

Some compounding pharmacies have become an industry in customized compounded hormones. Between 1 million and 2.5 million women in the United States are using these products with an approximate 26–32 million prescriptions a year, compared with 36 million prescriptions for hormones from Big Pharma. One estimate is 40 percent of hormones prescribed in the United States for MHT are compounded preparations. Compounded hormones are a $1 billion/year industry, with none of the regulatory hassles or expensive studies. Given these numbers it hardly seems accurate to call them Little Pharma, they're really Big Natural.

With a pharmaceutical hormone I know exactly how much hormone is in each dose, how much of that dose is absorbed and how quickly, and how that hormone behaves in the body. I also know how the hormone impacts the lining of the uterus. None of this is available for compounded products. This lack of data is especially concerning as customized recipes (for example, using a novel cream or different fillers in a pill), offered as a benefit of compounding can result in inaccurate doses (meaning the product contains more or less than claimed) or higher or lower levels in the blood due to inconsistencies in how the drug is absorbed. One study looking at estrogen levels in compounded products found that 30 percent contained more than advertised on the labeling—at times up to 200 percent more estrogen—a cause for concern.

FDA-approved prescription medications are followed for years after approval to identify concerns that may have been missed with the relatively short-term data that was used in the approval process. This is called postmarketing surveillance and is an essential component of ensuring the safety of pharmaceuticals. This doesn't occur formally with most compounded hormones. The lack of reporting of adverse events leads to the misperceptions that these medications are safer, just like me not looking under my fridge can give me the false reassurance that it's totally clean under there. Except with hormones what you don't know can hurt you. Compounded medications don't always display the same warning labels mandated by the FDA, also supporting the illusion of safety. Despite the lack of scrutiny, up to 67 percent of women believe compounded hormones are safer than pharmaceutical prescriptions.

Recently, the FDA became aware of 4,202 adverse events related to compounded estradiol and testosterone pellets marketed by BioTE Medical (BioTE) that were never reported to the FDA. These adverse events included cancers, strokes, heart attacks, and deep vein thrombosis (blood clots) and a myriad of other concerning issues. BioTE sourced their hormone pellets from Carie Boyd's Prescription Shop and AnazaoHealth Corporation.

Their widespread acceptance of compounded MHT shows the true marketing prowess of Big Natural, because the raw hormones used in compounded products are the same as used by Big Pharma. Compounding pharmacies don't know their yam farmer. If the product contains estradiol or progesterone or any other hormone (with the exception of conjugated equine estrogens), the hormone was synthesized in a lab, and whether the estradiol is from a pharmaceutical company or from a compounding pharmacy, it was made the same way.

Many women are told compounded hormones can be tailored to get a so-called custom, personalized fit by adding other hormones such as estriol, estrone, DHEA, and testosterone. The only indication for testosterone is lowered libido (see chapter 15 for more on testosterone). There is no data on the safety of pregnenolone in MHT.

Dehydroepiandrosterone (DHEA) is a hormone made by the adrenal gland. It can be converted into DHEA-S (a sulfate form) and together DHEA and DHEA-S are the most abundant steroid hormones in the body. DHEA is one of the precursor hormones converted in the body to estradiol, progesterone, and testosterone (see Appendix A, p. 342). DHEA levels decrease with age. As some studies have linked higher levels of DHEA with successful aging the idea that supplementation could have a health benefit is a valid hypothesis. However, studies show that DHEA is not associated with an improvement in sexual function, mood, or bone density. Higher levels of DHEA during the menopause transition and after menopause are associated with an increased risk of depression. For these reasons DHEA is not recommended in MHT. There is an FDA approved vaginal DHEA-S product for women with genitourinary syndrome of menopause (see chapter 14).

Estrone and estriol are often compounded with estradiol in formulations known as biest (sometimes 80 percent estriol and 20 percent estradiol, but other times 50 percent estriol and 50 percent estradiol) and triest (80 percent estriol, 10 percent estrone, and 10 percent estradiol). These products can be compounded into capsules, a lozenge, creams, and gels. Estrone and estriol are relatively weak estrogens, so more has to be given to get the same effect as estradiol. Estriol is primarily made by the placenta, so I've always found that passing this off as natural or specialized for women in menopause as odd. Claims that estrone and estriol are safer or more gentle (whatever that means) are unfounded.

In 2013 a group of researchers compared the blood levels of women taking biest to an FDA-approved estradiol patch, the first time such data was published (which is shocking considering how long these products have been available). A 2.5 mg dose of biest in Vanicream (the vehicle cream, and one of the most commonly used), which is 2 mg of estriol and 0.5 mg of estradiol, was tested and compared with a 0.05 mg estradiol patch, supposedly equivalent doses. The biest produced much lower blood levels of estradiol than the patch, and the estradiol levels were erratic versus steady for the patch. A 3 mg dose of biest produced higher levels than the 2.5 mg dose, but still less than the 0.05 mg estradiol patch.

Given the much lower blood levels with the 2.5 mg dose of biest there's a concern that improvement of symptoms on this product could be placebo and, more importantly, that it won't protect against osteoporosis. Interestingly, there was no significant rise in blood levels of estriol with the biest cream. As the accuracy of testing very low levels of estriol isn't known, it's hard to draw conclusions, but it's possible the estriol in this formulation isn't even absorbed across the skin or that it's rapidly metabolized or converted into other hormones.

But what about the women who say they feel better on compounded hormones? It can take a while to adjust to hormones, both the benefit and the side effects, and by the time someone seeks a different path of care with compounded alternatives, the period of adjustment may be close to passing. There's also the benefit of an expensive placebo, which

264 — THE MENOPAUSE MANIFESTO

studies tell us is more effective than less expensive placebos. Many providers of compounded hormones don't accept insurance, so in addition to the expense of hormones there's potentially a more expensive office visit. Operating outside of the insurance system also typically allows a provider to spend more time with their patients—a massive issue with the American health care system—and more time to listen and discuss options is almost certainly going to leave a person feeling better, possibly affecting outcome.

I can hear the insults now: Dr. Gunter is just a tool of Big Pharma (I haven't taken any money from a pharmaceutical company since 2004). It wouldn't surprise me if a variation of this appears on an online review. The truth about the safety and the science of so-called bioidentical, plant-based, and compounded products will affect a large revenue source for many.

There is a database that tracks whether doctors have taken money from Big Pharma called Dollars for Doctors. Unfortunately, there are no disclosures about the kind of money providers might get for promoting compounded products or for being associated with labs and recommending unindicated hormone levels.

One major issue with Big Pharma is how their studies almost always show a positive outcome. Take, for example, drugs for stomach ulcers. According to work done by Dr. Ben Godacre, a physician and researcher in the United Kingdom, 85 percent of studies funded by a drug company show these medications to be beneficial, but when that same medication is evaluated with government-funded research only 50 percent of studies have positive outcomes. Wall Street only rewards blockbusters, so data on failed drugs is rarely published as it negatively affects stock prices. This is really unfortunate, as learning a drug doesn't work is actually very valuable.

The answer to the litany of issues with Big Pharma isn't to send women to an unregulated industry with little to no research; the answer is to demand better from the industry. Compounded hormones aren't helping women avoid the gaps in medicine; they're exploiting them. If these products are so amazing the compounded industry should turn some of that $1 billion a year they make into quality studies to prove their claims.

That's the wonderful thing about science—if you prove a product is superior, I will accept it and change.

Compounded Hormones and Blood Tests

So-called hormone customization with compounded hormones has another dark side—blood tests to individualize therapy. It sounds appealing, but it's not based in what we know about hormones and menopause. Hormone levels aren't recommended as the aim isn't a specific hormone level. Hormones are started based on age, symptoms, and risk for osteoporosis. It's also important to note that hormone levels vary dramatically during the menopause transition (for example, levels in the morning can be different from the evening), so this is a highly unreliable barometer. Some providers recommend salivary hormone testing—I see this a lot from naturopaths. This "testing" is useless.

In studies where more elegant monitoring is performed over multiple days, hormone levels don't correlate well with symptoms. After menopause, the circulating estrogens in the blood don't reflect what the body needs; they're estrogen effluent or runoff from the tissues. In addition, blood levels may not reflect what's happening in the tissues as they can convert estradiol to estrone or estrone to estradiol as needed (see chapter 3).

Hormone tests also add unnecessary expense and provide the illusion that a provider is listening and is being responsive and they keep women coming back for office visits to discuss these levels and adjust them. These tests are rarely covered by insurance carriers. The tests are a waste of money...this is one area where insurance companies get it right.

How Did the Bioidentical/Plant-Based Myth Take Hold?

The terms "bioidentical" and "natural" for MHT have been around since at least the 1990s. These words tapped into the expanding practice of alternative medicine, which was already fairly mainstream by the mid-1990s. Proponents of these unstudied regimens didn't argue that women were being hormonally ignored by medicine. After all, 41 percent of menopausal women in North America in 1997 were taking MHT. What they argued was pharmaceutical MHT was unnatural—"horse hormones are natural for horses, not women," was a common quip. There was also an inaccurate assertion that compounded hormones were somehow better because they could be "balanced" to meet a woman's needs (think back to biest and triest), but no evidence ever materialized.

With the WHI the belief that CEE (Premarin)—so called horse hormones—was bad was seemingly vindicated as CEE was the estrogen studied in the WHI. As many women and providers were hesitant to prescribe pharmaceutical estrogens and there were few evidence-based nonhormonal alternatives, a vacuum of care was created and in walked Big Natural. The absence of data regarding risk with these products (you have to study something to identify risk) was parlayed into safety, and the certainty with which these hormones were promoted must have felt like a welcome alternative to the conflicting messages from medicine. The confidence surrounding bioidenticals was mistaken as competence.

Bioidenticals didn't really explode until celebrities got into the act. Suzanne Somers, the actress and celebrity endorser of fitness equipment and author of books such as *Eat, Cheat and Melt the Fat Away*, published her first book on hormones in 2004, *The Sexy Years: The Hormone Connection*. There is little difference between the theories advanced by Somers and those by Dr. Wilson in his 1966 *Feminine Forever*. Menopause is a disease and women can stay fit, feminine, and fantastic through the miracle of estrogen, which according to Somers was—yes, you guessed it, 100 percent safe. The only substantive difference between Wilson and Somers was the latter's claims about bioidenticals.

And then Oprah Winfrey stepped into the picture devoting two episodes to MHT in January 2009, one where she interviewed Robin McGraw (wife of Dr. Phil) and two weeks later with Suzanne Somers. Dr. Christiane Northrup, a longtime devotee of bioidentical hormones, was included as the medical voice of reason. The information presented by Somers was largely medically incorrect and generally went unchallenged. The doses and regimen used by Somers would be a joke, except that's what she was taking and recommending to other women. Somers claimed this was the regimen recommended by her own doctor, Dr. Prudence Hall.

According to *Newsweek*, who covered the episodes at the time, the fact that Suzanne Somers developed breast cancer as well as precancer of the uterus while taking her bioidentical hormones was never mentioned. Somers was simply the warrior woman forging a path for wellness.

It's no wonder Somers developed precancer of the uterus. She was using topical progesterone cream, which is ineffective at protecting the uterus from estrogen. This was never pointed out, then again Winfrey's expert, Dr. Northrup, recommends topical progesterone in her books. About these therapies Winfrey said, "Women have the right to demand a better quality of life for ourselves."

Yes, women *should* demand a better quality of life, but it's absurd and offensive to suggest an unstudied MHT regimen that promotes unsafe topical progesterone is empowerment. Never mind Somers's message about femininity as currency. I often wonder if this better quality of life that Oprah wanted women to demand also included refusing vaccines, because when Dr. Northrup was on the show she was already public about her opposition to the HPV vaccine. Cervical cancer hardly feels like a path to empowerment.

Winfrey apparently found Somers and Northrup so compelling that she decided to start what she called bioidentical estrogen, although whether she used a pharmaceutical or compounded product was not discussed. At the time approval from Winfrey was better than approval from God. Oprah recounted in *O, The Oprah Magazine* that immediately she "felt the veil lift." How can modern medicine with our stodgy studies and demands for data compete with Oprah Winfrey writing the following:

> After three days, the sky was bluer, my brain was no longer fuzzy, my memory was sharper. I was literally singing and had a skip in my step.

It is important to point out that MHT does not appear to be effective at treating menopausal brain fog, and dramatic improvements in menopause-related symptoms with MHT are not typically seen in three days.

Every misogynistic trope about hormones was successfully rebranded by Somers as feminism, and the absence of medical evidence and taking an unstudied hormone regimen were apparently advocating for oneself. According to Google trends, January 2009 remains the peak online search for the term "bioidentical hormones."

As for Somers's compelling research? Her personal doctor, Dr. Prudence Hall, who also wrote the foreword for Somers's 2013 book, *I'm Too Young for This!* is under probation by the Medical Board of California until August 2022 related to her use of hormones. Furthermore, while on probation—according to the Medical Board—she is prohibited from representing herself as a specialist in OB/GYN or endocrinology. She was charged with "gross negligence, repeated negligent acts, and failure to maintain adequate and accurate medical records in the care and treatment of two patients."

And Dr. Northrup? As of September 2020 she was promoting antivaccine beliefs and QAnon conspiracy theories as well as COVID-19 antimask propaganda to her more than 100,000 followers on Instagram and to her over 100,000 Twitter followers on Twitter.

It's not surprising to find conspiracy theories—the idea that people or a group are colluding in clandestine ways to influence outcomes—linked with bioidentical or so-called natural hormones. After all, there are common themes between this kind of alternative medicine and conspiracy theories. They both advance the concept that people have been lied to, be it by medicine, the media, the government, or the pharmaceutical industry. One popular conspiracy theory is bioidentical hormones were very popular until Wyeth/Ayerst developed Premarin, putting the makers of bioidenticals out of business. This is ludicrous. What women were getting before Premarin were injections of theelin, which was estrogens extracted from the urine or placentas of pregnant women or from hog ovaries. Theelin was likely awful by our standards today, producing wild swings in hormone levels. And the hormones of the 1920s and 1930s weren't made by the local self-trained wise-woman, they were made by pharmaceutical companies.

At its heyday Premarin had 41 percent of the MHT market, and compounded hormones currently have 40 percent of the market share. It's a strange tactic to parlay this success story into victimization by Big Pharma.

The menopause transition can be a time of anxiety for some women, and anxiety drives people to look for comfort. Claims of customization and the certainty of Big Natural provide the illusion of control and safety. And what better comfort than the healing balm of nature. The back and forth of studies on MHT—part of the scientific process—is chaos in comparison.

It's important to acknowledge that women have been lied to by medicine—they've had their hot flushes dismissed, been told pain with sex is normal and just have a glass of wine to relax, and their crumbling bones have been ignored. The pharmaceutical industry does selectively publish data, and some doctors are influenced by money from Big Pharma. These truths make the part of the message about so-called natural therapies being an answer to issues in medicine more believable.

I want to acknowledge how hard it will be for many women reading this information about so-called natural therapies and compounded hormones. It's a normal reaction to want to dismiss this information, because the alternative is to accept that you've been led astray. Keep in mind it was never possible to make an informed decision about these products without accurate information.

If custom compounded or so-called plant-based products were truly superior, there would be quality data to support their use, and consequently experts like me would be prescribing them and our professional societies would be recommending them. If these products are so safe and so effective, why hasn't this $1 billion industry provided the research to prove it?

BOTTOM LINE

- Compounded hormones are an untested, unregulated $1 billion/year market.
- The raw hormone used in MHT from a compounded pharmacy comes from the same sources as the hormones in pharmaceutical MHT.
- Compounded estrogen creams may not have enough estradiol to treat hot flushes and prevent osteoporosis.
- Topical progesterone is often recommended as part of bioidentical preparations, but progesterone is not absorbed well topically, so this is unsafe.
- There are safety concerns with testosterone pellets and they're not recommended.

Chapter 21

Meno-Diets:

What Makes a Healthy Menopause and Beyond

A HEALTHY DIET IS ONE of the cornerstones of optimizing health across the menopause continuum, and yet less than 20 percent of women in the United States maintain a healthy diet during their menopause transition and beyond. This is unfortunate, especially considering that a healthy diet has many benefits, from lowering the risk of heart disease (the number one cause of death for women), reducing the risk of type 2 diabetes, preventing constipation and hemorrhoids, lowering the risk of colon cancer, and reducing the risk of Alzheimer's disease to name a few.

Before we get started, let's dispel with that quote assigned to Hippocrates, "Let food be thy medicine." It appears everywhere—from medical journals to Instagram accounts promoting diets to a post on Gwyneth Paltrow's goop.com that was written to chastise me because I criticized their lack of science and fact checking. This quote is fake. It doesn't appear anywhere in the sixty or so volumes of the *Hippocratic Corpus* (the works attributed to Hippocrates and his peers). What was that about the value of fact checking goop?

The ancient Greeks distinguished food from medicine. Diet was an important part of good health and recommended based on symptoms, sex, and season (not exactly supported by science). Their diets were related to their understanding of the human body and diseases, much of which we now know to be wrong. For example, specific foods that were believed to be drying were recommended for women as women were overly moist. Also, the idea that the ancient Greeks unlocked dietary secrets that have not been, and never will be, published in a reputable medical journal, but will rather be disclosed to you on a site selling supplements, is rather suspect.

Food science is challenging enough, but add in appeals to ancient wisdom (our elders knew better, like the fake Hippocrates quote) and natural fallacy (nature is best) and sorting food fact from fiction is a significant challenge. While it's true that eating oranges can cure scurvy and a diet of red meat may reverse iron deficiency, those diseases are the result of dietary inadequacies, so the food isn't treating an underlying condition.

A healthy diet is an important foundation and should be thought of as preventative care. Despite this medical truth, discussions about diets often fall by the wayside in favor of interventions, such as menopausal hormone therapy (MHT) or supplements. The reasons are multiple and sometimes complex. While it's true many health care providers receive little to no training in nutrition, many are equipped to have these conversations but they don't have the time in a twenty-minute (or less) office visit to discuss changes of menopause and menopausal hormone therapy, never mind diet unless they can bend time to their will. It can also be difficult for people to access the real experts on nutrition—registered dietitians or appropriately credentialed nutritionists.

And then there is fat phobia, not just in society but in medicine. Most of the messaging women receive about food in a medical office is tied to their supposedly problematic bodies as opposed to the foundational benefits of a healthy diet. When women can't get answers from medicine or are dismissed or insulted, it's no wonder they look elsewhere. Enter the nutri-charlatans—from doctors, to registered dietitians, to nutritionists, to influencers—these are people with wild claims about the curative powers of this season's superfood and bold promises of a hormone reset or the supposed dangers of grain brain. And of course, their program and supplements or special tea can fix it all. For a price.

The Challenges of Food Science

In addition to communication and access issues for nutrition, food science is challenging. Studies can have bias due to funding, in the same way that Big Pharma influences studies on medications. Then there's the sheer volume of data produced, and much of it is contradictory. Almost every day it seems as if there is a new dietary do or don't. Are eggs good now or are they bad? It's easy to lose track as the consensus seems to change as often as hemlines.

Diet is also incredibly difficult to study. One can look at populations and note a dietary pattern that seems linked with a health outcome—this is known as an observational study. For example: after following a group of women living in East Asia, one might observe they have a lower incidence of hot flushes and they also eat more soy than women in the United States. Might the soy be the cause? Maybe, but all we have is an association. It could also be that soy is consumed in higher amounts throughout the lifetime, not just during the menopause transition. Or that diets high in soy are typically higher in vegetables and lower in saturated fat. Or perhaps people who live in East Asia have consumed soy for centuries and have co-evolved to use it more effectively, either by genetics or differences in intestinal bacteria, so the benefit can't be translated to other populations. Or maybe it has nothing to do with the soy per se, but that soy consumption is linked with education or another social determinant of health. The association with soy and a reduced risk of hot flushes could also be a purely spurious finding, meaning it's a statistical fluke.

What we eat and how our body uses that fuel is very complex and can rarely be boiled down to a single ingredient. Observational studies can generate interesting information and trigger hypotheses, but the data is rarely clean enough to make definitive conclusions.

There are also studies with food interventions, meaning a research study that enrolls women, randomly assigns a diet, and controls for as many variables as possible so the only thing different about the two groups is the diet. These studies can answer many more questions than observational studies, but they're very expensive, and getting a lot of people to follow a diet for a long period of time can be challenging. One good example is the dietary arm of the Women's Health Initiate (WHI), the same study that looked at MHT. The WHI randomly assigned over 48,000 women to either a low-fat eating pattern or their regular diet. This was supposed to be *the* study to determine if a low-fat diet could prevent breast cancer, colorectal cancer, and coronary heart disease in women after menopause. The problem? Adherence to the diet wasn't great and the women assigned to the low-fat arm had only a 9 percent reduction in breast cancer, which was within the margin of statistical error. These women also lost a few kilograms, likely from tracking what they ate, which could have explained their slightly lower rate of breast cancer. This doesn't mean we should blame the women who were unable to follow the diet. Rather, the lack of adherence means the study design was poor, not a sign of a problem with the participants.

To control for the fact that it's harder to follow a specific diet when people have access to their own kitchens and restaurants, there are studies where people live at a research facility and all the food is prepared and tracked and blood levels and other measurements are taken regularly. These studies produce high-quality data, but few people want to live in what amounts to a motel for months, so these studies are limited to several weeks. This short-term data may not necessarily pan out over the long term. These studies are also expensive, so they are generally limited to small numbers of participants. Even in this highly controlled situation, the results can be conflicting. For example, one such study compared a high-fat ketogenic diet with a high-carbohydrate vegetarian diet. These two diets are nutritional opposites, and yet each diet improved some variables and worsened others.

Basically, the science of nutrition is challenging, and sometimes studies raise more questions than they answer, but that is also the meandering path of science. The problem is most of us—doctors included—want a nice, tidy answer about food. Perhaps this desire explains the popularity of so-called super foods. Who doesn't want a food that can do it all? An apple a day was supposed to keep the doctor away. That is until açai berries, turmeric, quinoa, kale, oatmeal, pomegranate, coconut oil, and celery juice were all found to be super foods. How does a super food get replaced so quickly? Shouldn't it be super forever?

Nutrition 101

Macronutrients provide energy—protein: 4 calories per gram, carbohydrates: 4 calories per gram, and fat: 9 calories per gram. They also provide essential building blocks. For example, amino acids in protein are up-cycled into everything from enzymes to eyelashes, and the cholesterol in fat is repurposed into many things, ranging from cell membranes to estrogen.

Micronutrients are vitamins and minerals essential for the body to function. Unlike macronutrients, they're only needed in small amounts, hence the "micro." Some examples are iron, iodine, folate, zinc, and vitamins A and C.

Carbohydrates are chains of sugar molecules and are divided into two groups: simple and complex. Simple carbohydrates have one or two sugar molecules, so they are smaller and easier to digest. Examples include sugars found in food, such as sucrose and glucose in fruits and vegetables and galactose and lactose in dairy as well as refined sugars such as table sugar and high fructose corn syrup.

Complex carbohydrates are strings of three or more sugar molecules and include starches and fiber, but only starches can be digested. Starches include many vegetables (such as broccoli, carrots, and potatoes), legumes (think soybeans, lentils, beans, peas, and chickpeas), nuts, and whole grains (for example, oatmeal, whole wheat, brown rice, and quinoa). When a grain is refined, the parts with most of the fiber and nutrients have been removed (the bran and the germ). Whole wheat flour and brown rice are complex carbohydrates, whereas white flour and white rice are simple carbohydrates.

Simple carbohydrates and starches are broken down into glucose, which is either used immediately for energy, converted into a storage sugar called glycogen, or repackaged and stored as fat. Simple carbohydrates are easier to digest, so the glucose hits the bloodstream quickly, whereas with complex carbohydrates the glucose is delivered at a slower rate. Diets high in simple carbohydrates are linked with increased rates of cardiovascular disease and type 2 diabetes.

A diet high in refined carbohydrates has been linked with lower levels of sex hormone binding globulin (SHBG) and thus increased levels of active or unbound estrogen and testosterone. (Remember the Seats Handy on the Bus, Girl? mnemonic from chapter 3.) This may have a negative impact on hormonally responsive cancers, such as breast and endometrial (lining of the uterus).

Be a Fiber Evangelical!

I love talking about fiber with my patients. It has so many health benefits and it's a dietary intervention that can be discussed without ever mentioning weight. It involves adding something in, not the denial of taking a food away, and it can produce rapid results that can feel, well, cathartic.

Fiber is a nondigestible carbohydrate. There are two types: soluble, which is dissolvable in water, and insoluble—which isn't. They are both beneficial and are typically found together in the same food. Functional fiber is found in supplements.

Women need 25 g of fiber a day and men 38 g—I'm sure there is a great joke in here about men being more full of shit. The typical fiber intake in the United States in 17 g a day, and only 5 percent of people get the recommended daily amount—so lots of room for improvement. Dietary fiber has so many health benefits, so bumping up intake is a way for many women to improve their health. The only real downside is where there is fiber, there will be gas.

Why is fiber so amazing? It provides bulk, which increases the sensation of fullness after a meal, and the increased volume of stool stimulates the bowel, reducing constipation. Preventing constipation and softer stool reduce the risk of hemorrhoids, and no person ever in the history of humanity has said, "No, I'm good, I like my hemorrhoids." Fiber also slows the digestion of carbohydrates, reducing spikes in blood sugar after a meal, and it draws water from the contents of the colon into the stool, making the stool soft, so it passes more easily and is less hard or scratchy on its way out. Fiber is also associated with a reduction in total cholesterol and LDL cholesterol (the bad cholesterol), and postmenopausal women typically get a bigger reduction in cholesterol in response to fiber intake than women in their menopausal transition.

Fiber may also affect estrogen levels over the long term. Bile is a substance made by the liver and it's excreted via the gallbladder into the bowel to aid with digestion. It also contains some estrogen. In the small intestine much of the estrogen is reabsorbed and transported back to the liver (a process called enterohepatic circulation). Fiber reduces the reabsorption of estrogen from the bowel for premenopausal women. This is one proposed mechanism for fiber's association with a lower rate of hormonally responsive breast cancers. After menopause fiber doesn't have this impact on estrogen as levels of estradiol in the blood are incredibly low because most estrogen is produced locally in tissues, so there is little to no estrogen in bile. So don't worry, a high fiber meal isn't going to result in an evening of hot flushes on top of the gas. That would be the worst!

Fiber lowers the pH of stool, is anti-inflammatory, and inhibits the growth of potentially harmful bacteria while increasing absorption of some minerals. Some soluble fiber is also a prebiotic, meaning it encourages the growth of healthy gut bacteria. Two examples are inulin and fructooligosaccharides, found in onions, leeks, garlic, wheat, oats, asparagus, chicory root, and Jerusalem artichoke. The Jerusalem artichoke can have very high levels of inulin, earning it the well-deserved nickname fartchoke. I've had them once. I eat a lot of fiber so I felt my colon and I had trained for this moment. I was mistaken. It was the most painful gas I've ever experienced.

A high-fiber diet is also associated with lower rates of cardiovascular disease, type 2 diabetes, and colon cancer. Fiber may also help some people with weight maintenance, either from the sensation of fullness or other mechanisms. But I only discuss that in the office when people ask. Fiber has so many benefits there's no reason to bring weight into the discussion. Even reducing constipation and hemorrhoids makes fiber worthwhile! There is nothing quite like the happiness of a patient whose constipation has resolved courtesy of a dietary change.

Fiber is found in whole grains, legumes, and certain fruits and vegetables, so most foods that are high in fiber also have important micronutrients. Wheat bran is the outer portion of the wheat grain and is particularly effective at bulking stool. Functional fiber in supplements or added to food is effective for constipation, but is unlikely to have all of the health benefits of dietary fiber.

I encourage every woman regardless of where she is on the menopause continuum to record what she eats for several days and calculate the fiber intake and adjust accordingly. This is one of the easiest dietary changes you can make and it doesn't involve denial. For example, adding in a serving of high-fiber cereal a day or switching from white rice to brown rice are both simple changes that you can make.

I'm personally a fan of high-fiber cereals, and after taste-testing many, I have a list of several that I recommend. After all, it's not whether there's enough fiber, it's whether it has enough fiber and is palatable enough that one can eat it regularly that matters. I like cereals because they're readily available, it's easy advice for people to follow, they're often supplemented with micronutrients so can be nutritionally complete, and getting 25 g of fiber a day is difficult even for those who eat a lot of vegetables and legumes. My favorite high-fiber cereals are Kashi Go Rise (13 g of fiber and 12 g of protein, a good way to stay powered up all morning), Kellogg's All Bran (also 13 g of fiber per serving and makes a lovely homemade granola with ¼ cup of dried oatmeal, and some walnuts) and Post Foods Uncle Sam (10 g of fiber but unlike the others zero added sugar, just wheat berry and flax).

Food Processing

Natural food is unchanged from its form in nature—think a banana, chickpeas, chicken, or honey. Anything that changes the fundamental nature of the food, from freezing to pasteurization to adding sugar, is processing. Flour is processed as is cheese, tofu, and a can of kidney beans. Even baby carrots (they're just larger carrots that have been whittled down to bite size, I was so disappointed to learn that fact). Processed foods are often part of a nutritious diet, and many aspects of processing improve food safety and/or extends the shelf life.

Ultra-processed foods are the health issue. Although the definition has changed slightly over the years, these foods are typically thought of as industrial formulations, meaning they have ingredients other than salt, sugar, and fats not typically used in home cooking. Some definitions have also included food with five or more ingredients (my Uncle Sam Cereal only has four ingredients, just saying). Ultra-processed foods account for 58 percent of dietary energy consumed in America and 90 percent of the added sugar.

There are always some exceptions with diet, which only adds to the confusion. Most packaged breakfast cereals are ultra-processed foods, but there are some that provide a high amount of whole grains and fiber as well as added micronutrients with only a small amount of added sugar. Some store-bought potato chips are simply potatoes, salt, and oil, but most people would consider them ultra-processed as not many people have the equipment to produce these kinds of chips at home.

Ultra-processed foods, with the exception of some breakfast cereals, are typically nutritionally incomplete—they offer fuel but are deficient in micronutrients. They also lead people to eat more calories. In one study where people had all their meals prepared in a research facility and were asked to eat until they felt satisfied, those on a diet of ultra-processed foods ate 500 more calories a day. There are probably a variety of reasons—these foods are easier to chew, the lack of fiber means less of a feeling of fullness, greater changes in levels of glucose and insulin, and the added sugar, fat, and salt just taste so good.

Ultra-processed foods are associated with abdominal obesity, metabolic syndrome, type 2 diabetes, hypertension (high blood pressure), and cardiovascular disease. As these conditions are more common during the menopause transition and postmenopause, after maximizing fiber intake eliminating ultra-processed foods is probably the next best dietary recommendation.

Eliminating ultra-processed foods in America can be a privilege. Due to social determinants of health and structural racism, many people live in neighborhoods where access to fresh foods may be limited. In addition, working long hours—often at more than one job—to survive financially can leave little time for grocery shopping and food prep. Healthier foods are often more expensive than ultra-processed equivalents.

A Word on Fats

Fat is either saturated or unsaturated, which refers to how the carbon atoms bond with hydrogen atoms. This chemical definition isn't necessary to learn; the gist is saturated fats come from animal products (think meat, dairy, and poultry) and are typically solid at room temperature. Unsaturated fats come from fish, vegetables, nuts, and grains. There are some exceptions (always with the exceptions in nutrition); for example, coconut oil is high in saturated fat. Unsaturated fats can be further classified as monounsaturated and polyunsaturated—the latter often called PUFAs, but you may know them by their common name, omega-3 and omega-6 fatty acids.

Dietary fat is important for calories, improving absorption of fat-soluble vitamins, and fats are important building blocks for the body.

Excess fat is stored in adipose cells and can later be converted into glucose if needed; this process is called ketogenesis. After a meal, dietary fat is broken down into cholesterol and triglycerides (see chapter 8). Low-fat diets haven't shown to have health benefits, but all fat isn't created equal. The bulk of the evidence suggests a diet high in saturated fats is associated with an increased risk of cardiovascular disease and increased levels of LDL (the bad cholesterol). Unsaturated fats—mostly found in vegetable oils, nuts, and fish—have the opposite effect. Trans fats, which are fats modified in an industrial process, are universally bad and should no longer be in food in the United States due to regulatory changes.

Omega-3 fatty acids deserve a special mention. They are alpha-linolenic acid (ALA), eicosapentaenoic acid (EPA), and docosahexaenoic acid (DHA). ALA is found in flaxseed (to get the ALA from flaxseed it needs to be ground), walnuts, soybeans, canola oils, and omega-3 enriched eggs, but DHA and EPA are found only in fish and other seafood. The body can't make ALA so it has to come from diet. We can convert some ALA into small amounts of EPA and DHA, although typically this isn't enough so they also need to come from diet. This is likely one reason why diets rich in fatty fish are linked with so many positive outcomes as other dietary sources of EPA and DHA aren't available. Omega-3 fatty acids lower triglycerides, reduce atherosclerosis, and may lower blood pressure. Supplementation with omega-3 fatty acids is often indicated for postmenopausal women (see chapter 22 for more).

The major omega-6 fatty acid is linoleic acid and it's found in vegetable oils, such as corn, safflower, and flax seeds. Omega-6 fatty acids also lower the risk for diabetes and are also heart healthy, so efforts to increase omega-3 fatty acids shouldn't come at the expense of decreasing omega-6 fatty acids.

Caffeine

It's all good. *All Good.*

Okay, almost all good.

Perhaps you don't share my caffeine addiction, but like a diligent scientist I'm proclaiming my bias here up front. I know I'm not the only one; 85 percent of adults in the United States have caffeine daily, and coffee and tea are two of the most popular beverages worldwide. Caffeine can also be found in cacao beans (chocolate), sports drinks, and other plants and berries.

Overall, the data is reassuring—up to five cups of coffee a day isn't harmful and appears to be associated with a reduction in all causes of mortality, a reduced incidence of liver disease, gallbladder disease, and Parkinson's disease. Caffeine may also reduce the risk of depression, reduce the pain of headaches, and increase alertness. However, for some there can be a negative effect on sleep and an increase in anxiety. Caffeine poisoning would require seventy-five to a hundred cups in a short period of time, so it's not really a possibility with food and drink; however, caffeine supplements are another matter and should be avoided.

There is one coffee caveat—a chemical in coffee called cafestol can raise cholesterol. Levels of cafestol are highest in unfiltered coffee, like French press, lower in espresso, and the lowest levels in drip and instant coffee. More than six cups a day of unfiltered coffee or espresso is linked to higher levels of LDL cholesterol, so women with an elevated LDL who drink a lot of unfiltered coffee or espresso may wish to switch to drip. For reference, I'm a "four to five cups of espresso a day" gal.

Alcohol

I was looking online for a recent study I'd remembered reading, but had forgotten where I'd left my digital bread crumbs so I Googled, "new study alcohol." The second and third results—from the same health news site no less—were as follows:

"Light drinking may protect brain function," and "Even low-risk drinking can be harmful."

I mean come on.

Alcohol can affect many organ systems, impacting sleep, hot flushes, libido, the brain, bones—this will be addressed in the relevant chapters. From an overall health standpoint, alcohol and its toxic metabolites can damage the liver, heart, bone, and stomach. Alcohol also plays a role in car accidents, other accidents, and homicides. Alcohol use is linked with several cancers, such as breast, esophageal cancer, and liver.

There may be several ways that alcohol increases the risk for breast cancer. Some metabolites may be carcinogenic; alcohol is linked with obesity, a risk factor for breast cancer; alcohol affects the liver's ability to metabolize estrogen, thus raising levels; and alcohol impacts the liver's ability to produce the carrier protein SHBG (sex hormone binding globulin, remember Seats Handy on the Bus, Girl?—see chapter 3), so more estrogen and testosterone are unbound and free to impact tissues.

In contrast, there's data that links low levels of alcohol intake, especially red wine, with a reduced risk of heart attack. This is admittedly frustrating, but alcohol having both risks and benefits is a good example of how a single food does not a diet make. A small amount of alcohol when part of one kind of diet may well offer benefit and in other contexts or amounts may not.

For an otherwise healthy woman who doesn't have alcoholism or liver disease and isn't going to drink and drive, less than 17 g a day of alcohol may offer some health benefits, meaning all things considered there's a net benefit. In the United States, 12 ounces of regular beer (5 percent alcohol), 5 ounces of wine (12 percent alcohol), and 1.5 ounces of distilled spirit (40 percent alcohol) is 14 g, which is equivalent to 1.75 units. These seven to nine drinks a week should be divided over at least the course of three days, not saved up for one night.

Eating Plans and Menopause

With this basic nutritional advice, what are the best dietary plans for the menopause continuum?

The healthiest diet for menopause will typically be the one that's heart healthy, as heart disease is the number one cause of death for women. Ideally, this diet should also include special attention to prevention of osteoporosis, Alzheimer's disease, and breast and endometrial cancer.

It's easy to cherry-pick data from studies and weave a compelling tale about the supposed superiority of one diet over another, but many diets have both pluses and minuses, and the reality of food science means there are a lot of "well, maybes" and "it depends." There's also context. For example, it's best to limit saturated fats to less than 10 percent of your daily calories and down to 5 percent or 6 percent for a heart-healthy diet.

And yet if someone loses and maintains a 25 kg weight loss following a low carbohydrate diet that is high in animal fat (which is saturated fat), as long as their triglycerides and LDL are in the normal range, then that diet is likely healthy for that person. Any negative effect on triglycerides and LDL is offset by the health benefits of the weight loss. Perspective here is important.

It's also important to remember humans are creative omnivores. Before mass migration and emigration were possible, humans thrived in wildly diverse sources of food, so there seems to be significant adaptability. This means there are many ways to eat healthy.

There are three diet plans that appear to be beneficial for heart and brain health as well as lowering the risk of diabetes, which are three of the biggest health concerns for women as they age. The DASH diet (dietary approaches to stop hypertension), the Mediterranean diet (based on traditional diets in Greece, Southern Italy, and other Mediterranean regions), and the MIND diet (Mediterranean-DASH Intervention for Neurodegenerative Delay), which combines aspects of DASH and the Mediterranean diet with an emphasis on foods that have been shown to be neuroprotective or brain healthy. All three diets focus on lean meats, fish, whole grains, fruits and vegetables, and olive oil, and they limit salt, sweets, and eliminate ultra-processed foods and sugar-sweetened beverages. Women interested in learning more about these diets can find quality information at the American Heart Association (go to heart.org) and the National Institute of Aging (go to nia.nih.gov/health) and search internally on the sites. See appendix B for a summary of these plans.

Plant-based diets (vegetarian and vegan) can also be very heart healthy and are good options, but will require supplementation with omega-3 fatty acids and vitamin B12, and possibly with other micronutrients such as iron.

Precision Nutrition

The concept of precision nutrition involves developing targeted dietary recommendations based on individual factors, for example, genetics or the microbiome (bacteria in the intestinal tract). In theory this is intriguing. However, given the overall low quality of the American diet—38 percent of women ages forty to fifty-nine and 23 percent of women age sixty and older eat fast food every day— instead of genetic and micro-biome testing, something that will likely only be accessible and practical based on socioeconomic status, might it be better to research ways to im-plement what we know works on a larger scale—less fast food, more vegetables, more fiber, eliminating sugar-sweetened beverages and fruit juice? Instead of precision nutrition for a select few we need good nu-trition for all.

BOTTOM LINE

- The foundation for healthy eating is whole grains, plenty of vege-tables, and fruit.
- Women should have 25 g of dietary fiber a day.
- Ultra-processed foods are associated with many negative health outcomes, so reducing or eliminating these foods can be very beneficial.
- Fish and seafood are the only source of the essential omega-3 fatty acids.
- The DASH, Mediterranean, and MIND diets are three excellent plans for overall nutritional health during the menopause con-tinuum.

Chapter 22

Menoceuticals:

Supplements and Menopause

ALMOST 60 PERCENT OF ADULT WOMEN in the United States are taking at least one supplement. These products are often taken for general health reasons or preventative care, but many women cycle through a variety during their menopause transition and during post menopause in search of relief from symptoms or for menopause-related concerns—I refer to this latter group of supplements "menoceuticals."

I dedicated two chapters to the biological, chemical, and financial evolution of hormone therapies for menopause, so it's only fair that I turn that same eye to the supplement business. The manufacturers of these products aren't local healers brewing small batches in their kitchens; this is an industry. And what an industry it is—in the United States supplements enjoy a business of more than $30 billion a year. Increasingly supplements are branded as wellness promoting—achieve healthy lifestyle from the outside in! But tying supplements to wellness is no different from linking Premarin in the 1950s with glamour. The ugly truth is lifestyle marketing works.

A wide range of over-the-counter (OTC) products are found under the umbrella of supplements, such as vitamins, minerals, botanicals, amino acids, hormones, phytoestrogens, fish oils, probiotics, desiccated animal parts, and dietary supplements. These products are rarely studied and are essentially unregulated.

In 1994 the United States passed the Dietary Supplement Health and Education Act (DSHEA), removing multiple safeguards for consumers. For example, companies don't have to prove the product contains what's advertised on the label. Consequently, adulterated products are common. Sometimes the main ingredient is swapped out for a less expensive product, there may be no active ingredient at all, or instead of a botanical there may be an actual pharmaceutical drug. For example, a supplement of black cohosh sold for hot flushes could contain, among other things, the herb pictured on the bottle, estradiol (a prescription hormone), an antidepressant, or a completely untested designer steroid. It may even be rice powder. It's a lottery and the odds are never in the consumer's favor. In 2015 the New York State attorney general investigated herbal products sold at GNC, Target, Walmart, and Walgreens, and 80 percent of the products didn't contain any of the herbs on the labels. Yes, 80 percent. Another study in 2013 from the University of Guelph found up to one-third of supplements didn't contain the botanicals claimed on the labels.

Imagine the outrage if we allowed companies to play content roulette with other products? What if each time we opened a can of kidney beans, never mind a bottle of antibiotics, it was a game of Is It or Isn't It? With supplements the motto is truly *buyer beware.*

The harm in substituting ingredients goes beyond the fact that a person may be taking a pharmaceutical or a potentially harmful botanical. Lack of quality control means the supplements used in a specific study may not be uniform or may contain an entirely different compound, meaning it's not even possible to know what's really being tested. It's also possible that the batch provided for the study might not be consistent ingredient-wise with what people buy at the store. There are many issues with Big Pharma, but at least I know that every pill, patch, or cream I prescribe contains the dose that it claims.

Another issue with supplements in the United States is the lack of safety testing; these products are presumed safe unless the Food and Drug Administration (FDA) is provided with evidence of harm. The American public pays a hefty price for the lack of safety studies, as supplements send approximately 23,000 people to the emergency room each year and are a growing cause of liver failure. Even when the FDA is notified, the response is often a tepid warning letter to remove the product. What does a 30-billion-dollar-a-year industry care about a few slaps on the wrist?

These products are largely untested, so there is no research and development pipeline to slow them down, and another product seems readily available if one gets pulled from the market. Supplements are like shark's teeth, there's always another one.

Advertising regulations for supplements are similarly lax. The DSHEA allows vague claims about body parts and physiology, known as "structure/function claims," as long as the following disclaimer is included:

> These statements have not been evaluated by the Food and Drug Administration. This product is not intended to diagnose, treat, cure, or prevent any disease.

A manufacturer can legally advertise a supplement helps "maintain hormone health" or provides "ovary support" or "memory support" without defining those terms or providing evidence of, well, anything. These quasi-scientific terms are very effective marketing. Who doesn't want to support their ovaries or their memory?

Unsurprisingly, the supplement industry has grown significantly since the regulations were relaxed. In 1994 there were approximately 4,000 supplements on the market in the United States, and by 2012 there were 55,000. While advertising plays a big role, supplements are often recommended by medical practitioners, and like with Big Pharma there may be financial ties. For example, naturopathic medicine claims to use the power of nature to help the body heal itself. Much of this healing happens courtesy of supplements. In 2016 STAT news reported the lobby to increase the licensing of naturopaths in several states was heavily funded by vitamin manufacturers.

There is no database that links providers who get financial support from the supplement industry, so it may not be clear if a provider has been paid to post about supplements on Instagram or to speak about them at an event. Providers who sell supplements in their office will get money from sales, and some doctors and naturopaths even sell their own brand of supplements, further increasing their profit from the sale of these products.

Selling supplements in a medical office, especially branded supplements, creates an imbalanced power dynamic that is definitely not in any woman's favor. How do you tell a doctor or naturopath while you are sitting in their office that you don't want to buy their special formulation? Gunter's first rule of health care information is you can't get quality information from someone selling that product, because they clearly have bias. If you wouldn't learn about medications for depression from the company selling your antidepressants, you shouldn't learn about supplements from a provider selling them. They can be your drug store or your doctor, but they can't ethically be both.

The American College of Obstetrics and Gynecology has the following to say about OB/GYNs and selling supplements:

- Obstetrician-gynecologists should not sell or promote agents or devices as being therapeutic without an adequate evidence base for medical benefit.
- Obstetrician-gynecologists should not use their professional influence or clinical environment to sell or promote nonmedical products or services or to enroll participants into multilevel marketing schemes.
- The sale of prescription or nonprescription medication or devices directly to patients from obstetrician–gynecologists' offices is discouraged when reasonably convenient, alternative vendors exist.

It's important to acknowledge the confusion and fear surrounding estrogens that was created by the Women's Health Initiative in 2002 left a void that supplements, just like bioidentical and compounded hormones (discussed in chapter 20), helped fill. There were fewer nonhormonal options for symptoms of menopause pre-2002, so turning to supplements isn't surprising. Many women also turn to supplements because they've been dismissed and/or disenfranchised by the medical system. If the person recommending supplements is listening and validating your concerns, why would you return to see the providers who dismissed your drenching hot flushes or periods that soak your clothes as *not that bad?*

Supplements have also exploited fears about hormones with claims of being inherently natural, which is mistaken as safety. But supplements aren't natural. The most natural thing is to get micronutrients from food. Vitamins and minerals are absorbed much better from diet as they're combined with fiber and other factors that enhance absorption. Like estradiol or progesterone, whether something is found in nature is marketing not medicine, what matters is whether a product is indicated and if it's safe and effective.

ANOTHER ISSUE WITH supplements are the studies—when they exist, that is. Like with Big Pharma, the industry-funded studies almost always show a beneficial effect, although the study design with supplements is frequently poor. A low-quality study with positive results is very unhelpful because medically speaking it doesn't say much of anything. A good analogy is trying to identify a person in poor light and from a distance. The answer is, "Well, maybe" at best. Conclusions just aren't possible.

Adding to the confusion, supplements are sometimes medically indicated. Some notable examples are folic acid preconception and during pregnancy, vitamin D for those unable to get enough through diet and sun exposure, or multivitamins for people who may have difficulties absorbing micronutrients, such as women who have had bariatric surgery (weight loss surgery). Some vegans and vegetarians may need iron and/or vitamin B12 supplements, as the only source of those are animal products.

And then there are headlines from frequently visited medical sites, like this one from WebMD, "These Vitamins and Supplements Fight Inflammation." This is a vague claim that means nothing medically, but it gives the false impression that these products are helpful.

Sigh.

The Semi-Secret History of Women, Medicine, Midwifery, and Plants

Many supplements for menopause tie into the belief that there are ancient recipes that were once widely known and effective only to be extinguished by patriarchal medicine, the pharmaceutical industry, or both.

There is a tendency to exoticize or romanticize the vast recipe literature of remedies in ancient Egyptian, Greek, Persian, Hindu, and Chinese texts, but most were based on disease models we know today to be untrue. For example, if a woman in ancient Egypt had a sore ear and jaw, the treatment was vaginal pessaries of herbs and fumigation, whereas a doctor today might want to consider an ear infection, a sinus infection, or a dental abscess as the potential cause, and none of those are treated vaginally. Many ancient Greek therapies for women involved substances believed to be drying, because one of the root causes of women's health issues were that they were overly moist. It would be incorrect to base any woman's treatment for any condition based on the ancient concept of excessive moisture. There's also a lot of cherry-picking with ancient therapies that involves selecting the parts that sound palatable and rejecting the rest. Vaginal fumigation was a therapy in ancient Greece, rebranded by modern wellness as vaginal steaming, but in truth many recipes were revolting. A disemboweled puppy or dog (it varied depending on the ailment) stuffed with the herbs was often burned to get the steam.

Ingredients may also have been chosen for cultural or religious significance, as medicine frequently reflected the world around. For example, pomegranate is often recommended in recipes for abortion, but it's also the fruit of the dead in Greek mythology. Many ingredients may also have been costly on purpose, perhaps our elders knew what we know today—expensive medications have a greater placebo effect. This is one explanation for castoreum—secretion from the scent glands of beavers—appearing in so many European therapies during medieval times and the Renaissance.

Western medical remedies from the 1500s until the early 1900s were often based on the mistaken belief that the lack of menstruation meant dangerous humours were accumulating, so therapies often involved bloodletting or purgatives (substances that cause vomiting or diarrhea). Another root cause of women's health concerns was that women had too hot a temperament, so sudorifics—therapies that cause sweating—were prescribed for a variety of symptoms. Opium and alcohol appear in many remedies, and in the 1800s onward cannabis was recommended—although the latter was recommended at least by one of the most academic OB/GYNs of the 1800s to temper the hyper sexual nature of women in menopause.

Some claim there are herbal therapies for menopause that come directly from ancient Chinese medicine, but according to Charlotte Furth in *A Flourishing Yin: Gender in China's Medical History: 960–1665*, the modern diagnosis of menopause has been transferred to traditional Chinese medicine (TCM) from nineteenth-century medicine. In TCM, menopause wasn't viewed as different from old age and so historically, there are no specific remedies for symptoms we associate today with menopause. Any TCM recommended for menopause is a nineteenth-century recipe. That doesn't make it bad or good; it's just important to understand the origins as some people are drawn toward these therapies as they mistakenly believe they are ancient or at least much older than they are.

Given what we now know about phytoestrogens, many have wondered if some ancient recipes may have worked because they contained these plant substances that can act like estrogens (see chapter 19 for more). Modern phytoestrogen supplements are marginally effective at best for a variety of menopause-related symptoms, and these modern supplements contain far more active compounds than any ancient recipe could hope to achieve, so unlikely.

It's possible the plants used in ancient recipes were contaminated with mycotoxins, substances made by fungus with very potent estrogen-like activities (see chapter 19). This would mean the therapy worked not because the recipe was effective, but rather there was an unknown contaminant. Estrogenic mycotoxins can be very potent, so a minuscule amount could theoretically have a medicinal effect. Mycotoxins can also have serious health implications. For example, ergot is a mycotoxin produced by rye contaminated with *Claviceps purpurea* and can produce serious illness, premature labor, abortion, and even be fatal. So potent is ergot that European standards only allow 1 mg per kg of grain. If an ancient remedy worked because of a mycotoxin, we wouldn't wish to replicate that today.

Many people mistake my insistence on proving if and how botanicals work as well as their safety with being dismissive. But if a plant is helping medically it's having a physiological effect and we should understand what that is and also if the product is safe. Don't women deserve that? Plants can be more dangerous than pharmaceuticals, so why insist on drug safety and not extend that safety requirement to botanicals? Also, if a therapy proves effective we can use that knowledge to help women. To me studying all therapies regardless of source is an act of feminism, because women can only be empowered about their health with accurate information.

Many substances found in nature and originally used as ancient medicines or folk remedies have been incorporated into medicine when they were proven to be useful. Physicians and midwives connected ergot poisoning with abortion, and then someone wondered if ergot might also trigger uterine contractions after delivery to stop postpartum hemorrhage. Word of mouth led to increased usage, and reports gradually made their way into the medical literature. Eventually, the pharmaceutical industry took notice and ergot was purified into reliable doses with known effects, and as a result ergotamine is still used in medicine today. Willow bark became aspirin and opium from poppies was used for thousands of years until technology allowed for morphine to be isolated, allowing for standardized dosing thus improving safety. Today, as was the case hundreds of years ago, medicine is on the lookout for active compounds in nature. Many botanicals have been investigated and dismissed because there wasn't an effective ingredient or sometimes because the compound was unsafe.

I believe ancient healers were doing the best they could with their given circumstances. Asking for scientific proof to offer our patients safe and effective therapy is simply medicine. We don't accept the Hippocratic understanding of a woman's body being too moist, so why wouldn't we turn that same critical eye to all of historical medicine?

Supplements as the New Patent Medicines

Proprietary elixirs and concoctions have been around for a long time. They were originally called *nostrum remedium,* our remedy in Latin eventually becoming known as nostrums. The term "patent medicine" comes from products that found favor with royalty and were subsequently issued a royal letter or *patent* as endorsement. They were heavily advertised with wild claims and patient testimonials. Exactly like many supplements today.

Patent medications were popular in the 1800s. It's understandable why women approaching menopause turned to them as many medical therapies of the day were crude and ineffective at best. Common prescriptions were bloodletting, leeches to the vulva, purgatives, sudorifics, sedatives, belladonna, and vaginal injections with a solution of acetate of lead. Even removing the ovaries was recommended, even though mortality from the surgery was high.

Advertisements for patent medicines were aimed specifically at women. The same product was typically recommended for almost every medical condition, from uterine prolapse to infertility, to missed periods (often code for pregnancy and hence the insinuation the product could induce an abortion), and to menopause. Some contained pennyroyal, an extract from an herb in the mint family that has long been used as an abortifacient. It's highly toxic and should not be taken in any dose. While it may induce uterine contractions, side effects are liver failure and death. Other common ingredients in these elixirs were quinine, boric acid, and oil of theobroma—which you might know as cocoa butter.

Yes, some patent medicines contained chocolate.

One of the most successful patent medicines was Lydia Pinkham's Vegetable Compound for ailments peculiar to women, and it was specifically geared toward the change of life or menopause. According to Rainey Horwitz, who took a deep dive into Lydia Pinkham and her Vegetable Compound for the Embryo Project Encyclopedia (it's well worth a read), Lydia Estes Pinkham invented this concoction of alcohol, roots, and herbs in her kitchen in 1873 in Lynn, Massachusetts. Pinkham started small, but as requests increased her business expanded. The product was heavily advertised as *A Woman's Cure for Women's Ills*. It could apparently do all of the following:

> give quick relief and effect a permanent cure in all cases of irregularity, faintness, headaches, chlorosis, megrims, displacements, periodic bearing down pains, dizziness, palpitations, depression, pains in the back, and those dull and listless days when you feel fit for nothing.

Chlorosis is anemia or a low blood count, megrims is low spirits, displacements is prolapse, the bearing down pain I suspect is menstrual cramps. This was gynecology in a bottle! And yes, if something sounds too good to be true it is. We now know that all of these conditions are caused by vastly different biological processes, and there isn't one therapy to rule them all.

Each bottle came with an eighty-page free book on women's health titled *Lydia E. Pinkham's Private Textbook Upon Ailments Peculiar to Women*. Women were even encouraged to send in questions to be answered by Pinkham, and they received handwritten replies…even for years after her death. That became a minor scandal, with the Pinkham brand claiming no one ever suggested Pinkham herself wrote all the replies. There were also Pinkham postcards (basically trading cards). With no one else talking publicly about women's health, of course women turned to Lydia Pinkham.

Pinkham's original recipe included black cohosh, life root, unicorn root, pleurisy root, and fenugreek seed—the black cohosh was apparently the ingredient for menopausal symptoms. The original recipe contained alcohol, although this wasn't disclosed for many years. Pinkham's Vegetable Compound was tested in 1911 and the results published in the *British Medical Journal*—it was 19.3 percent alcohol, which is the same alcohol content of most port wine for reference. (I know, right?!) No evidence of any active substances was identified. While it's possible the testing of the day may not have been capable of detecting an active ingredient (that's being generous to Pinkham on my part), given the recipe and Pinkham's method of extraction, it's very likely there was no active ingredient except the alcohol.

I decided to perform a trial of a home version of Pinkham's tonic—well, the alcohol part. I wanted to see if 30 ml (1 tbsp) of 19.3 percent alcohol every four hours—the dose of the supposedly inactive ingredient in Pinkham's vegetable compound—might improve a dull and listless day. I chose a good quality port with a 19.5 percent alcohol content (look, I wasn't going to drink nasty port before my coffee). Between the COVID-19 pandemic and the smoke-filled skies of California's fire season, it wasn't hard to find a day where I felt fit for nothing, so one Sunday morning I began with a shot of port after brushing my teeth and continued to dose myself regularly until bedtime. For science. Let's just say it smoothed the day a little, and no, I am not recommending it as therapy. Clearly there was an active ingredient, just not quite as advertised.

Omega 3 Supplements

The importance of omega-3 fatty acids were discussed in chapter 21. A large clinical trial that followed over 13,000 women ages fifty-five years and older found taking a 1 g omega-3 supplement (the brand Omacor, a prescription fish oil supplement) reduced heart attacks by 40 percent for White women who had less than one and a half servings of fish per week in their diet and by 77 percent for African American women regardless of fish intake. Omacor was used in the study as it's an FDA-approved prescription, so the dose and purity were known. There are vegan omega-3 supplements made from seaweed, although if it's not prescription, contents and dose can't be assured. Side effects of 1 g of omega-3 fatty acids a day are uncommon, but can include bad breath, heartburn, nausea, diarrhea, headache, and sometimes even smelly sweat.

Higher doses of prescription omega-3 fatty acids are used to treat elevated triglycerides—up to 4 g a day. In these doses they can lower triglycerides by 20 percent to 30 percent, but they can also affect the blood's ability to clot and interact with anticoagulant medications. These doses should only be used under medical supervision.

For many women, an omega-3 supplement of 1 g a day makes good sense.

Vitamin B12

Vitamin B12 is important for making red blood cells, a functioning nervous system, as well as a variety of metabolic processes and synthesis of DNA. Low levels are associated with many symptoms including fatigue, depression, irritability, mouth ulcers, and tingling in the hands and feet. The recommended daily amount of vitamin B12 is 2.4 mcg, and there is more than that in a 3-ounce serving of salmon and a cup of milk has 1.1 mcg. Vitamin B12 is not found in plants.

Absorbing vitamin B12 is a complicated process that gets less efficient with age, consequently, approximately 20 percent of people ages sixty and older are deficient. Women ages fifty and older and those who follow a vegan diet should pay close attention to their vitamin B12 intake and supplement as needed. Many vegan foods are fortified with vitamin B12, including several breakfast cereals, nutritional yeasts, and plant-based milks such as soy. Some medications, for example, metformin for type 2 diabetes and medications for acid reflux, and weight loss surgery can reduce absorption of vitamin B12, so supplements may be needed here as well.

Vitamin B12 injections have long been promoted as a miracle cure for fatigue and are popular in the world of wellness. The liquid is bright red and looks more like an elixir than a medication we give in the office, but women need a health care provider not a potions master. When I attended the "goop health" conference in New York, I was astounded to see a long line of women eagerly pulling down their pants to expose the top of their buttocks to receive an intramuscular injection of bright red vitamin B12 from a doctor they'd never met—all in the name of wellness. Injections of vitamin B12 should only be prescribed by your health care provider and are only indicated for people who are unable to absorb sufficient vitamin B12 from supplements.

It's fascinating how injections of vitamin B12 are branded as natural, immune boosting (not a thing), and wellness promoting, and other interventions or medications, such as vaccines, are stuck with the Evil Pharma label. This is especially dumbfounding with vitamin B12, as the injections are made by a pharmaceutical company and they contain small amounts of aluminum, one of the ingredients that some people falsely claim make vaccines unsafe or unnatural. While the amount of aluminum in B12 is less than the amount in vaccines (and the amount in both is very safe), people don't get a vaccine once a month for years.

Vitamin E

Vitamin E is a group of fat-soluble compounds called tocopherols and tocotrienes. These compounds are antioxidants and are important for the immune system and heart health. Vitamin E deficiency in North America is very rare. It's found in a variety of foods including leafy green vegetables, nuts, seeds, vegetable oils, and fortified cereals. Several studies have evaluated vitamin E supplements for preventative health care, and they haven't been shown to protect against heart disease, cancer, or cognitive decline with aging. Some studies have raised concerns about vitamin E supplements showing a small but increased risk in dying among those taking doses of 400 IU a day and possibly even for those taking as little as 150 IU a day.

Over-the-Counter Hormones

OTC hormones are available seemingly everywhere, even on Amazon. Avoid them. They may not even contain hormones, but there are many other reasons to also give them a pass. Here are the four most common products marketed to women in the menopause continuum:

- **PROGESTERONE CREAM:** It's not absorbed well (if at all) through the skin, so it's ineffective even if the product does contain progesterone. If a woman is taking estrogen and relies on a progesterone cream to protect her uterus she could get endometrial cancer. This is actually one of my tips on how to know you are getting bad menopause advice—if the provider recommends topical progesterone get up and walk out the door.

- **ANYTHING THAT CLAIMS TO CONTAIN ESTROGEN:** The amount of estrogen matters regarding risk of blood clots and endometrial cancer, so nonpharmaceutical products could be unsafe. However, most OTC products that claim to be estrogen are actually something else. For example, Life Extension sells Estrogen for Women. The description reads as follows: *This plant-based estrogen supplement is designed to support healthy estrogen metabolism and support against common menopausal discomforts, such as hot flashes and night sweats.* Estrogen supplement sure sounds like it contains estrogen, but it's really a mixture of herbal products that are largely ineffective for menopause symptoms. This is a good example (or really an enraging example, because this type of labeling shouldn't be allowed) of how labels can be misleading.

- **DEHYDROEPIANDROSTERONE AND DEHYDROEPIANDROSTERONE SULFATE (DHEA AND DHEA-S):** Made by the adrenal gland and ovaries and together DHEA and DHEA-S are the most abundant steroid hormones in the body. Levels decline about 2 percent a year, but for some women they may temporarily increase during the menopause transition. DHEA and DHEA-S are enigmatic hormones, and the full scope of their function in the body isn't well understood, but they're believed to have an effect on brain function and on inflammation. DHEA is also a step in the pathway that converts cholesterol into testosterone, estrogens, and progesterone (see chapter 3), hence the recommendation from some for menopause. At least twenty-three studies have evaluated DHEA for a variety of menopause-related indications, and there was no benefit for sexual function, overall well-being, cognitive function, or benefits on lipids or blood sugar. Admittedly the quality of the studies is poor, but based on this data there is no evidence to support DHEA for women in their menopause transition or postmenopause or for issues with desire. DHEA-S is an effective vaginal therapy, prescription only, for genitourinary syndrome of menopause (GUSM, see chapter 13)).

- **PREGNENOLONE:** Another precursor hormone in the cholesterol to progesterone/estradiol/testosterone pathway (see Appendix A). There is a myth that in times of stress the adrenal gland will siphon pregnenolone to make stress hormones, such as cortisol, short-changing the ovaries and thus lowering the levels of estradiol and progesterone. It's often referred to as pregnenolone steal. There is no evidence for it in the medical literature, and the hypothesis is not biologically plausible based on how the body works. While it's true stress can temporarily halt menstruation for some women and chronic stressors can affect reproductive function, this is due to complex interactions that affect the hormone signaling and has nothing to do with the ovaries having insufficient pregnenolone. The false hypothesis of pregnenolone steal is often paired with another nondiagnosis, adrenal fatigue— the idea that stress depletes the adrenal gland. When people are given these false diagnoses it doesn't mean they don't have symptoms, it means they've been misdiagnosed. Skip pregnenolone supplements and ignore anyone who makes the diagnosis of pregnenolone steal or adrenal fatigue.

Probiotics

Probiotics are live microorganisms that confer a health benefit to the host. Basically, they're bugs that do a body good. In the 1990s probiotics were the new thing in women's health and we recommended them for prevention of vaginal infections and for bladder health, but now they're marketed for a wide variety of medical concerns and conditions. Despite the probiotic hype, there is scant science to support their widespread use in women's health. The gastrointestinal and vaginal microbiomes (communities of bacteria) are complex, dynamic, and our understanding of them is in its infancy, so the idea they can easily be manipulated for only positive benefit with a probiotic pill is more science fiction than science. There is data, however, that suggests probiotics can help prevent a potentially dangerous kind of antibiotic-associated diarrhea called *Clostridium difficile* enterocolitis.

For women in the menopause continuum, probiotics are most likely to be recommended for preventing urinary tract infections or UTIs (bladder infections). The few studies that exist are low quality, and a 2015 Cochrane review that looked at the body of evidence concluded the following:

> No significant benefit was demonstrated for probiotics com-
> pared with placebo or no treatment, but a benefit cannot be
> ruled out as the data were few, and derived from small studies
> with poor methodological reporting.

There is research with a strain called *Lactobacillus crispatus,* the domi-nant beneficial bacteria in the vagina for many women, to reduce recurrence of vaginal infections such as bacterial vaginosis. Adding *Lacto-bacillus crispatus* to standard therapy for bacterial vaginosis reduced the risk of recurrence from 45 percent to 30 percent. If further studies with this bacteria show benefit over the long term it will be a helpful addition, but it's clearly *not* a cure-all. This probiotic isn't currently available over the counter. Other data for probiotics and vaginal health is underwhelming.

Probiotics also suffer from the same quality control issues as other sup-plements. One study found 33 percent of probiotics contained fewer bacteria colonies than claimed on the label, and 42 percent of products tested were mislabeled, meaning they didn't have the bacteria they claimed or they had other species. These products are also typically quite expensive.

Other Supplements

Here are some other supplements often targeted to women during meno-pause:

- **ANTIOXIDANTS:** These are substances that may prevent cell dam-age from free radicals, which are unstable molecules either created naturally by the body or found in the environment (ex-amples include cigarette smoke and sunlight). Some examples are vitamins E and C, selenium, and carotenoids (which many of us know as substances that give pigment to foods, such as carrots, pumpkin, and tomatoes). Vegetables and fruit are excellent sources of antioxidants, but there is no evidence supporting the use of antioxidant supplements for the general population and there is some data suggesting risks (for example, as previously discussed with vitamin E). In one study women who took antioxidant supplements during chemotherapy for breast cancer had an increased risk of recurrence of their cancer. There is ongoing research on antioxidant therapy and until there is quality data, it's generally best to get antioxidants from food.

- **BIOTIN:** Also known as vitamin B7 and it's often recommended for hair and nails, although there is no proof it works for people who don't have a biotin deficiency. It's plentiful in most diets, and some good sources are salmon, egg yolks, and sweet potato. It is even made by bacteria in the bowel, so diet-related deficiency is uncommon in otherwise healthy individuals. Many biotin supplements contain 650 times more than needed, although it's a water-soluble vitamin so the excess just becomes expensive urine. High levels of biotin can interfere with several lab tests, including hormone levels such FSH and LH (see chapter 3), thyroid tests, cortisol, vitamin D, and troponin—a test used to help diagnose heart attacks.

- **GREEN TEA EXTRACT:** Sounds healthy, right? After all, green tea is good for you! Green tea extract is an extract of the plant, not the tea. It's associated with liver failure, so that's a no.

- **IODINE:** Thyroid conditions increase as women age, so iodine is often marketed to women over forty as a necessary supplement to protect both the thyroid and the immune system. Nonpregnant adults need 150 µg of iodine per day, the amount in ½ teaspoon of iodized table salt. Dairy, eggs, and fish are also good sources of dietary iodine. The primary function of iodine is production of thyroid hormones. Iodine only supports the immune system because a functioning thyroid is necessary for a healthy immune system. Taking excessive iodine with a normal thyroid can paradoxically cause hypothyroidism (low thyroid function). In fact, endocrinologists use high doses of iodine for women with hyperthyroidism (an overactive thyroid) to "stun" it to buy time to treat it by more permanent means. Some women take so much OTC iodine in supplements they develop hypothyroidism. In these situations people often can't believe they were led astray, and it can take multiple visits to convince them otherwise. There are also studies linking excessive iodine intake with autoimmune thyroiditis and papillary thyroid cancer.

- **MULTIVITAMINS:** These products have been reimagined for women over fifty to provide support from within—don't fall for it! The only reimagining here is to figure out how to target women's fears as they age. Multiple studies have addressed multivitamins and they have no benefit for otherwise healthy women, and some data even suggests harm. One theory with harm from is the antioxidants in the supplements may not just protect healthy cells, but also cancer cells as well. There may also be other mechanisms; for example, some vitamins and minerals affect the ability to absorb others, so high doses in the intestine from a multivitamin may affect the ability to absorb important nutrients from food. Although excess water-soluble vitamins are simply flushed out with your urine (yes, as mentioned with biotin above, it turns out many vitamins just make expensive urine), excess fat-soluble vitamins are stored in fat, possibly accumulating and causing potential harm. Unless a woman has had weight loss surgery, or has other reasons that affect her ability to absorb micronutrients from her diet, multivitamins are a no.

- **VITAMIN A:** This is a group of compounds also knows as the retinoids. Doses of 10,000 IU a day or more are associated with an increased risk of osteoporosis. Vitamin A deficiency is rare, yet several supplements aimed at women often contain 10,000 units of vitamin A. This is all risk and no benefit. Topical retinol and prescription vitamin A is a different story, as these products have been shown to reduce the appearance of wrinkles as they promote the growth of collagen.

- **VITAMIN B6 AND B12:** I often encounter women taking this combination, but supplements of vitamin B6 combined with B12 together are associated with an increased risk of osteoporosis and fracture—in one study there was a 50 percent increased risk of a hip fracture. The higher the dose of the vitamins the greater the risk.

- **YAM CREAMS:** They capitalize on the fact that pharmaceutical hormones are made from a substance found in yams, diosgenin. The body can't convert diosgenin or other substances in yams into hormones, however, and yams don't contain any hormones or substances with medicinal properties. A store near me sells a wild yam cream that claims to relieve cramps, moodiness, provide adrenal support, and balance estrogen and progesterone. All for $24.80 a jar. Sounds just like a patent medicine, right? A study of a topical wild yam cream compared with a placebo showed no benefit, as predicted. These products are predatory and a scam. Yams are food, not medicine.

How to Do Your Own Research

Menoceuticals deserve the same scrutiny as prescription medications. This can be challenging given the low quality of much of the research, so here are some questions to consider:

- **HOW CAN THIS PRODUCT HELP ME IN A MEANINGFUL WAY?** Don't accept vague terms such as "ovary support" or "adrenal support"; demand an expected outcome and precision about dose. For example, 1 g of omega 3 fatty acids a day reduces the risk of heart attacks.
- **BE WARY OF PRODUCTS THAT CLAIM TO DO IT ALL:** Hot flashes, moodiness, cramps, headaches, backache—these are diverse medical conditions and the idea there is one universal therapy isn't biologically plausible. If a supplement sounds too good to be true, it's too good to be true (also, Big Pharma would have scooped it up years ago).
- **WHAT DO MEDICAL PROFESSIONAL ORGANIZATIONS SAY ABOUT THIS SUPPLEMENT?** Specifically the North American Menopause Society (NAMS), the International Menopause Society (IMS), the American College of Obstetrics and Gynecology (ACOG), or the Society of Obstetricians and Gynecologists of Canada (SOGC). Enter the name of the supplement or product and then the name of the society into the search engine.

- **WHAT DOES THE OFFICE OF DIETARY SUPPLEMENTS AT THE NATIONAL INSTITUTE OF HEALTH RECOMMEND?** You can find out at ods.od.nih.gov.

- **WHAT ARE THE POTENTIAL RISKS INCLUDING FINANCIAL?** Unlike prescription medications, supplements don't have product inserts that list side effects, complications, and potential interactions with medications. Never assume a product is benign or that it doesn't have an interaction with another medication just because it isn't a pharmaceutical or because the labeling claims it is natural. The National Center for Complementary and Integrative Health (www.nccih.nih.gov) is a good place to start a search for safety and always tell your provider if you are taking any supplements or are planning to start. Another excellent resource is your pharmacist. As for the financial risk, supplements range from $20 a month to $90 or more. Over time that's a lot of money.

- **CAN I CHANGE MY DIET SO I DON'T NEED THE SUPPLEMENT?** Making these changes may not be possible for some women, but it's always worth a try. A registered dietician or a nutritionist may be able to help, and most can make their recommendations economical. In America this may be covered by health insurance (in countries with universal health care it may be no cost), but even for those who have to pay for a consultation it is likely worth it in the long run as supplements can be twenty to forty dollars a month or more and often people end up taking more than one. One visit with such a professional could potentially pay for itself in supplements not taken in far less than a year.

- **DOES THE PERSON RECOMMENDING THE PRODUCT PROFIT FROM THE SALE?** Talk with a medical professional who doesn't profit from the supplement to get unbiased information.

- **DOES THE PERSON RECOMMENDING THIS SUPPLEMENT USE TERMS SUCH AS PREGNENOLONE STEAL OR ADRENAL FATIGUE?** If so, get another opinion.

- **IF YOU DO TAKE A SUPPLEMENT, LOOK FOR ONE THAT HAS BEEN VERIFIED BY AN INDEPENDENT AGENCY FOR PURITY:** Look for products with a seal of approval from one of three independent agencies—NSF International, US Pharmacopeia (USP), or ConsumerLab—that test these products for purity. This will reduce the chance that a product is adulterated and the product contains what the label claims.

P.S. I expect *a lot* of hate mail for this chapter.

BOTTOM LINE

- Supplements are an unregulated multibillion-dollar-a-year industry, and many companies have financial ties with the providers and influencers who recommend their products.
- With the exception of omega-3 fatty acids and vitamin B12, the majority of supplements for otherwise healthy women who do not have a nutritional deficiency have weak supporting data (see chapter 11 for information on calcium and vitamin D).
- Many supplements are adulterated; this makes them challenging to study and raises safety concerns.
- Multivitamins are only recommended for women who have a reduced ability to absorb vitamins; food remains the best and most natural way to get micronutrients.
- Avoid over-the-counter hormones.

Chapter 23

Contraception and the Menopause Transition:

Pregnancy Prevention and Menstrual Management

WOMEN MAY USE CONTRACEPTION DURING their menopause transition for several reasons: for contraception, to manage medical conditions that predated their menopause transition (for example, painful periods or pain from endometriosis), and to help bothersome symptoms of their menopause transition, such as irregular or heavy menstrual periods. Reviewing the options helps women make evidence-based decisions not only during their menopause transition, but knowing how certain contraceptives may help during the menopause transition may alter choices women make in their thirties or even earlier as planning for menopause should be part of the contraception conversation.

As women age, they are more likely to accumulate medical conditions that increase their risk of complications with certain forms of hormonal contraception. The main risks relevant to the menopause transition will be discussed shortly, but a full rundown of all the medical conditions that impact contraception safety is beyond the scope of this book. The Centers for Disease Control and Prevention (CDC) and World Health Organization (WHO) are excellent resources for this information. Enter "CDC" or "WHO" and "medical eligibility criteria for contraception" into your search engine of choice to get to the relevant site. Both the CDC and WHO have free apps with the same detailed information about contraceptive safety.

Do I Really Need Contraception in My Forties?

Woman not at risk of getting pregnant don't need contraception. This includes women who don't partner with men, women who partner with men but are abstinent by choice or circumstances, and women who partner with men and their male partner has had a vasectomy or is a trans man. Women not in these groups should consider what getting pregnant might mean for them. In other words, how much do they not want to be pregnant?

Every woman looks at the risk of pregnancy differently. Women who would continue with a surprise pregnancy should know maternal complications, including maternal mortality, increase with age as does the risk of birth defects. For example, 1 in 20 or 5 percent of all pregnancies for a woman aged forty-five will have Down syndrome. Women who would not want to continue their pregnancy—for whatever reason they choose—may wish to consider the availability and cost of abortion where they live.

At the age of forty a sexually active heterosexual woman has approximately a 5 percent chance of getting pregnant each menstrual cycle. Different models have been developed to try to determine the odds of pregnancy by age, and it's estimated by age forty-five approximately 55 percent of women are no longer able to get pregnant, by age forty-seven that number is 79 percent, and by fifty it's 92 percent. Pregnancies without assisted reproduction are uncommon over the age of forty-five, but they happen and they are incredibly rare between the ages of fifty and fifty-five. The oldest woman to conceive without the assistance of reproductive technology is Dawn Brooke of Guernsey, Channel Islands, who was fifty-nine when she delivered her son in 1997!

I've cared for several women between the ages of forty-five and fifty who thought three months with no period was simply their menopause transition, so their positive pregnancy test was definitely unexpected. Pregnancies after age forty-five are more common among women who have already had multiple children, suggesting perhaps increased fertility overall. There is an old saying that some women can get pregnant if their partner throws his pants on the bed. While hyperbole, there are definitely some women who, for lack of a better word, seem to have super fertility. However, if a woman has used contraception all of her life, she wouldn't know if she were in that super fertile group or not.

Contraception and the Menopause Transition: When to Stop?

No blood test or ultrasound can tell a woman that she no longer needs contraception. Some practitioners suggest testing the hormone FSH (follicle stimulating hormone, see chapter 3), because it's elevated in menopause. These practitioners believe an FSH level ≥30 IU/l on two occasions measured at least six to eight weeks apart and at least fourteen days after the last birth control pill/patch/ring for women using these methods means contraception is no longer needed. This approach has never been tested in large studies. Ovulation is erratic during the menopause transition, especially during the one to two years before the final menstrual period, and some women can have menopausal levels of FSH for several months and then ovulate the next cycle. Meaning, a woman can have an elevated FSH level eight weeks apart and still get pregnant. Most major medical societies advise against this testing given the unreliability.

The guidelines for stopping contraception are based on age and the last menstrual period. While waiting to see if the last period was the final one, backup contraception is recommended:

- **WOMEN UNDER THE AGE OF FIFTY:** Continue contraception until two years after the final menstrual period. Even though menopause is diagnosed when there hasn't been a period for a year, guidelines recommend this extra year to be certain. There are other medical reasons a woman may not have a period for two years, so women in their early forties especially should be certain their lack of a period isn't due to something other than menopause.
- **WOMEN AGES FIFTY YEARS AND OLDER:** Continue contraception for one year after the final menstrual period.
- **WOMEN AGES FIFTY-FIVE YEARS AND OLDER:** Stop contraception.

I'd *like* to say that stopping a method for one to two years to commence the Great Menstrual Wait is a *fine* strategy, but I think it sucks for many women. Not all women on the birth control pill (or the patch or the ring) want to keep taking it until they're fifty-five if they don't need the medication. The doses of estrogen are higher than that found in menopausal hormone therapy (MHT), so many women might transition to

MHT sooner if they knew they no longer needed the contraception. Also, using condoms for an additional year or two or taking the morning after pill in a panic five months after the last period adds expense, inconvenience, and stress.

I don't have a better option; I just want to acknowledge the suckitude.

Hormonal IUDs

Hormonal intrauterine devices (IUDs) contain levonorgestrel, which is a progestin (see chapters 17 and 18). The pregnancy rate with the levonorgestrel IUDs (LNG-IUD) is 0.2 percent to 0.3 percent, so they're an excellent option for women who definitely don't want to be pregnant. Progestin IUDs work by making cervical mucus inhospitable to sperm—basically, they create a chemical sperm blockade. They aren't abortifacients, meaning there's no evidence they prevent implantation of a fertilized egg or disrupt an existing pregnancy.

There are currently four hormonal IUDs available (as of July 2020) in the United States (see supplemental table 8, p. 341). They vary by the amount of levonorgestrel, how much is released each day, and the duration of contraception. Two of these IUDs can be used beyond the recommended guidelines. When the Mirena is inserted at the age of forty-five or later it's considered effective until the age of fifty-five, making it a very popular IUD for women during the menopause transition.

Hormonal IUDs reduce the amount of menstrual bleeding each cycle by more than 75 percent and 30 percent of women will have no periods, so they're often an appealing choice for women with irregular and/or heavy periods. The lowest dose IUD, Skyla, has the least impact on bleeding. This reduction in bleeding/no bleeding with LNG IUDs is due to the progestin and isn't harmful. The downside is irregular spotting or light bleeding for at least thirty days during the first three months after insertion (50 percent of women will have irregular bleeding for more than thirty days). This is a nuisance (you can ruin a lot of underwear if unprepared), and for women who consider one to two months of spotting unacceptable the LNG-IUD may not be the best option. Other benefits of these IUDs include reducing period cramps, treating pelvic pain from endometriosis (a condition where tissue similar to the lining

of the uterus grows in the pelvic cavity), and reducing the risk of both endometrial and ovarian cancer.

The Mirena is the real standout. Not only can it prevent or treat
bleeding issues, it can be used for endometrial protection in MHT (see
chapter 18), making the transition from contraception to MHT seamless.
Estrogen can be started if symptoms, such as hot flushes, become
bothersome or when the decision is made to start estrogen to protect
against osteoporosis. Women who don't start MHT can have their IUD
removed when they are fifty-five.

Major complications with the LNG-IUD are uncommon. The risk of
the body expelling the IUD is 2 percent to 10 percent. Infection happens
in 1.4 cases out of 1,000 insertions (antibiotics don't lower the risk) and
the risk of perforation (meaning the IUD goes through the uterus into the
abdominal cavity and a serious complication) is <0.5 percent. There is
some data that suggests the LNG-IUD may slightly increase the risk of
breast cancer, meaning for every 7,690 women using this method an
additional one woman will develop breast cancer. A small percentage of
women may experience headaches, nausea, breast tenderness, and
ovarian cysts as side effects.

Copper IUD

Highly effective with a failure rate of 0.8 percent. It's hormone-free and
works because copper is toxic to sperm. Only one copper IUD is currently
available in the United States—the ParaGuard or Cu380A. However, there
are multiple copper IUDs of different sizes and shapes in many other countries. How the United States fell so far behind IUD-wise would be an entire
chapter in another book, perhaps a future *Gunter's Guide to Gynecology*.
Like the LNG-IUD, the copper IUD also reduces the risk of ovarian cancer.

The Paraguard is approved for ten years, but when inserted at the age
of thirty-five or older it can be relied upon for contraception until
menopause. Several other copper IUDs are also effective beyond their
approval date. The copper IUD doesn't affect the menstrual cycle, so
women can use their period to determine when they are postmenopausal.
Unless there are other issues, it's best to leave in until a woman is over
the age of fifty and hasn't had a period for a year.

There's one downside with the copper IUD—a potential for heavier periods. "I'd like heavier periods please," has been said by no woman ever! Heavy periods don't happen to everyone and if they do they can often be managed (see chapter 10 for more information), but it's something to consider for women who already have heavier periods since they're *not* going to improve with a copper IUD. Like the LNG-IUD there is the risk of pain with insertion, as well as the low risks of expulsion, infection, and damaging the uterus with insertion.

An IUD Sounds Great, but Doesn't Insertion Hurt? A lot?

The average pain score with an IUD insertion is 5 on a 10-point scale (where 0 is no pain and 10 is the worst pain imaginable). Many women rate the insertion of an IUD similar to period pain—this should not be used to downplay the pain with insertion, because many women have significant pain from menstrual cramps. Women who are concerned the pain will be bad, have not previously been pregnant, or who have painful periods are more likely to have more pain with IUD insertion. Older data suggested the Mirena may have been slightly more painful than the copper IUD due to the Mirena insertion tube being slightly wider in diameter than the Paraguard—4.8 mm versus 4.39 mm. However, the Mirena is now 4.4 mm so that no longer seems to be an issue.

The pain for an IUD insertion can be caused by several things including the speculum (the instrument inserted vaginally to keep the vaginal walls apart so the cervix can be visualized), an instrument that may be needed to stabilize the cervix, dilating the cervix to pass the IUD, and cramping from the uterus as the IUD is placed. There has been a lot of research on medications and procedures to try to reduce this pain and unfortunately many things have been tried, but nothing has been overly successful. This is probably because there are likely several different sources of the pain, and there's no easy way to treat pain from stimulating the cervix and the uterus. This is why there is no easy pain relief in labor.

There is a common belief if men could get IUDs they would get a general anesthetic in the operating room, but a comparable procedure for a man is a cystoscopy (looking in the bladder with a rigid telescope), and that procedure is performed in the clinic, like an IUD. This doesn't mean it's acceptable for women to have painful procedures if men do, rather just to point out that men aren't getting more pain relief than women for this comparable procedure.

It's best to discuss concerns with your provider about pain in advance of the procedure, so there are expectations and a plan. As anticipating pain can increase pain, consider some deep breathing and even some affirmations and reminding yourself that if the average pain score is 5, that means 50 percent of women have pain scores of 5 or less and that most women who have an IUD would recommend having an IUD to a friend. Oral pain medication thirty minutes or so before the procedure may help some women. Various numbing or anesthetic medications for the cervix have been tried, and they may help some women a little, but the results of these studies aren't overwhelming. Another option is sedation, meaning intravenous medication to reduce pain. After all, we have modern anesthesia for a reason. This adds expense to the procedure for many women, decreases convenience as sedation requires a special room and monitoring equipment or possibly even an operating room, and anesthesia carries a very small risk of complications, but for some women this may be the best option. Everyone has a different risk benefit ratio, meaning what kind of pain is tolerable for them versus the hassle of needing someone to drive them home from an anesthetic for an IUD. It's not wrong to need more pain control. You need the pain control you need. More options allow for a more informed choice. Unfortunately, more pain control may mean more cost and sadly many women are not offered these options.

Combined Hormonal Contraception

Commonly referred to as "The Pill." Combined hormonal contraception is an estrogen, typically ethinyl estradiol *combined* with a progestin. They're available as a pill, a patch, or a vaginal ring, and they work by suppressing ovulation and by making cervical mucus inhospitable.

Estrogen-containing birth control pills have anywhere from 10 to 35 mcg of ethinyl estradiol per pill. Older pills contained 50 mcg per pill, but are no longer in general use. A pill that contains estradiol valerate is also now available. There are several different progestogens in use, and with the exception of desogesterel (see below), they are all very similar. The patch and the ring both contain ethinyl estradiol, but the patch has the progestin norelgestromin and the ring has the progestin etonogestrel.

The typical failure rate with combined hormonal contraception for women less than forty-five years old is 9 percent, but it's 0.3 percent when used exactly as directed. This difference between typical and ideal use reflects the fact that remembering to take a pill every day, or changing a patch or ring, can be hard for a lot of people (even OB/GYNS). During the menopause transition the failure rate of these methods drops as fertility drops. Basically, if a forty-seven-year-old misses two pills she is much less likely to ovulate during that window than a twenty-seven-year-old.

Combined contraception has some definite advantages during the menopause transition:

- **CONTROL OF ABNORMAL BLEEDING:** Regulating periods and reducing the amount of menstrual blood. The medication can be used continuously, meaning no placebo or off week, and for many women this will stop periods altogether. This isn't harmful; it means the lining of the uterus is thin from the hormones, and as there is no withdrawal of a progestogen there's no trigger for bleeding.
- **PREVENTING SYMPTOMS OF MENOPAUSE:** Courtesy of the estrogen.
- **PROTECTING THE BONES:** The estrogen delays menopause-related bone loss and may be helpful for women at higher risk of osteoporosis.
- **REDUCES THE RATE OF OVARIAN CANCER AND ENDOMETRIAL CANCER:** Definitely an added bonus.

There are some risks with combined contraception, and many of them increase with age, so it's important to make sure these medications are safe for you:

- **CARDIOVASCULAR EFFECTS:** The estrogen increases the risk of blood clots, stroke, and heart attacks (see table 5). Cofactors that increase the risk of these complications include age, smoking, high blood pressure, and a history of migraine headaches.

Women who don't smoke and who don't have conditions that raise their risk of stroke or heart attack generally can take combined hormonal contraception until age fifty to fifty-five years.

- **DEPRESSION:** There's been a fair amount of research in this area, so concerns raised by women have been evaluated. The largest study on depression and hormonal contraception from 2016 suggested a small correlation between the pill and depression for teens (one additional case of depression for every two hundred teens prescribed the pill; for perspective teens also have a higher risk of postpartum depression), but there was no impact of hormonal contraception on depression for adults. Some studies have even shown hormonal contraception improves mood. It's important to acknowledge some women do report a change in mood on the pill, but it isn't known whether there is a small group who are uniquely vulnerable, the negative association of mood and contraception is recall bias (looking back and trying to link what is happening to an event), or some women have other risk factors for depression that are associated with starting the pill but not caused by the pill (for example, the menopause transition, acne or a new sex partner). A history of depression or being on antidepressants is not a contraindication to starting the pill, but if any woman notices concerning changes in her mood, then obviously she needs to discuss that with her medical providers.

- **BREAST CANCER:** There is some data to suggest a very small increased risk for women who are current users of combined hormonal contraception, but many of these studies have limitations. Overall, the risk of breast cancer is at most 1 increased case for every 7,690 women (just as with the hormonal IUD). Women who have had breast cancer shouldn't use any form of hormonal contraception.

Other tips about combined hormonal contraception:

- **AIM FOR THE LOWEST EFFECTIVE DOSE OF ESTROGEN:** While there isn't good data to suggest a 10–20 mcg estrogen-containing pill is safer than a 35 mcg, many women prefer to be on the lowest dose when possible. As the recommendation for MHT is to take the lowest

Table 5: Risk of Blood Clots with Hormonal Contraception, MHT, and Pregnancy

	RISK OF BLOOD CLOTS*
Baseline risk	1–5/10,000 women per year
MHT oral therapy	8–9/10,000 women per year
Estrogen-containing contraception	3–15/10,000 women per year
Pregnancy	5–20/10,000 women per pregnancy
Postpartum	40–65/10,000 women per 12 weeks

* As risk increases with age, women ages forty to forty-five are typically at the higher end of each risk category.

dose, it seems intuitive to apply that same principle with the estrogen in contraception. There's only one dose of patch and ring.

- **HOT FLASHES DURING THE PLACEBO PILL WEEK:** Take the pill every day so there is no hormone-free interval.
- **MINIMIZE RISKS OF BLOOD CLOTS:** Some data suggests these risks may be slightly higher with a birth control pill that contains the hormone drospirenone and the patch. When there is no compelling reason for these products, they may be best to avoid.
- **THE PILL DOESN'T CAUSE WEIGHT GAIN:** This is a fairly common myth and can lead some women away from this method, but multiple studies have not found a link. Women taking the birth control pill have been compared with those who chose a copper IUD and the weight gain was small, but the same in both groups. As women who selected a copper IUD also gained the same amount of weight, the cause couldn't be hormones. It is possible that the life changes that lead women to choose contraception, such as a change in relationship, could be a cause of weight gain.

Progestin-Only Pill

These pills only contain a progestin, so they won't increase blood pressure and don't have the slightly increased risk of blood clots, stroke, and heart attack seen with estrogen-containing contraception. There is only one progestin-only pill or POP on the market in the United States and Canada (as of July 2020), and it contains norethindrone. Unlike the combined oral contraceptive, the primary mechanism of action is hostile cervical mucus just like the progestin IUD (hostile cervical mucus would be a great name for a punk band). About 40 percent of cycles on the norethindrone pill are ovulatory.

The typical failure rate of progestin-only pills is 9 percent, but the failure rate is <1 percent for women over the age of forty, likely due to the reduction in fertility. Progestin-only pills have a narrow margin of error; for example, they need to be taken within three hours of the same time each day for optimal effectiveness. The reduction in fertility with age likely offers additional protection. There's a newer POP available in the UK, Europe, and other countries that contains the progestin desogesterel. One brand name is Cerzaette. The advantage of this formulation is it has a twelve-hour window for pill taking each day and it is also effective at blocking ovulation, reducing the failure rate.

POPs are generally very safe, although for some women with cardiovascular disease or a history of stroke the risks may outweigh the benefits, so if these conditions are present whether a POP is safe requires consultation with a health care provider. There is no age-specific limit for progestin-only contraceptive pills, and so these are a fine choice for women who prefer the oral contraceptive pill but for whom estrogen is contraindicated.

Symptoms of menopause may happen on the POP, such as hot flushes, but sometimes progestins can help so the picture may be confusing. The POP may help with heavy or irregular periods during the menopause transition, but in general it is less effective at controlling periods than methods that also have estrogen.

Injectable Hormonal Contraception

Depot medroxyprogesterone acetate or DMPA is a progestin also known by the brand name DepoProvera. It's an injectable contraception administered every twelve weeks with a pregnancy rate of 3 percent. DMPA can be effective treatment for heavy menstrual bleeding as 50 percent of women who have been using it for a year or more will stop having periods. However, one issue with DMPA for women as they age is a potential effect on bone density, and in the United States the product insert has a Black Box Warning, which states that prolonged use is associated with a reduction in bone density that may not be completely reversible. The warning also states that DMPA should only be used for longer than two years when there is no other adequate form of contraception. This is based on one small study of teens and bone health.

The World Health Organization (WHO) reviewed the data on DMPA and bone density and concluded there should be no restrictions for women ages eighteen to forty-five. At ages forty-five and older, the benefits of DMPA are believed to outweigh the potential risk of bone loss, but admittedly there isn't much data on bone loss and recovery for women in the menopausal transition. Women at higher risk of osteoporosis will need to weigh a potential negative impact on bone versus other benefits of DMPA. For perspective, pregnancy and breastfeeding also result in bone loss, but it's reversible.

DMPA may increase the risk of cardiovascular disease and stroke for some women, so women with high blood pressure that isn't controlled by medication or other risk factors for heart disease will need to have an in-depth discussion with their provider if DMPA is safe for them. DMPA is associated with an average of a 2 kg (4.4 lbs) weight gain. Many people erroneously think depression is a common side effect with DMPA; however, studies haven't proven this connection and so, like the pill/patch and ring depression is not a contraindication to starting. If an individual woman feels the method is affecting her mental health, then of course she should stop.

Etonogestrel Implant

The most effective form of contraception is an implant of a rod containing etonogestrel, a progestin with the trade name Nexplanon. It has a failure rate of 0.01 percent and is approved for three years, but is effective for five. Irregular bleeding from the implant, especially in the first year of use, is common. Overall, it isn't as good an option for controlling irregular periods as other hormonal methods. It isn't associated with bone loss or cardiovascular complications, like DMPA.

Sterilization

Vasectomy and female sterilization are nonreversible forms of contraception. Vasectomy is the safest method, but it isn't an option for all women, either due to the lack of a regular partner, multiple partners, or women with a partner unwilling to have a vasectomy. Conversations with a couple where the man is refusing to have a vasectomy while his partner has endured all the physical changes that come with pregnancy are always discouraging. Given how few couples rely on condoms long term, most women have borne the burden of contraception for the duration of their heterosexual relationships and frankly, it's time for the men to step up. The failure rate with a vasectomy is 0.15 percent.

Tubal ligation is the most popular method of permanent contraception. The rates vary considerably by country. In the United States tubal ligation is the fifth most common surgical procedure, and the rates are much higher than in Europe. Female sterilization is also a very popular method in India, Colombia, and El Salvador. Failure rates are <0.5 percent. The procedure requires a general anesthetic, which is one of the major drawbacks as that increases the risk, the expense, and the resources needed. The other issue is it requires surgically entering the abdomen, so there is a risk—albeit small—of inadvertently damaging other organs or major blood vessels. The risk of a major complication is <1 percent.

A tubal ligation is most commonly done via laparoscopy (operating telescope), with typically two small incisions, but it can also be performed soon after a delivery with an incision under the belly button (postpartum tubal ligation). Via laparoscopy the options are removing the entire tube or permanent clips to block the tube (removing the tube lowers the risk of ovarian cancer by 50 percent). It's technically more challenging to remove the tubes immediately after delivery, so with a postpartum tubal ligation the fallopian tubes are tied or cut instead.

Some women report changes in their menstrual cycle after a tubal ligation, a so-called post–tubal ligation syndrome, but studies have not found this association and a tubal ligation doesn't affect the age of natural menopause. The difference in periods after a tubal ligation may be due to the fact that, following the procedure, many women stop their estrogen-containing contraception pills and without the cycle control provided by the pill, their menstrual pattern—irregular periods—emerges. Remember, the menopause transition is the time when menses become abnormal, so menstrual irregularity within a few years of a tubal ligation in the late thirties or early forties is expected. A woman considering a tubal ligation should also weigh how she might feel if she were to develop heavy and/or irregular periods later in life—or even within a few years of her surgery—and the recommended treatment is hormonal contraception. If this would bother her, then she may wish to reconsider her options.

Condoms

Both male and female (also called internal condoms) are excellent options. The male condom has a failure rate of 13 percent and the female condom of 21 percent over one year. Condoms also protect from sexually transmitted infections (STIs), which are on the rise among *all* age groups. Rates of chlamydia have almost doubled among adults ages fifty-five to sixty-four years and the rate of trichomonas for women over forty is higher than among women ages twenty-five to thirty-nine. The reasons are complex. Many people falsely assume STIs aren't a concern over forty. The lower estrogen levels in the vagina in the forties and beyond may increase the risk of acquiring some STIs. People who have been in a long-term relationship who are newly dating may underestimate their risk of STIs, feel uncomfortable buying condoms, or may be unfamiliar with condom etiquette. (It's not forward to bring your own or rude to insist; also, do you really think someone who doesn't care about your health is going to be invested in your orgasm?)

Erectile dysfunction or ED for men increases with age—by the age of forty about 40 percent of men have some degree of erectile dysfunction and it increases by 10 percent each decade (so 50 percent at age fifty, 60 percent at age seventy, and so on). Many men with ED are not capable of wearing a male condom. In one study 46 percent of heterosexual men aged fifty and older reported that a condom could result in the loss of an erection. A good way around age-related condom concerns, besides direct conversation about expectations and safety as well as seeking treatment for ED, is a female condom. These condoms are inserted vaginally and are independent of erectile quality. A female condom can also be used anally.

Condoms also protect the vaginal ecosystem, and multiple studies show they reduce the incidence of bacterial vaginosis, which is a disturbance of the vaginal ecosystem that results in discharge, irritation, and odor. Bacterial vaginosis also increases the risk of acquiring many STIs, such as HIV or gonorrhea, if exposed.

Contraceptive Gel

There is a new contraceptive gel on the market called Phexxi—rhymes with sexy. Women insert an applicator of the product before sex. The gel is acidic and prevents ejaculate from temporarily raising the pH of the vagina (that's what allows the sperm to thrive in the vagina so they can swim to the cervix and up into the uterus).

Phexxi is $250 to $275 for a box of twelve without insurance. "Sure he's nice, but is he Phexxi-worthy?" could replace the Elaine Benes sponge-worthy meme from the TV show *Seinfeld*. Jokes aside, it's great to have another on-demand contraceptive that is woman controlled. Phexxi has a failure rate of approximately 27 percent over one year, so worse than condoms. In the initial study about 18 percent of women developed vaginal or vulvar burning, and it shouldn't be used by women with recurring UTIs.

Postcoital Contraception

There are two oral medications for postcoital contraception, commonly referred to as the morning after pill: 1.5 mg of levonorgestrel (a progestin, has been marketed under the name Plan B) and 30 mg of ulipristal acetate (a medication that blocks progesterone, trade name Ella). These methods both work by delaying or inhibiting ovulation long enough that the sperm dies. Levonorgestrel method delays/inhibits ovulation for two days and the ulipristal method for five days. Those differences, and the fact that ulipristal may be less affected by body weight, likely explain why ulipristal is more effective. The copper IUD is also excellent emergency contraception, because it's immediately toxic to sperm and the inflammatory response may also affect egg quality. It's the most effective method.

If ovulation has already happened the oral medication won't be effective, but as the copper IUD damages sperm it's still useful regardless of ovulatory status. There's no medical contraindication to either of the

Table 6: Postcoital Contraception

METHOD	DAYS AFTER SEX	RISK OF PREGNANCY	ACCESS	IMPACTED BY WEIGHT
None (for reference)	n/a	10* %	n/a	n/a
Levonor-gestrel	Within 72 hours	2.2%	OTC in the US, Canada, UK, Australia and many other countries	Less effective for BMI ≥25
Ulipristal	Up to 5 days	1.4%	Prescription in US and Canada, OTC in many other countries	Less effective for BMI ≥30
Copper IUD	Up to 5 days, some studies suggest up to 10 days	0.1%	Requires a doctor's visit	No

* Chance of conception on the most fertile day of the cycle.

morning-after pills. Common side effects are temporary nausea and headache. Irregular bleeding may also happen.

Having a package of postcoital contraception on hand is a great strategy for women using any method subject to user error (think pills, patch, ring, injection, condoms, etc.) as well as for women who don't think they need contraception and then plans change. Sprinting to the closest pharmacy on the Las Vegas Strip at the age of forty-four in a cold sweat despite the oppressive heat is not a fun experience. #JustSaying #BeenThere.

Fertility Awareness—Based Methods

Fertility awareness–based methods or FABM are often called natural family planning (NFP) or the rhythm method. They encompass a variety of methods that track biological markers, such as menstrual cycle length, cervical mucus, body temperature, cervical position, and urinary hormone levels, to predict fertile windows when conception is most likely to occur. To avoid pregnancy during the fertile window, abstinence or another method is used. Failure rates range from 2 percent to 34 percent, although many of these methods haven't been adequately tested. The effort of tracking the various markers, the unpredictability of these markers for some women, and the need for periodic abstinence or back up contraception all contribute to the failure rate.

The menstrual cycle irregularity and fluctuation in hormone levels of the menopause transition can make it challenging to track these biological markers. There's only a single study of 160 women ages forty to fifty-five using FABM—the pregnancy rate was 6 per 100 women per year or 6 percent. There were no pregnancies for women ages forty-four and older, but given the low number of study participants it isn't possible to know if that's simply due to the lower pregnancy rate at that age or the effectiveness of the method, therefore no conclusions can be made about effectiveness.

BOTTOM LINE

- Women should consider themselves capable of conceiving until they've been two years without a period and are younger than fifty, or one year without a period for those fifty years old or older.
- When inserted at age forty-five or older the Mirena IUD is highly effective contraception until age fifty-five and can transition from contraceptive to the progestin in MHT.
- A copper IUD inserted at the age of thirty-five or older is effective until menopause.
- A low-dose estrogen-containing oral contraception can be used by many women until age fifty-five and can treat many symptoms of the menopause transition.
- On-demand contraception, condoms (both male and internal condoms), Phexxi, and postcoital contraception are also excellent options.

Part 4

Taking Charge of the Change

Chapter 24

Welcome to My Menoparty:

How an OB/GYN Tackles Menopause

WHILE WRITING THIS BOOK I often thought of my mother, which considering our awful relationship seemed odd. Many women look to their mothers, sometimes for information or guidance but also as a mirror for divination—does their mother's experience portend their own future or no? But growing up I wanted to be the opposite of my mother and as we never discussed anything reproductive health related—she didn't like that I was a gynecologist and wondered if perhaps instead I could do something good for women's health and be a radiologist and read mammograms—I wondered why this book was triggering me to look back. It was much more than her osteoporosis.

I began to think more about her menopause transition, which I described previously as volcanic. Her mood swings, anger, and cruelty towards me during that time is painful, even today. My mother suffered from depression her whole life and developed severe postpartum depression after I was born, so it would make sense, biologically-speaking, that she may have suffered more with her mental health during her menopause transition. It doesn't excuse her cuelty, but it does give me more empathy toward her than I believed I was capable of feeling. She had no one to talk with about her symptoms and even though hornones were available in the 1970s and might have helped, they weren't offered.

Her family lived in England and she had no close friends. While writing this book I often thought of how lonely she must have felt with a changing body and the fear that maybe the blackness that enveloped her after my birth was barely at arm's length.

In so many ways menopause is about perpsective.

I started my menopause transition around the age of forty-five. I was frankly surprised it was this late because my mother was already well through menopause when she was that age. I chalked it up to not smoking and a long time on the birth control pill. But of course, who knows.

My final menstrual period was at a very average fifty years old. I had a few hot flushes, mostly at night, until about a year before my last period, when they rapidly became bothersome. I tried creative layering with my clothing, but needing to rip off less clothing only succeeded in making me slightly less angry when I had a hot flush.

Like many women my hot flushes and night sweats are worse in the summer months. In fact this summer—which was blisteringly hot—I had more hot flushes than I'd had in a long while. I kept pressing my estrogen patch to see if that might help, but they don't work that way (the estrogen absorbs slowly), so it was as effective as pushing the walk button at a street light.

One interesting observation I've made about my hot flushes is they don't seem to happen outside, even when it's hot. I've never had a hot flush running or riding my bike either, even when I'm hot and sweaty. I am curious if I'm having them and I'm not aware or if they are truly happening less often. I also wonder if this is something other women experience and if it could be an explanation for regional variations in hot flushes. It could just be me and my wonky thermostat—menopause is like that. I also experience nausea with my hot flushes, something I have yet to read about. At times my flushes make me feel as if I have had too much to drink and I need to pray to the porcelain God. I thought I was the only one, but once I mentioned it in a blog post several years ago many women have messaged me to say they also thought they were the only ones.

As this book gestated I began to wonder how many other questions haven't been asked because for so long people who experience menopause and who are best able to say what is happening haven't had a seat at the medical table? Or because talking about menopause was considered impolite or something not done because who wants to draw attention to the fact they are aging? The patriarchy has been controlling menopause for too long—demanding our silence and when we speak they have governed the very words that we use—and we are continuing to pay the price.

I'm often asked why I started hormones, and it fascinates me how clandestine that decision seems. I remember telling one reporter I was on MHT and she gasped, as if I'd just told her I had sex on the roof of the British Museum with a hot guy I'd just met in a London club whose name I didn't know. I guess her response was a reflection of the significant reduction in women using menopausal hormone therapy (MHT), but also I think the false idea that estrogen is a dangerous way to conjure youth played a role.

At this point in the conversation I remind whoever has asked that estrogen is just a medication and then I bring up risk-benefit ratio. I've alluded to it throughout the book, but it's worth mentioning again as I feel the concept is poorly taught and it's very important. By the risk-benefit ratio I mean the risk we are willing to tolerate for the chance of a benefit, and it varies person to person. I would never go sky diving; there is no benefit I could achieve from that pursuit that could counter any risk, because I hate heights. In fact I feel slightly unwell even now imagining myself jumping out of an airplane. So with no possible benefit, I don't need to consider the risk. But others who want the thrill may feel differently. Those who have a good understanding of parachute safety likely feel the risk is much lower than I—a frightened nonexpert.

When considering the risk I think its important to consider how you might feel if you have that bad side effect. Most of us consider the upsides more than the downsides. However, even a rare risk, for example 1 in 10,000, isn't zero, and so when I discuss risk with my own patients I always ask them how they will feel if they are that one person who has the complication?

Women deserve safe medications, but risks in the 1/10,000–1/100,000 a year range are likely not preventable. The rarity of these events means they're almost impossible to identify in studies used for drug approval. This is a major reason the Food and Drug Administration (FDA) requires post-marketing surveillance, which are larger studies after the medication is approved to identify safety signals missed in the original studies. It's also important to put these rare risks in perspective and to discuss the consequences of not using a medication. One analysis suggests between 18,000 and 91,000 women may have died prematurely because either they or their doctors feared estrogen in the ten years after the WHI was published.

Given my mother's osteoporosis—her early age and the severity of her osteoporosis—estrogen seemed like the option for me. I decided if I had a fracture and had never started MHT, I would never forgive myself. I looked at the small risk of breast cancer and decided that it was worth it for me.

I chose transdermal estradiol as it is clearly the winner safety-wise. That doesn't mean oral medications are unsafe, but when there is no competing reason for oral therapy why assume the increased risk of blood clots with oral therapy, no matter how small? I am using a patch that is changed twice weekly (the weekly patch just didn't stay on longer than four days for me). The biggest issue for me is the leftover adhesive, which has a similar consistency with tar, and getting it off my skin is hard. I'm always running late so I'm not sure I have the time to apply an estradiol lotion or gel and wait for it to dry. These quality of life issues matter, because for a therapy to be useful you have to be able to use it.

Before I started the estrogen, sex in my late forties required a silicone-based lube, but I seem to be in the 50 percent of women for whom MHT treats genitourinary syndrome of menopause. The vaginal therapies are also excellent options, so if I hadn't needed transdermal estrogen I would probably have tried the ring. I have a hard time remembering to take medications, so the more user-friendly the better.

I didn't have any false beliefs about estrogen, and that is a very important point. There are people who push the concept that every woman needs estrogen and that there is no cancer risk. If there was good data showing that every woman should take estrogen after menopause, then the professional societies, like the North American Menopause Society (NAMS) or the American College of Obstetrics and Gynecology (ACOG), would be recommending it.

As an OB/GYN I was also able to navigate the competing claims from different medical organizations. Knowing what the menopause experts at NAMS had to say about estrogen was important, because the American College of Physicians calls estrogen a high risk medication. If this were the first thing someone read on estrogen, why would they consider it for hot flushes or for any reason? Obviously, I disagree with the American College of Physicians as do many others, but if this is where a woman's provider is getting their information about MHT it may well affect how they counsel their patients.

And of course there are people who are in the never estrogen camp because menopause is a normal phase of life. But this ignores conditions like osteoporosis and menopause-triggered depression—and also quality of life. Why should a woman who has twenty hot flushes a day and hasn't slept well in weeks not try estrogen if it's safe so she can have a better life? Pregnancy is a normal phase of life, but we wouldn't consider it acceptable to deny care for morning sickness, not to provide pain medication in labor, or to refuse a blood transfusion after delivery if indicated due to blood loss. After all, some women hemorrhage after a completely typical delivery.

The truth is many women do better with estrogen, for a variety of reasons, and many don't need it. That's why it's important to know as much about menopause as possible so each woman can make choices that work for her.

I changed some things in my life as the result of research for this book. I have recommitted to a regular exercise plan. Honestly, study after study listed exercise in the "helps" category. Like every study. It's a work in progress, life gets so busy, but it's amazing preventative care. I have also fine-tuned my diet a bit. I've upped my legumes and dropped my milk consumption to one to two cups a day and am exploring a combination of the Mediterranean and MIND diets discussed in earlier chapters. Finding good recipes on a regular basis is a chore, so I get most of mine from the *New York Times* food section, but I am also creating some recipes that emphasize the nutritional needs for women in menopause. I am eating fatty fish at least twice a week and that takes effort, but if I couldn't make this happen I would take an omega-3 supplement. I've also started a vitamin D supplement—vitamin D production drops with age and I'm trying to do better with sunscreen.

Like many of my friends I felt menopause was a magnet for what felt like a rapid and unwelcome change in shape. I'd like to blame my hormones, but I also have to be truthful. This was a period of time where I stopped exercising and ate a lot of meals in restaurants. This is an important point and deserves emphasis—it's very easy to blame menopause when it can be *waves hands all around* everything else. Just as it's important not to dismiss women who are having menopause-related concerns, it's equally as important to not blame all concerns on menopause and assume that estrogen is the answer.

I'm mindful that MHT is just one part of my menopuzzle. In addition to diet, exercise, and balance training, I'm working on CBT to help with hot flushes and being vigilant with annual blood pressure screening, checks on lipids and blood sugar every two to three years (based on my values), my bone density screening, and mammograms. It takes a fair bit of maintenance in your fifties and beyond.

I am aware as an OB/GYN I have a lot of privilege—including my knowledge of medicine, the medical system, and the fact that I trained when fear of estrogen hadn't been overly hyped. But menopause shouldn't be a mystery to women and it's not a marginal concern—this is women's health care.

Chapter 25

Final Thoughts:
Putting It All Together

KNOWING WHAT IS HAPPENING TO your body and that there are options is itself powerful medicine. One of the common experiences I hear with menopause is loneliness. Think back to the canoe analogy at the beginning of this book—many women feel as if they are on a journey by themselves. I hope this book has provided a guide to the waters that lie ahead or an explanation of a journey already started.

So what next?

The first thing for any woman struggling with symptoms that she feels may be menopause-related is to record what is happening. I call these symptoms the "bother factor." Maybe it's hot flushes or feeling low energy, but for others it could be forgetfulness or heavy periods. It may be all of these or something else. But I find it's best to have specifics, especially if you are heading to a medical provider for help. I personally love when my patients bring in these lists. I would rather know everything up front as that may help me guide therapy and of course I want my patients to be heard.

When women ask me about their menopause and what they should do, I know many are wondering if they should take hormones. Hopefully this book has helped answer many questions about what hormones can and can't do, as well as raised awareness about the risks that may be part of menopausal hormone therapy (MHT). Equally as important, I hope this book has helped people step back from MHT and take in the bigger picture of menopause, not only to reframe the experience but also to consider all the ways to optimize health along the menopause continuum. When we focus on hormones we miss many other important interventions, like quitting smoking, diet, and exercise. Or the value of CBT for hot flushes, insomnia, and low desire.

But there is other harm in being estrogen-exclusive. When people imply all women need estrogen during their menopause transition or during their postmenopause, it's simply a rebranding of what we heard with hormone marketing in the 1950s and 1960s. It's just now instead of estrogen being packaged as glamorous, it's sold as natural and self-care. MHT isn't a Get Out of Menopause Jail Free Card, it's one puzzle piece. For some women a big piece of the puzzle and for others not at all.

Instead of thinking in terms of natural or unnatural, menopause is best navigated with facts. After all, it's natural to get osteoporosis during menopause and even natural for the estrogen produced by the ovaries to cause breast cancer. It's not natural for women who are postmenopausal to have the levels of estradiol in their blood that come with MHT. None of these facts make MHT good or bad.

The best way to approach menopause is to be informed so women can understand if what is happening is menopause-related; what diseases she may face due to her combination of genetics, health, and menopausal status; and what is the best way to achieve quality of life and health and how to best balance those goals against any risks. This can only happen with accurate information and without the prejudice of the patriarchy.

How Do You Know if You Are Seeing the Right Provider?

Whether a woman is getting information from her provider in the office, from a book, a magazine, or an online source, it's important to know some basics about how to determine whether that information is trustworthy or not. If it's found online at the North American Menopause Society (NAMS), the American College of Obstetricians and Gynecologists (ACOG), the Society of Obstetricians and Gynecologists of Canada (SOGC), the Australasian Menopause Society (AMS), or the International Menopause Society (IMS) then it has been vetted by experts and typically those experts have been required to disclose any biases.

A good way to start looking for information online isn't to just use a search engine, rather to search internally on NAMS or ACOG or to enter a search, such as "hot flushes" and add "NAMS" or "ACOG" or any other medical professional society. This will filter results from those organizations, so they should appear at the top of the search.

NAMS also has a menopause certification for providers. While many providers who are not NAMS certified are excellent, looking for one if you are in North America who has that certification will help a woman find someone who has demonstrated an increased interest in the area, has passed a proficiency exam on the subject, and is required to stay up to date with continuing medical education to maintain their certification.

What do you do about information you receive or find on your own? Without reading the paragraph in question it's not possible to me to say something is trustworthy or suspect, but here are some red flags about information sources and content that women should be mindful of in their search for quality information on menopause:

- **SALIVARY HORMONE LEVELS:** These are never indicated. Ever. If any friend of mine were seeing a provider who recommended salivary hormone levels, my advice would be ask for her money back, walk out the door, and forget everything that person told her. I often see women who have paid a lot of money for these tests and they are understandably upset when I tell them they are of no value. Most frequently I speak with women who paid for this testing on the advice of a naturopath. It's always a difficult conversation explaining how the results are useless—people have a hard time accepting how something done by a lab with results on paper is medically meaningless. Also, no one likes to hear they paid money for something that is unhelpful.
- **HORMONE LEVELS TO GUIDE THERAPY OR "SEE WHERE YOU ARE":** Some providers recommend blood tests for hormone levels, typically estradiol and FSH (follicle stimulating hormone) although there may be others, to diagnose menopause, to see if a woman is close to menopause, or to manage MHT. This is not indicated.

Just as we don't need hormone levels to diagnose puberty, we don't need them for the menopause transition or postmenopause. Hormone levels are indicated when women are younger than forty, but otherwise they aren't helpful and are a waste of money and resources. This isn't fringe medical knowledge only known to a few providers, but this is the standard recommendation from NAMS and ACOG. If my provider recommended hormone levels I would always be wondering, "What else that is common knowledge do they have wrong?"

- **HORMONE HEAVY THERAPY:** Some providers only recommend hormones and women are either not told about the nonhormonal options, are told they don't work, or are frightened by the side effects. I see this most often with hot flushes—the nonhormonal therapies can be very effective for many women. If it's Hormones! Hormones! Hormones! get another opinion.

- **DO THEY SPEAK OF ESTROGEN AS IF IT'S A WONDER DRUG AND 100 PER-CENT SAFE?** Estrogen can help many women with some symptoms, but even where estrogen is very helpful—for example hot flushes—it doesn't eliminate 100 percent of symptoms for 100 percent of women. For me, the idea of estrogen as wonder drug needed by all women is an echo of misogynistic ideas that menopause means decay. Estrogen is a therapeutic tool—there are some specific things it can do. Like any medication, if it isn't needed then it shouldn't be started. All medications have risks, even estrogen. And while the risks are small, they exist.

- **RECOMMEND COMPOUNDED HORMONES OVER PHARMACEUTICALS:** These are untested, unregulated, and studies have raised concerns about dosing. This includes testosterone pellets. Not recommended at all.

- **RECOMMEND TOPICAL PROGESTERONE:** This is another "get up and walk out the door and/or block online" moment. Progesterone is not absorbed topically, and relying on it could lead a woman taking estrogen to develop endometrial cancer. Hard pass.

- **THE PROVIDER IS ANTIVACCINE OR ENGAGES IN OTHER MEDICAL CON-SPIRACY THEORIES:** Google their name and the word "vaccines" and then repeat with the word "fluoride" (antifluoride in water is another common medical conspiracy theory). Many aren't shy about this—in fact, it's often a badge of honor. Vaccines are safe and save lives. Fluoride in the water is safe. Medical conspiracy thinking is the opposite of rational, measured thought and has no place in medicine. There is a big overlap between wellness and natural medicine and conspiracy theories, so be very careful here.

- **DO THEY RECOMMEND SPECIAL SUPPLEMENTS?** This isn't about vitamin D or omega-3 fatty acids or about replacements when there may be a deficiency (for example, iron). These are "special" multivitamins for menopause or concoctions to "support" the thyroid or adrenal gland or ovary. There is no such thing. Organs don't need support. Some doctors even have branded supplements with their face and/or name plastered on the bottle. Talk about bias. These products are medically untested and could be adulterated. If they worked they would be recommended by medical professional societies.

- **DOES THEIR WEBSITE SELL PRODUCTS?** You can't get quality information about a product from the person who profits from the sale. Don't take advice on menopause from people who have online stores with products aimed at menopause. They can be your care provider or your store, but they can't be both. Shops and science don't mix.

Don't Blame Everything on Menopause: Remember the M Diagram

I was watching the Oprah episode on hormones featuring Robin McGraw (Dr. Phil's wife). They were in the first ten minutes of an episode about her book, which was just published at the time, and Oprah wanted to discuss the section on menopause. Oprah explained to the audience that in her book McGraw detailed how she had been neglecting her own care—like many women—at the expense of caring for others. While she was ensuring her children ate healthy meals and had their medical appointments on time, she was eating cake for breakfast, gummies for lunch in the car, and was very sad one of her sons was heading to college. She felt terrible. This is not an uncommon story and until this point I was very interested. How did Robin McGraw solve that equation of too many demands and endlessly giving of herself to meet them?

Bioidentical hormones.

No, really.

My partner, who I affectionately call Dr. Jen Adjacent, yelled at the screen, "Of course you feel bad. You are eating cake for breakfast and gummies for lunch and are sad that your kid is going to college. How is that the fault of menopause?"

The point is well taken. Think back to our M diagram from chapter 1. Menopause doesn't happen in a vacuum. Patriarchy has made it so many of us are quick to blame hormones for everything. Look, we all want easy answers—even doctors—but for women who feel they are fatigued or at the end of their rope there is likely more to it than simply menopause.

Be Wary of New or Novel Therapies

It's common for people—doctors especially—to over interpret small signals in studies in a positive way. Women have been harmed by therapies not being thoroughly evaluated and so they deserve the highest quality data. The problem is that can take time and of course we all want our answers today.

A Reproductive Reckoning

I felt a simmering rage as I passed through my menopause transition, and it has only increased in intensity. I've seen it in other women and it made me curious as to why? It's taken a while to organize my thoughts, because admittedly for the longest time it felt as if I wanted to utter one long primal scream. While measurable in the moment, screaming into the ether is eventually exhausting and isn't a particularly good agent for self-care or change. I needed to understand the source of my anger, because it was only then that I would be able to stop it from living rent-free in my head and be able to use that force constructively. While writing this book it finally slid into focus.

To be a woman is to coexist with a unique reproductive gauntlet imposed by biology. For me there were heavy periods, menstrual diarrhea, and devastating pregnancy complications. Other women face different obstacles and suffering, all the consequences of a biology wired to improve reproductive outcomes. The system isn't perfect, so some women bleed too much, others have immune systems that turn on them and produce diseases such as rheumatoid arthritis, some develop high blood pressure during their pregnancy or postpartum depression, and that's "okay" on the grand scale because evolution only has to be good enough. But good enough means good enough for many, not all.

The kludgy equation of large brains and the ability to walk upright—the very wellspring of humanity—only works because women physically suck it up, some more than others. The price of evolution and all that we have achieved due to brains and mobility literally depend on women bearing an unequal physical burden. That women have more challenging biology compared with men isn't exactly a secret; after all, before the Affordable Care Act was passed in the United States, being a woman was essentially a pre-existing condition.

In addition, women are also the ones who typically bear more financial consequences of their biology, whether they have children or not. They are more likely to have lower paying jobs, and even when they are doing equal work as men they are often paid less. The best/worst example of this is OB/GYNs—largely women—getting paid less to do a vulvar biopsy than urologists—largely men—receive for doing a scrotal biopsy. Same procedure, same equipment, same pain level, same sexual consequences. Different reimbursement.

Women are also more likely to do unpaid work: household things like cooking, cleaning, and childcare, and also the emotional labor in a household and the office.

Taxing our bodies to fix the gaps seems to be encoded in our DNA.

Women are gaslit into believing that their bodies—the very thing that allows them to hack the big brain-small pelvis equation—are problematic and that consequently they themselves are problematic. We're dirty, silly, fat, gross, weak, or we're simply just complainers. We are forced to make do with a medical system largely designed around the needs of men and we have our medical concerns dismissed as "not that bad" or we are told they are fabricated.

Entering the menopause transition, I was already pissed about the unequal medical and societal burden created by a uterus, ovaries, vagina, and vulva—as if they are the barbed wire on a mud-filled obstacle course. But after running that gauntlet instead of emerging to menopausal fields of glory, what awaited was a reboot to Woman 2.0. A less desirable upgrade and with another set of medical hurdles to tolerate. More ways to suck it up and to be judged as lesser than men. It's as if you get to do it all over again. But worse, because now you are considered old.

And there it was. The source of my rage was this reproductive reckoning. The realization that menopause was just one more way that the burden of perpetuating the species is unequally borne by women and one more way that our biology is weaponized against us. It is the ultimate gaslighting because it's this biology—from puberty to grave—that literally birthed humanity as we know it.

Many women have been conditioned to fear menopause as an expiration date for relevance and as a sign of weakness only because that is what men thought. In fact, we have this amazing data that tells us that menopause is the opposite—a time when historically women contributed great things to society because of their knowledge and their age. Yes, menopause has symptoms and is associated with medical concerns, but there is help and it's certainly not a pre morbid state.

When told by a patriarchal society the story of menopause is one about deserted youth, frailty, and diminished worth. The story I want you to remember is about value, agency, and voice and the knowledge to keep yourself in the best of health while demanding an equal seat at the table.

That's my manifesto.

Supplementary Material

Supplemental Tables

Supplemental Table 1: Typical Bleeding Patterns and Associated Conditions for Women Ages 40 to Their Final Menstrual Period (assuming pregnancy had been excluded)

BLEEDING PATTERN	QUALITY OF BLEEDING	COMMON CAUSES
Regular periods	Spotting between periods	Polyp Cancer/precancer Infection
Regular periods	Heavy or lasting >7 days	Fibroids Adenomyosis Cancer/precancer Medications/supplements that affect clotting
Irregular periods	Heavy or light flow	Menopause transition Hormonal contraception Menopausal hormone therapy Hypothalamic amenorrhea Thyroid disease Elevated Prolactin Cancer/precancer
Bleeding after sex	Can range from spotting to a heavy flow	Polyp in the cervix Infection Cancer/precancer Inflammation of the cervix

Supplemental Table 2: Common Vaginal Moisturizers: pH and Osmolality Where Applicable

PRODUCT	BASE	pH	OSMOLALITY
HyaloGyn	Hyaluronic acid	4.8	1,336
K-Y Liquidbeads	Silicone	N/A	N/A
Moist Again	Water	5.68	187
Replens	Water	3.0	1,177
Vagisil Prohydrate Natural Feel	Hyaluronic acid	N/A	N/A
Yes Vaginal moisturizer	Water	4.15	250

Supplemental Table 3: Pharmaceutical Grade Vaginal Hormones

PRODUCT	MAINTENANCE DOSING	NOTES
Estradiol cream 0.01 mg/g	0.5–1 g twice a week	May be a better option for women with irritation and pain at the vestibule and on the vulva.
CEE cream 0.625 mg/g	0.5–1 g twice a week	May be a better option for women with irritation and pain at the vestibule and on the vulva.
Estradiol ring 7.5 mcg/day	1 ring exchanged every 3 months	May fall out for some women with prolapse. May be painful to insert for some women, and others, especially with arthritis, may have difficulties inserting and removing. Ultra-low dose*
Estradiol 4 mcg gel cap	1 twice a week	No applicator and minimal mess. Ultra-low dose.*
Estradiol 10 mcg gel cap	1 twice a week	No applicator and minimal mess. Ultra-low dose.*

PRODUCT	MAINTENANCE DOSING	NOTES
Estradiol 10 mcg tablet	1 twice a week	Preloaded in plastic applicator, some women bothered by the environmental impact.*
DHEA-S 6.5 mg	1 daily	

* Ultra-low-dose options don't appear to result in any measurable absorption of estradiol into the bloodstream, and estradiol levels remain in the menopausal range, which is <20 pg/ml.

Supplemental Table 4: Dose Equivalents of Different Estrogens and Delivery Systems

	DOSE EQUIVALENT	SOURCE
ORAL		
Estradiol	1 mg	Semi synthetic
CEE	0.625 mg	Natural
CE	0.625 mg	Semi synthetic
Ethinyl estradiol	0.005 mg (or 5 mcg)	Semi synthetic or synthetic
Estropipate	0.625 mg	Semi synthetic
Esterified estrogens	0.625 mg	Semi synthetic
TRANSDERMAL		
Estradiol patch (matrix)*	0.05 mg	Semi synthetic
Estradiol patch (reservoir)*	0.05 mg	Semi synthetic
Estradiol gel	3 different brands with different delivery systems, see supplemental table 5	Semi synthetic
Estradiol emulsion	2 packets	Semi synthetic
Estradiol spray	3 sprays	Semi synthetic
VAGINAL		
Estradiol ring	0.5 mg	Semi synthetic

* With a matrix patch the estradiol is in the adhesive, with the reservoir patch it is in a reservoir above the adhesive.

Supplemental Table 5: Dose Equivalents of Estradiol Gels

	DOSE	APPLICATION SITE	ESTRADIOL LEVELS
EstroGel	1 pump	Arm, from wrist to shoulder	35 mcg
Divigel	1 g packet	Upper thigh	34 mcg
Elestrin	2 pumps	Upper arm/shoulder	37.5 mcg

Supplemental Table 6: Progestogens in the United States and Canada

PROGESTOGEN	CLASS	ROUTES OF ADMINISTRATION
drospirenone	spironolactone derivative	oral
levonorgestrel	testosterone derivative	oral, intrauterine (IUD), transdermal
medroxyprogesterone acetate	progesterone derivative	oral
norethindrone acetate	testosterone derivative	oral, transdermal
norgestimate	testosterone derivative	oral
progesterone	progesterone	oral, vaginal gel

Supplemental Table 7: Progestogen Regimens

	PROGESTOGEN	ADDITIONAL NOTES
Continuous	Daily	• Menopause transition: may worsen bleeding irregularities • Postmenopause: shouldn't restart periods (most women prefer no bleeding)
Cyclic	12–14 days/month	• Menopause transition: Least likely to worsen bleeding patterns • Postmenopause: 80% of women will have some bleeding each cycle

	PROGESTOGEN	ADDITIONAL NOTES
Intermittent	3 days on and 3 days off	• Can be helpful for women who have persistent bleeding postmenopause on continuous therapy who wish to have no bleeding
Long cycle	14 days every 2–6 months	• Heavier bleeding, but less often • Least preferred approach as may not be enough exposure to reduce the cancer risk, requires in depth consultation and special monitoring

Supplemental Table 8: Levonorgestrel IUDs in the United States (as of August 2020)

BRAND NAME	HORMONE TOTAL	DAILY HORMONE RELEASED	DURATION OF USE (FDA APPROVED)	EXTENDED USE (STUDIES SUPPORT USE BEYOND FDA RECOMMENDATIONS)
Mirena	52 mg	20 mcg	5 years	7 years
Lilette	52 mg	18.6 mcg	4 years	5 years
Kyleena	19.5 mg	17.5 mcg	5 years	No data
Slya	13.5 mg	14 mcg	3 years	No data

Appendices

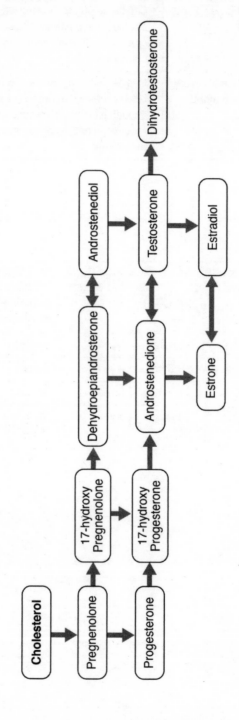

Appendix A: Synthesis of Estradiol, Estrone, and Testosterone from Cholesterol

Appendix B: DASH, Mediterranean, and MIND diets

DASH	MEDITERRANEAN	MIND
Whole grains, daily	Whole grains, 1–2 servings/meal main meal	Leafy green vegetables, ≥6 servings/week
Vegetables daily	Vegetables ≥2 servings/meal	Other vegetables, ≥1 serving/day
Fruits daily	Fruits, 1–2 servings/meal	Berries ≥2 servings/week
Dairy, low fat or nonfat 2–3 servings/day	Olives/nuts/seeds, 1–2 servings/day	Whole grains ≥3 servings/day
Poultry, 2 servings/week	Potatoes ≤3 servings/week	Fish ≥1 serving per week
Fish and seafood, 1–2 servings/week ≤2 servings/day	Legumes ≥2 servings/week	Poultry ≥2 servings per week
Legumes, 2 servings/week	Fish, seafood ≥2 servings/week	Beans ≥3 servings/week
Nuts, seeds, 4–5 servings/week	Poultry/white meat 2 servings/week	Nuts ≥5 servings/week
Fats and oils, 2–3 servings a day	Egg 2–4 servings/week	Wine 1 glass/day
Sweets, ≤5 servings a week	Low fat dairy 2 servings/day	Butter <1 tbsp/day
	Red meat ≤1 serving/week	Cheese <1 serving/week
	Processed meat ≤1 serving/week	Red meat <4 servings/week
	Sweets ≤2 servings/week	Pastries and sweets <5 servings/week
	Red wine, in moderation	Olive oil

Selected References

Chapter 1: A Second Coming of Age

Menopause Practice: A Clinician's Guide, 6th ed. C.J. Crandall, Editor-in-Chief. North American Menopause Society, 2019.

El Khoudary, S.R., Greendale, G., Crawford, S.L., et al. The menopause transition and women's health at midlife: A progress report, from the Study of Women's Health Across the Nation (SWAN). *Menopause* 2019; 26: 1213.

Epperson, C.N., Sammel, M.D., Bale, T.L., et al. Adverse childhood experiences and risk for first-episode major depression during the menopause transition. *Journal of Clinical Psychiatry* 2017; 78.

Chapter 2: The History and Language of Menopause

Dean-Jones, L. Menstrual bleeding according to the Hippocratics and Aristotle. *Transactions of the American Philological Association* 1989; 119.

Bonnard, J.-B. Trans, L.E. Doherty, V. Sebillotte Cuchet. Male and female bodies according to ancient Greek physicians. *Clio* 2012; 37.

Gentle, K.M. *Reclaiming the Role of the Old Priestess: Ritual Agency and the Post-Menopausal Body in Ancient Greece.* Dissertation, Graduate Program in Greek and Latin, Ohio State University, 2009.

Stolberg, M. A woman's hell? Medical perceptions of menopause in preindustrial Europe. *Bulletin of the History of Medicine* 1999; 73.

Physician, A. *The Ladies Physician Directory, 1727.* Printed and sold by the author's appointment, at the gentlewoman's at the Two Blue Posts in Haydon-Yard, in the Minories.

Fothergill, J. On the management proper at the cessation of the menses. *Medical Observations and Inquiries* 5 (1776): 160–86. Reprinted in F. Churchill, ed. *Essays on the Puerpal Fever and Other Diseases Peculiar to Women.* Selected from the writings of British authors prior to the close of the eighteenth century (1849), 503–16. Sydenham Society Publications, London.

De Gardanne, C.P.L. Sur les avis à donner aux femmes qui entrent dans l'âge critique. Dissertation, 1812.

De Gardanne, C.P.L. *Avis aux femmes qui entrent dans l'lge critique,* 1st ed. Paris: De J. Moronval, 1816.

De Gardanne, C.P.L. *De la menopause, ou de l'age critique des femmes,* 2nd ed. Paris: Meguig non-Marvis, 1821.

Tilt, E.J. *The change of life in health and disease,* 2nd ed. London: John Churchill, 1857.

Tillier, An. Un âge critique. La ménopause sous le regard des médecins des XVIIIe et XIXe siècles. *Clio Histoire, femmes et sociétés* 2005; 21.

Minkin, M.J., Reiter, S., Maamari, R. Prevalence of postmenopausal symptoms in North America and Europe. *Menopause* 2015; 22.

Chapter 3: The Biology of Menopause

Burger, H.G., Hale, G.E., Dennerstein, L., Robertson, D.M. Cycle and hormone changes during perimenopause: The key role of ovarian function. *Menopause* 2008; 15 (4): 603–12.

Taylor, H.S., Pal, L., Sell, E. *Speroff's Clinical Gynecologic Endocrinology and Infertility,* 9th ed. New York: Lippincott Williams & Wilkins, 2019.

Menopause Practice, A Clinician's Guide, 6th ed. C.J. Crandall, Editor-in-Chief. North American Menopause Society, 2019.

Broekmans, F.J., Soules, M.R., Fauser, B.C. Ovarian aging: Mechanisms and clinical consequences. *Endocrine Reviews* 2009; 30; *Journal of Clinical Endocrinology and Metabolism* 2012; 97.

El Khoudary, S.R., Greendale, G., Crawford, S.L., et al. The menopause transition and women's health at midlife: A progress report from the Study of Women's Health Across the Nation (SWAN). *Menopause* 2019; 26: 1213.

Tepper, P.G., Randolph, J.F., Jr., McConnell, D.S., et al. Trajectory clustering of estradiol and follicle-stimulating hormone during the menopausal transition among women in the Study of Women's Health across the Nation (SWAN).

The use of Antimüllerian hormone in women not seeking fertility care. ACOG Committee Opinion No. 773. American College of Obstetricians and Gynecologists. *Obstetrics & Gynecology* 2019; 133.

de Kat, A., van de Schouw, Y.T., Eijkemans, M.J.C., et al. Can menopause prediction be improved with multiple AMH measurements? Results from the Prospective Doetinchem Cohort Study. *Journal of Clinical Endocrinology and Metabolism* 2019; 104.

Chapter 4: The Evolutionary Advantage of Menopause

Amundsen, D.W., Diers, C.J. The age of menopause in classical Greece and Rome. *Human Biology* 1970; 42.

Pollycove, R., Naftolin, F., Simon, J.A. The evolutionary origin and significance of menopause. *Menopause* 2011; 18.

Thompson, M.E. Comparative reproductive energetics of human and nonhuman primates. *Annual Review of Anthropology* 2013; 42.

Pliny the Elder, The Natural History. http://perseus.tufts.edu/hopper/text?doc=Perseus%3Atext%3A1999.02.0137%3Abook%3D7%3Achapter%3D49

Social Security Actuarial Life Tables. Accessed 5/16/20, https://ssa.gov/oact/STATS/table 4c6.html

Gurven, M.D., Gomes, C.M. Mortality, senescence, and life span. In M.N. Muller, R.W. Wrangham, D.R. Pilbeam, eds. *Chimpanzees and Human Evolution.* Cambridge, MA: Belknap Press of Harvard University Press; 2017: 181–216.

Shanley, D.P., Kirkwood, T.B.L. Evolution of the human menopause. *BioEssays* 2001; 23.

Hawkes, K., O'Connell, J.F., Jones, B. Hadza Women's time allocation, offspring provisioning, and the evolution of long postmenopausal life spans. *Current Anthropology* 1997; 38.

Croft, D.P., Johnstone, R.A., Ellis, S., et al. Reproductive conflict and the evolution of menopause in killer whales. *Current Biology* 2017; 27.

Schubert, C. Benefits of menopause: Good fishing. *Biology of Reproduction* 2015; 92.

El Khoudary, S.R., Greendale, G., Crawford, S.L., et al. The menopause transition and women's health at midlife: A progress report from the Study of Women's Health Across the Nation (SWAN). *Menopause* 2019; 26: 1213.

Arnot, M., Mace, R. Sexual frequency is associated with age of natural menopause: Results from the Study of Women's Health Across the Nation. *Royal Society Open Science* 7: 191020.

Chapter 5: The Timing of Menopause

Morris, D.H., Jones, M.E., Schoemaker, M.J., et al. Familial concordance for age at natural menopause: Results from the Breakthrough Generations Study. *Menopause* 2011; 18.

Bjelland, E.K., Hofvind, S., Byberg, L., et al. The relation of age at menarche and age at natural menopause: A population based study of 336,788 women in Norway. *Human Reproduction* 2018; 33.

Klonoff-Cohen, H.S., Natarajan, L., Chen, R.V. A prospective study of the effects of female and male marijuana use on in vitro fertilization (IVF) and gamete intrafallopian transfer (GIFT) outcomes. *American Journal of Obstetrics and Gynecology* 2006; 194: 369–76.

Gargiulo, A.R. *Yen & Jaffe's Reproductive Endocrinology E-Book.* New York: Elsevier Health Sciences. Kindle Edition.

Song, T., Kim, M.K., Kim, M.L., et al. Impact of opportunistic salpingectomy on anti-Müllerian hormone in patients undergoing laparoscopic hysterectomy: A multicentre randomised controlled trial. *BJOG* 2017; 124.

Mahal, A.S., Rhoads, K.F., Elliott, C.S., Sokol, E.R. Inappropriate oophorectomy at time of benign premenopausal hysterectomy. *Menopause* 2017; 24(8): 947.

Infertility workup for the women's health specialist. ACOG Committee Opinion No. 781. American College of Obstetricians and Gynecologists. *Obstetrics & Gynecology* 2019; 133: e377–84.

Parker, W.H., Broder M.S., Liu Z., et al. Ovarian conservation at the time of hysterectomy for benign disease. Obstet Gynecol 2005;106.

Hammer, A., Rositch, A.F., Kahlert, J., et al. Global epidemiology of hysterectomy: Possible impact on gynecological cancer rates. *American Journal of Obstetrics & Gynecology* 2015;7.

Ding, N., Harlow, S.D., Randolph, J.F., et al. Associations of perfluoroalkyl substances with incident natural menopause: The Study of Women's Health Across the Nation. *Journal of Clinical Endocrinology and Metabolism* 2020; June 3.

Ainsworth, A.J., Baumgarten, S.C., Bakkum-Gamez, J.N., et al. Tubal ligation and age at natural menopause. *Obstetrics & Gynecology* 2019; 133.

Gold, E.B., Crawford, S.L., Avis, N.E., et al. Factors related to age at natural menopause: Longitudinal analyses from SWAN. *American Journal of Epidemiology* 2013; 178.

Chapter 6: When Periods and Ovulation Stop Before Age Forty

Hormone therapy in primary ovarian insufficiency. Committee Opinion No. 698. American College of Obstetricians and Gynecologists. *Obstetrics & Gynecology* 2017; 129.

Primary ovarian insufficiency in adolescents and young women. Committee Opinion No. 605. American College of Obstetricians and Gynecologists. *Obstetrics & Gynecology* 2014; 123.

Menopause Practice, A Clinician's Guide, 6th ed. C.J. Crandall, Editor-in-Chief. North American Menopause Society, 2019.

Andany, N., Kaida, A., de Pokomandy, A., et al. Prevalence and correlates of early-onset menopause among women living with HIV in Canada. *Menopause* 2019; 27.

Pan, M.-L., Chen, L.-R., Tsao, H.-M., Chen, K.-H. Polycystic ovarian syndrome and the risk of subsequent primary ovarian insufficiency: A nationwide population-based study. *Menopause* 2017; 24.

Christ, J.P., Gunning, M.N., Palla, G., et al. Estrogen deprivation and cardiovascular disease risk in primary ovarian insufficiency. *Fertility and Sterility* 2018; 109.

Chapter 7: Metamorphoses of Menopause

Strings, S. *Fearing the Black Body: The Racial Origins of Fat Phobia.* New York: NYU Press, 2019.

Hetemäki, N., Savolainen-Peltonen, H., Tikkanen, M.J., et al. Estrogen metabolism in abdominal subcutaneous and visceral adipose tissue in postmenopausal women. *Journal of Clinical Endocrinology and Metabolism* 2017; 102.

Menopause Practice, A Clinician's Guide, 6th ed. C.J. Crandall, Editor-in-Chief. North American Menopause Society, 2019.

Ambikairajah, A., Walsh, E., Tabatabaei-Jafari, H., et al. Fat Mass changes during menopause: A metanalysis. *American Journal of Obstetrics and Gynecology* 2019.

Christakis, M.K., Hasan, H., De Souza, L., et al. The effect of menopause on metabolic syndrome: Cross-sectional results from the Canadian Longitudinal Study on Aging. *Menopause* 2020; 27.

Davis, S.R., Castelo-Branco, C., Chedraui, P., et al. Understanding weight gain at menopause. *Climacteric* 2012; 15.

Pollock, R.D., Carter, S., Velloso, C.P., et al. An investigation into the relationship between age and physiological function in highly active older adults. *Journal of Physiology* 2015; 3.

van Gemert, W.A., Peeters, P.H., May, A.M., et al. Effect of diet with or without exercise on abdominal fat in postmenopausal women—a randomised trial. *BMC Public Health* 2019; 19.

Chapter 8: The Heart of the Matter

Zheng, Y., Wen, T.S., Shen, Y., et al. Age at menarche and cardiovascular health. *Menopause* 2020; September (published ahead of print).

Wang, D., Jackson, C.A., Karvonen-Gutierrez, M.R., et al. Healthy lifestyle during the midlife is prospectively associated with less subclinical carotid atherosclerosis: The Study of Women's Health Across the Nation. *Journal of the American Heart Association* 2018; 7.

Menopause Practice, A Clinician's Guide, 6th ed. C.J. Crandall, Editor-in-Chief. North American Menopause Society, 2019.

Norris, C.M., Yip, C.Y.Y., Nerenberg, K.A., et al. State of the science in women's cardiovascular disease: A Canadian perspective on the influence of sex and gender. *Journal of the American Heart Association* 2020; 9.

Al-Salameh, A., Chanson, P., Bucher, S., et al. Cardiovascular disease in type 2 diabetes: A review of sex-related differences in predisposition and prevention. *Mayo Clinic Proceedings* 2019; 94.

Chapter 9: Is It Hot in Here or Is It Just Me?

Tepper, P.G., Brooks, M.M., Randolph, J.F., et al. Characterizing the trajectories of vasomotor symptoms across the menopausal transition. *Menopause* 2016; 23.

Avis, N.E., Crawford, S.L., Greendale, G., et al. Duration of menopausal vasomotor symptoms over the menopause transition. *JAMA Internal Medicine* 2015; 175.

Zeserson, J.M. How Japanese women talk about hot flushes: Implications for menopause research. *Medical Anthropology Quarterly* 2001; 15.

Brown, D.E., Leidy Sievert, L., Morrison, L.A., et al. Do Japanese American women really have fewer hot flashes than European Americans? The HiLo Health Study. *Menopause* 2009; 16.

Menopause Practice, A Clinician's Guide, 6th ed. C.J. Crandall, Editor-in-Chief. North American Menopause Society, 2019.

Management of Menopausal Symptoms ACOG. Practice Bulletin No. 514. *American College of Obstetricians and Gynecologists* 2014.

Nonhormonal management of menopausal-associated vasomotor symptoms: 2015 position statement of the North American Menopause Society. *Menopause* 2015; 22.

Kickey, M. Non-hormonal treatments for menopausal symptoms. *BMJ* 2017; 359.

Leach, M.J., Moore, V. Black cohosh (*Cimicifuga spp.*) for menopausal symptoms. *Cochrane Database of Systematic Reviews* 2012; Issue 9. Art. No. CD007244.

Liu, Zh., Ai, Y., Wang, W., et al. Acupuncture for symptoms in menopause transition: A randomized controlled trial. *American Journal of Obstetrics and Gynecology* 2018; 219.

Depypere, H., Timmerman, D., Doders, G., et al. Treatment of menopausal vasomotor symptoms with fezolinetant, a neurokinin 3 receptor antagonist: A phase 2a trial. *Journal of Clinical Endocrinology and Metabolism* 2019; 104.

Chapter 10: Menstrual Mayhem

Management of acute abnormal uterine bleeding in non-pregnant reproductive-aged women. Committee Opinion No. 557. American College of Obstetricians and Gynecologists. *Obstetrics & Gynecology* 2013; 121.

Management of Abnormal Uterine Bleeding Associated with Ovulatory Dysfunction. Practice Bulletin No. 136. American College of Obstetricians and Gynecologists, 2013.

Middleton, L.J., Champanera, R., Daniels, J.P., et al. Hysterectomy, endometrial ablation, and levonorgestrel releasing system (Mirena) for treatment of heavy menstrual bleeding: Systemic review and meta-analysis of data from individual patients. *BMJ* 2010; 341.

Beelen, P., Reinders, I.M.A., Scheepers, W.F.W., et al. Prognostic factors for the failure of endometrial ablation. *Obstetrics & Gynecology* 2019; 134.

Bulun, S.E. Uterine fibroids. *New England Journal of Medicine* 2013; 369.

Manyonda, A.-M., Belli, M.-A., Lumsden, J., et al. Uterine-artery embolization for myomectomy for uterine fibroids. *New England Journal of Medicine* 2020; 383.

Schaff, W.D., Ackerman, R.T., Al-Hendry, A., et al. Elagolix for heavy menstrual bleeding in women with uterine fibroids. *New England Journal of Medicine* 2020; 382.

Chapter 11: Bone Health

Osteoporosis in menopause. *Journal of Obstetrics and Gynaecology Canada.* 2014; 36.

Jha, S., Wang, Z., Laucis, N., et al. Trends in media reports, oral bisphosphonate prescriptions, and hip fractures 1996–2012: An ecological analysis. *Journal of Bone and Mineral Research* 2015; 30.

Menopause Practice, A Clinician's Guide, 6th ed. Crandall C.J., Editor-in-Chief. North American Menopause Society, 2019.

Guidelines for Women's Health Care, A Resource Manual, 4th ed. American College of Obstetricians and Gynecologists, 2014.

Chapter 12: This Is Your Brain on Menopause

El Khoudary, S.R., Greendale, G., Crawford, S.L., et al. The menopause transition and women's health at midlife: A progress report from the Study of Women's Health Across the Nation (SWAN). *Menopause* 2019; 26: 1213.

Bromberger, J.T., Kravitz, H.M. Mood and menopause: Findings from the Study of Women's Health Across the Nation (SWAN) over ten years. *Obstetrics and Gynecology Clinics of North America* 2011; 38.

Greendale, G.A., Wight, R.G., Huang, M.H., et al. Menopause-associated symptoms and cognitive performance: Results from the Study of Women's Health Across the Nation. *American Journal of Epidemiology* 2020; 171.

Cohen, L.S., Soares, C.N., Vitonos, A.F., et al. Risk of new onset depression during the menopausal transition. *Archives of General Psychiatry* 2006; 63.

Greendale, G.A., Karlamangla, A.S., Mali, P.M. The menopause transition and cognition. *Journal of the American Medical Association* 2020; doi:10.1001/jama.2020.1757.

Miller, V.M., Naftolin, F., Asthgana, S., et al. The Kronos Early Estrogen Prevention Study (KEEPS): What have we learned? *Menopause* 2019; 26.

Savolainen-Peltonen, H., Rahkola-Soisalo, P., Hoti, F., et al. Use of postmenopausal hormone therapy and risk of Alzheimer's disease in Finland: Nationwide case-control study. *BMJ* 2019; 364: l665.

Chapter 13: The Vagina and Vulva

Suh, D.D., Yang, C.C., Cao, Y., Garland, P.A., et al. Magnetic resonance imaging anatomy of the female genitalia in premenopausal and postmenopausal women. *The Journal of Urology* 2003; 170: 138–44.

The 2020 genitourinary syndrome of menopause position statement of the North American Menopause Society. *Menopause* 2020; 27.

Lindau, S.T., Dude, A., Gavrilova, N., Hoffman, J.N., Schumm, L.P., McClintock, M.A. Prevalence and correlates of vaginal estrogenization in postmenopausal women in the United States. *Menopause* 2017; 24: 536–45.

Edwards, D., Panay, N. Treating vulvovaginal atrophy/genitourinary syndrome of menopause: How important is vaginal lubricant and moisturizer composition? *Climacteric* 2016; 19.

Gunter, J. *The Vagina Bible,* Chapters 1 and 2. New York: Kensington, 2019.

Shifren, J.L. Genitourinary syndrome of menopause. *Clinical Obstetrics and Gynecology* 2018.

Ghandhi, J., Chen, A., Dagur, G., et al. Genitourinary syndrome of menopause: An overview of clinical manifestations, pathophysiology, etiology, evaluation, and management. *American Journal of Obstetrics and Gynecology* 2016; Dec.

Rahn, D.D., Carberry, C., Sanses, T.V., et al. Vaginal estrogen for genitourinary syndrome of menopause. A systemic review. *Obstetrics & Gynecology* 2014; 124; 5: 1147–56.

Hickey, M., Szabo, R.A., Hunter, M.S. Non-hormonal treatments for menopausal symptoms. *BMJ* 2017; 359.

The Use of Vaginal Estrogen in Women with a History of Estrogen-Dependent Cancer. ACOG Committee Opinion Number 659, March 2016.

Paraiso, F.M.R., Ferrando, C.A., Sokol, E.R., et al. A randomized clinical trial comparing vaginal laser therapy to vaginal estrogen therapy in women with genitourinary syndrome of menopause: The VeLVET Trial. *Menopause* 2019; 27.

Chapter 14: Bladder Health

Krause, M., Wheeler, T.L., II, Snyder, T.E., et al. Local effects of vaginally administered estrogen therapy: A review. *Journal of Pelvic Medicine and Surgery* 2009; 15.

Brubaker, L., Carberry, C., Nardos, R., et al. American Urogynecologic Society Best-Practice Statement: Recurrent urinary tract infection in adult women. *Female Pelvic Medicine and Reconstructive Surgery* 2018; 24.

Urinary incontinence in women. Practice Bulletin No. 155. American College of Obstetricians and Gynecologists. *Obstetrics & Gynecology* 2015; 126: e66–81.

Nicolle, L.E. Cranberry for prevention of urinary tract infection? Time to move on. *Journal of the American Medical Association* 2016; 16141.

Pelvic organ prolapse. Practice Bulletin No. 185. American College of Obstetricians and Gynecologists. *Obstetrics & Gynecology* 2017; 130.

Chapter 15: Let's Talk About Sex

Brotto, L.A., Bitzer, J., Laan, E., et al. Women's sexual desire and arousal disorders. *Journal of Sexual Medicine* 2010; 7.

Brotto, L. Evidence-based treatments for low sexual desire in women. *Frontiers Neuroendocrinology* 2017; 45.

Moynihan, R. Evening the score on sex drugs: feminist movement or marketing masquerade? *BMJ* 2014; 349:g6246.

Female sexual dysfunction. ACOG Practice Bulletin No. 213. American College of Obstetricians and Gynecologists. *Obstetrics & Gynecology* 2019; 134.

Meixel, A., et al. *Journal of Medical Ethics* 2015; 41.

Reed, B.G., Bou Nemer, L., Carr, B.R. Has testosterone passed the test in premenopausal women with low libido? A systemic review. *Journal of Women's Health* 2016; 8.

Bremelanotide (Vylessi) for hypoactive sexual desire disorder. *Medical Letter on Drugs and Therapeutics* 2019; 61.

Flibanserin (Addyi) for hypoactive sexual desire disorder. *Medical Letter on Drugs and Therapeutics* 2015; 57.

Brotto, L.A., Basson, R. Group mindfulness-based therapy significantly improves sexual desire in women. *Behavior Research and Therapy* 2014; 57.

Segraves, R.T., Clayton, A., Croft, H., et al. Bupropion sustained release for the treatment of hypoactive sexual desire disorder in premenopausal women. *Journal of Clinical Psychopharmacology* 2004; 24.

Nurnberg, H.G., Hensley, P.L., Heiman, J.R., et al. Sildenafil treatment of women with antidepressant-associated sexual dysfunction: A randomized controlled trial. *Journal of the American Medical Association* 2008; 300.

Shifren, J.L., Davis, S.R. Androgens in postmenopausal women: A review. *Menopause* 2017; 24.

Davis, S.R., Baber, R., Panay, N., et al. Global consensus position statement on the use of testosterone therapy for women. *Journal of Clinical Endocrinology and Metabolism* 2019; 104.

Davis, S.R., Moreau, M., Kroll, R., et al. Testosterone for low libido in postmenopausal women not taking estrogen. *New England Journal of Medicine* 2008; 359.

Chapter 16: Will I Ever Feel Rested Again?

Baker, F.C., Lampio, L., Saaresranta, T., et al. Sleep and sleep disorders in the menopause transition. *Sleep Medicine* 2018; 13.

Menopause Practice, A Clinician's Guide, 6th ed. C.J. Crandall, Editor-in-Chief. North American Menopause Society, 2019.

Xu, M., Bélanger, L., Ivers, H., et al. Comparison of subjective and objective sleep quality in menopausal and non-menopausal women with insomnia. *Sleep Medicine* 2011; 12.

Kravitz, H.M., Janssen, I., Bromberger, J.T., et al. Sleep trajectories before and after the final menstrual period in the Study of Women's Health Across the Nation (SWAN). *Current Sleep Medicine Review* 2017; 3.

Lampio, L., Polo-Kantola, P., Polo, O., et al. *Sleep in midlife women: Effects of menopause, vasomotor symptoms, and depressive symptoms. Menopause* 2014; 21.

Zolfaghari, S., Yao, C., Thompson, C., et al. Effects of menopause on sleep quality and sleep disorders: Canadian Longitudinal Study on Aging. *Menopause* 2019; 27.

Chapter 17: Menopausal Hormone Therapy

The "Marker Degradation" and Creation of the Mexican Steroid Hormone Industry 1938–1945. The Historic Chemical Landmarks Program. American Chemical Society.

Wilson, R.A. *Feminine Forever.* New York: M. Evans and Company, 1966.

Reza, A. *Marketing Menopause: An Analysis of How the Marketing of Premarin Changed as Societal Perception of Menopause Changed.* Ottawa: Carleton University, 2009.

Menopausal hormone therapy and health outcomes during the intervention and extended poststopping phase of the Women's Health Initiative randomized trials.
Executive Summary. *Journal of the American Medical Association* 2013; October.

Langer, R.D. The evidence base for HRT: What can we believe? *Climacteric* 2017.

Vinogradova, Y., Coupland, C., Hippisley-Cox, J. Use of hormone replacement therapy
and risk of venous thromboembolism: Nested case-control studies using the QRe-
search and CPRD databases. *BMJ* 2019; 364.

Menopause Practice, A Clinician's Guide, 6th ed. Crandall C.J., Editor-in-Chief. North American Menopause Society, 2019.

Manson, J.E., Bassuk, S.S., Kaunitz, A.M., et al. The Women's Health Initiative trials of
menopausal hormone therapy: Lessons learned. *Menopause* 2020; 27.

Chapter 18: The Cinematic Universe of Hormones

The 2017 hormone therapy position statement of the North American Menopause Society.
Menopause 2017; 24.

Minami, C.A., Freedman, R.A. Menopausal hormone therapy and long-term breast
cancer risk. Further data from the Women's Health Initiative trials. *Journal of the
American Medical Association* 2020; 324.

Reame, N.K. Estetrol for menopause symptoms: The Cinderella of estrogens or just
another fairy tale? *Menopause* 2020; 27.

Menopause Practice, A Clinician's Guide, 6th ed. Crandall C.J., Editor-in-Chief. North American Menopause Society, 2019.

Postmenopausal estrogen therapy: Route of administration and risk of venous thromboembolism. Committee Opinion No. 556. American College of Obstetricians and
Gynecologists. *Obstetrics & Gynecology* 2013; 121: 887–90.

Bagot, C.N., Marsh, M.S., Whitehead, M., et al. The effect of estrone on thrombin generation may explain the different thrombotic risk between oral and transdermal
hormone replacement therapy. *Journal of Thrombosis and Haemostasis* 2010.

Stute, P., Wildt, L., Neulen, J. The impact of micronized progesterone on breast cancer
risk: A systematic review. *Climacteric* 2018; 21.

Chapter 19: Phytoestrogens, Food, and Hormones

Rowland, I., Faughnan, M., Hoey, L. Bioavailability of phytoestrogens. *British Journal of
Nutrition* 2003: 89.

Patisaul, H.B. Endocrine disruption by dietary phyto-oestrogens: Impact on dimorphic
sexual systems and behaviours. *Proceedings of the Nutrition Society* 2017; 76.

Shappell, N.W., Berg, E.P., Magolski, J.D., et al. An in vitro comparison of estrogenic equivalents per serving size of some common foods. *Journal of Food Science* 2019.

Zamora-Ros, R., Knaze, V., Luján-Barroso, L., et al. Dietary intakes and food sources of
phytoestrogens in the European Prospective Investigation into cancer and nutrition
(EPIC) 24-hours dietary recall cohort. *European Journal of Clinical Nutrition* 2012; 66.

Steinberg, F.M., Murray, M.J., Lewis, R.D., et al. Clinical outcomes of a 2-year soy isoflavone
supplementation in menopausal women. *American Journal of Clinical Nutrition* 2011; 93.

Michaëlsson, K., Wolk, A., Langenskiöld, S., et al. Milk intake and risk of mortality and
fractures in women and men: Cohort studies. *BMJ* 2014; 349.

Chapter 20: Bioidenticals, Naturals, and Compounding

Bhavnani, B.R., Stancyk, F.Z. Misconception and concerns about bioidentical hormones used for custom-compounded hormone therapy. *Journal of Clinical Endocrinology and Metabolism* 2012; 97.

The Clinical Utility of Compounded Bioidentical Hormone Therapy: A Review of Safety, Effectiveness, and Use. Washington, DC: The National Academies Press, 2020.

Experts slam Oprah and Somers' take on menopause. *Newsweek* 2/8/09. Accessed 11/19/20 from https://newsweek.com/experts-slam-oprah-and-somers-take-menopause-82463

FDA statement on improving adverse event reporting of compounded drugs to protect patients. Accessed 11/19/20 from https://fda.gov/news-events/press-announcements/statement-improving-adverse-event-reporting-compounded-drugs-protect-patients

Disciplinary order, Prudence Hall, MD, Medical Board California. Accessed 11/19/20 from http://4patientsafety.org/documents/Hall,%20Prudence%20Elizabeth%202018-08-03.pdf

Liss, J., Santoro, N. Stand firm with science: The compounded bioidentical hormone industry needs major changes in oversight to keep consumers safe. *Contemporary OB/GYN* 2020; 65.

Chapter 21: Meno-Diets

Position of the Academy of Nutrition and Dietetics: Health implications of dietary fiber. *Journal of the Academy of Nutrition and Dietetics* 2015; 115.

Boutot, M.E., Purdue-Smith, A., Whitcomb, B.W. Dietary protein intake and early menopause in the Nurses' Health Study II. *American Journal of Epidemiology* 2017; 187.

Dunneram, Y., Greenwood, D.C., Burley, V.J., et al. Dietary intake and age at natural menopause: Results from the UK Women's Cohort Study. *Journal of Epidemiology and Community Health* 2018; 72: 733–40.

Marcason, W. What are the components to the MIND diet? *Journal of the Academy of Nutrition and Dietetics* 2015; 115.

Dinu, M., Pagliai, G., Casini, A., et al. Mediterranean diet and multiple health outcomes: An umbrella review of meta-analyses of observational studies and randomised trials. *European Journal of Clinical Nutrition* 2018; 72.

Martínez, Steele E., Galastri Baraldi, L., Laura da Costa Louzada, M., et al. Ultra-processed foods and added sugars in the US diet: Evidence from a nationally representative cross-sectional study. *BMJ Open* 2016; 6: e009892.

Hall, K.D., Ayuketah, A., Brychta, R., et al. Ultra-processed diets cause excess calorie intake and weight gain: An inpatient randomized controlled trial of ad libitum food intake. *Cell Metabolism* 2019; 19.

Chapter 22: Menoceuticals

Nonhormonal management of menopause-associated vasomotor symptoms: 2015 position statement of the North American Menopause Society. *Menopause* 2015; 22.

The composition of certain secret remedies *BMJ* 1911; 2.

Horwitz, R. *Lydia Pinkham's Vegetable Compound (1873-1906)*. Embryo Project Encyclopedia (2017-05-20). ISSN: 1940-5030, retrieved from http://embryo.asu.edu/handle/
10776/11506.

Manson, J.E., Cook, N.R., Lee, I-Min, et al. Marin n-3 fatty acids and prevention of cardiovascular disease and cancer. *New England Journal of Medicine* 2019; 380: 23–32.

Yao, P., Bennett, D., Mafham, M., et al. Vitamin D and calcium for the prevention of fracture: A systematic review and meta-analysis. *JAMA Network Open* 2019; 2.

Manson, J.E., Bassuk, S.S. Vitamin and mineral supplements. What clinicians need to
know. *Journal of the American Medical Association* 2018; 319.

Menopause Practice, A Clinician's Guide, 6th ed. Crandall C.J., Editor-in-Chief. North American Menopause Society, 2019.

Chapter 23: Contraception and the Menopause Transition

Use of hormonal contraception in women with coexisting medical conditions. ACOG
Practice Bulletin No. 206. American College of Obstetricians and Gynecologists. *Obstetrics & Gynecology* 2019; 133: e128–50.

Allen, R., Cwiak, C.A., Kaunitz, A.M. Contraception in women over 40 years of age. *Canadian Medical Association Journal* 2013; 185.

The ESHRE Capri Workshop Group. Female contraception over 40. *Human Reproduction
Update* 2009; 15.

Combined hormonal contraception and the risk of venous thromboembolism: A guide-
line. Practice Committee of the American Society for Reproductive Medicine. *Fertility
and Sterility* 2016.

Menopause Practice, A Clinician's Guide, 6th ed. Crandall C.J., Editor-in-Chief. North American Menopause Society, 2019.

Pergallo, R., Polis, C., Jenses, E.T., et al. Effectiveness of fertility awareness-based methods
for pregnancy prevention. *Obstetrics & Gynecology* 2018; 132.

Fehring, R.J., Mu, Q. Cohort efficacy study of natural family planning among perimeno-
pausal women. *Journal of Obstetric, Gynecologic, & Neonatal Nursing* 2014; 43.

Acknowledgments

The two people who deserve the biggest thank you are my sons, Oliver and Victor. "I can't, I'm writing," became so common a refrain that you stopped asking and instead found ways to be supportive while also keeping me in my place. You are owed a lot of deferred maintenance. Ears can get pierced. Shows can be binged. New desserts can be baked. And I hope eventually there are trips we can take. Do not lose your newfound ability to do your laundry and clean the kitchen.

Tania Malik, thank you for your suggestions and insight. I am eternally grateful for the time and effort that you graciously gave to help me shape this book. You are a talented writer and a gift of a friend.

Thank you Maya Creedman, Dr. Lori Brotto, Dr. Yoni Freedhoff, and Dr. Ethan Weiss for your invaluable feedback and questions.

To my family at Kensington. So many of you worked so hard to bring this book to life and I appreciate your devotion to both my vagenda and my manifesto. Special thanks to Esi Sogah for being such a wonderful and patient editor and for keeping me on track. That last one is hard, but you are more than up to the task! And Ann Pryor, you are all around awesome and thank you for getting my books into the hands of so many people. And thanks once again to Lisa Clark for her beautiful illustrations.

Thank you to Penguin Random House in Canada, especially Amanda Betts and Sharon Klein.

To everyone who reads and shares my posts, columns, and musings on social media. I appreciate your support and your questions and when you hold me accountable.

I would never be in this position if thousands of women hadn't trusted me with their care. It has been a gift to be your doctor and I hope to continue to earn that privilege.

And finally, Todd. If someone told me a few years ago that at fifty-three I would meet the love of my life, I would have snickered. Mr. Okay, sure. But I had long given up on the idea that there was a match for me. And then this? This!!!! I feel as if I am in some Mary Poppins universe where my list of wishes for my person were deemed ridiculous, so I tore it up and threw it in the fireplace and forgot about it only to have you arrive and pull my taped together list out of your pocket. You are my champion, my lover, my best friend and you do not let me get away with shit.

Index